An Overview of the Human Services

An Overview of the Human Services

Kristi Kanel

California State University, Fullerton

Lahaska Press
Houghton Mifflin Company
Boston • New York

This is dedicated to my mother, Joyce

Publisher, Lahaska Press: Barry Fetterolf
Senior Editor, Lahaska Press: Mary Falcon
Senior Marketing Manager, Lahaska Press: Barbara LeBuhn
Associate Project Editor: Kristen Truncellito
Art and Design Manager: Gary Crespo
Cover Design Manager: Anne S. Katzeff
Senior Photo Editor: Jennifer Meyer Dare
Composition Buyer: Chuck Dutton
New Title Project Manager: Susan Brooks-Peltier
Editorial Assistant: Evangeline Bermas

Cover image: (c) Ron Waddams, The Bridgeman Art Library

For instructors who want more information about Lahaska Press books and teaching aids, contact the Houghton Mifflin Faculty Services Center at

Tel: 800-733-1717, x4034

Fax: 800-733-1810

Or visit us on the Web at **www.lahaskapress.com**.

Lahaska Press, established as an imprint of Houghton Mifflin Company in 1999, is dedicated to publishing textbooks and instructional media for counseling and the helping professions. Its editorial offices are located in the small town of Lahaska, Pennsylvania. Lahaska is a Native American Lenape word meaning "source of much writing."

Printed in the U.S.A.

Library of Congress Control Number: 2006934902

ISBN-10: 0-618-60760-9

ISBN-13: 978-0-618-60760-0

23456789-EB-11 10 09 08 07

Contents

CHAPTER **4**   **Communication Skills and Personal Characteristics of Human Service Workers   76**

CHAPTER **8**   **Micro-and Mezzo-Level Assessments and Interventions   209**

CHAPTER **10**   **Stress Management   283**

CHAPTER **11**   **Ethical Issues in the Human Services   309**

CHAPTER **12**   **Organizational Structures of Human Services Agencies and Macro-Level Practice   330**

Preface

General Overview of the Book

Human services has evolved tremendously as a distinct discipline over the past 30 years. It was first studied in colleges and universities in response to societal changes in the 1960s and 1970s (changes that had already been evolving over the previous century) regarding the value of helping the disadvantaged, and it succeeded in creating an increased willingness on the part of both individuals and the government to become involved in providing services for those in need.

This book has been written for students who are just beginning to study the field of human services. It is intended to be an easy-to-read, practical guide to the field, it provides students with a nuts and bolts overview of the myriad facets that make up the field, and it offers students a glimpse of what they can expect to experience as they continue their education and begin working in the field.

Because the field of human services encompasses so many career opportunities, skills, client populations, and job duties, this book was written not only to introduce students to the field, but also to help them find their place in the field by guiding them toward a specific area of human services that might interest them. By the end of the book, students should have a clearer idea what they want to do, whom they want to help, and where they want to work.

Having taught introduction to human services for over 14 years and having heard consistent student complaints about not feeling connected to the often dry and impersonal textbooks used, I felt compelled to write a textbook that would inspire a sense of involvement with the subject matter. Written with that goal in mind, *An Overview of the Human Services* avoids pure lecture by providing numerous opportunities for students to engage in role-plays and other in-class activities. I believe that students who are genuinely interested in the course and actively engaged with the material will gain more from the course than they will if they feel distanced from the text, teacher, and other students. This text challenges students to become active learners via self-reflection, case studies, real-world scenarios, applied activities, and inventories. All of these applied and experiential activities bring theoretical concepts to life for students and help prepare them to serve in agency settings as beginning interns and volunteers.

Chapter-by-Chapter Walk Through

Organized into 12 chapters, *An Overview of the Human Services* proceeds in a cumulative manner from basic concepts and history to specific aspects of the human services field and finally to in-practice considerations such as delivery to clients, stress management, and ethics. Although students interact with and internalize the material throughout the text, the "Human Services Career Inventory" appendix asks students to give themselves a final self-assessment of their aptitude toward and interests within the field.

CHAPTER 1, *What Are Human Services?*

This chapter provides a succinct definition of the term *Human Services,* offers an overview of the different types of human service workers, defines the key terms used in the field, outlines the various places human service workers are employed, and explores the reasons why people should or should not choose a career in the human services. In addition, the chapter provides several case examples to help students begin to understand the practical nature of the book.

CHAPTER 2, *A Brief History of Human Services*

In order to show students the evolution of human services to its present-day incarnation, this historical overview chapter discusses how early societies dealt with behaviors that were seen as deviant and how eventually human compassion came to take the place of punishment. The chapter begins as far back as early humans and traces the evolution of human services through ancient civilizations, the early Christian era, and the Dark Ages, the Age of Reason, the nineteenth century, the twentieth century, and finally the twenty-first century. Throughout the chapter, students are shown how the values of the time greatly influence who receives help and how and how mental health, social welfare, correctional services, and educational services have evolved over time.

CHAPTER 3, *Human Service Workers*

Expanding upon a list first proposed by the Southern Regional Education Board, this chapter begins with definitions and examples of typical functions and roles that human service workers play, then outlines the educational levels of human service workers and the four types of human service agencies. Finally, the chapter ties together the above sections by listing career options within each type of agency based on educational level. Critical Thinking/Self-Reflection questions and a table of actual job postings help students to begin the process of deciding in what capacity they might want to work and what education level they will need to attain to achieve their goals.

CHAPTER 4, *Communication Skills and Personal Characteristics of Human Service Workers*

The purpose of this chapter is to introduce students to basic helping skills, what personal qualities can often lead to successful helping, and how to achieve assertive communication skills. The chapter begins with an outline of the general goals of effective communication, then defines and provides examples of specific effective communication skills, and finally defines and provides examples of personal characteristics human service workers should have. A table summarizing the various effective communication skills and personal characteristics is provided along with numerous real-world scenarios and critical thinking/self-reflection boxes to help students internalize the material.

CHAPTER 5, *Biological and Psychological Theories of Causality*

The first of two chapters that focus on theories of causality of social problems and deviant behaviors, Chapter 5 discusses the biological (or medical) and psychological models. The biological model is discussed first and includes brief descriptions of some of the biological determinants of deviant behaviors and how these may influence human service delivery. The majority of the chapter focuses on the psychological model, outlining the psychological theories of psychoanalysis, existential-humanist therapies, behaviorism, and cognitive therapies, and explains the implications of each theory in terms of human service delivery. A table summarizing the key elements of all of the psychological models of causality is provided, and students are asked to reflect upon and internalize the material throughout the chapter.

CHAPTER 6, *Sociological Theories of Causality*

This second of two chapters that focus on theories of causality begins with foundational definitions of the social, political, and cultural factors that influence human behaviors. The chapter then presents the specific needs and issues facing various cultural groups in our society, including women, LGBT individuals, racial and ethnic minorities, religious groups, the elderly, the economically disadvantaged, and persons with disabilities. A Personal Bias Inventory provides an opportunity for students to assess their own biases toward certain groups, while a Personal Causality Theories and Reaction Inventory at the end of the chapter asks students to assess their emotional reactions to various client populations and determine whether they feel biology, psychology, and/or sociology is the root of problems faced by those populations.

CHAPTER 7, *Populations That Utilize Human Services*

This chapter discusses the needs and issues of client populations that utilize human services, including individuals and families living in poverty; children, disabled persons, and the elderly; victims of abuse; perpetrators of crime and violence; substance abusers; people with mental disorders; AIDS and HIV patients; and at-risk adolescents. In addition to discussing the needs and issues of these groups, the chapter also explores prevalence and causality. Two tables summarize various drugs and their effects and various types of mental disorders. As in all chapters, students are asked to internalize and actualize the material as they read via Critical Thinking/Self-Reflection boxes and real-world examples.

CHAPTER 8, *Micro- and Mezzo-Level Assessments and Interventions*

This assessment chapter opens with brief discussions of primary, secondary, and tertiary interventions and the importance of client assessment. The bulk of the chapter focuses on various interventions in the community at the micro and mezzo level, including suicide prevention and crisis intervention. Additionally, the chapter describes and illustrates with examples how to write intake assessments, case notes, progress notes, and reports.

CHAPTER 9, *Human Services Delivery to Client Populations*

The client populations discussed in Chapter 7 and the intervention strategies presented in Chapter 8 come together in Chapter 9. Each section of this chapter describes specific interventions (emergency situations and interventions, secondary intervention, tertiary intervention, and primary prevention) for each population along with real-world examples, giving students a window through which to view how clients are actually treated in the community in various situations.

CHAPTER 10, *Stress Management*

Because stress is a major part of the human services field, this chapter focuses on this important topic. The chapter begins with brief definitions of stress and burnout. Thereafter, the chapter focuses on the symptoms and impacts of stress and burnout and how to reduce and manage stress and burnout by using cognitive re-framing, maintaining a healthy lifestyle, improving interpersonal communication, learning how to be assertive, and maintaining a sense of humor. Numerous examples throughout the chapter illustrate these methods of stress management.

CHAPTER 11, *Ethical Issues in the Human Services*

Because ethics are crucial in the field of human services, this chapter not only defines ethics but also presents a number of ethical dilemmas for students to navigate. The chapter begins with a general definition of ethics and a discussion of the importance of ethics in the human services field, and then it presents specific ethical issues such as confidentiality, dual relationships, countertransference, and values clarification, which are illustrated with many examples of appropriate and inappropriate ethical behaviors. A concluding discussion about continuing education emphasizes the importance of ongoing training to maintain ethical standards throughout one's human services career.

CHAPTER 12, *Organizational Structures of Human Services Agencies and Macro-Level Practice*

The final chapter examines two topics. The first half of the chapter examines the general characteristics of human service agencies, including norms, leadership styles, staffing patterns, and economic realities, and then it outlines the various types of public and nonprofit human services agencies. The second half of the chapter deals with macro-level practices, such as creating new programs and macro-level interventions. As part of the macro-level practice discussion, the chapter includes an example of a grant.

Special Features

As mentioned earlier, the primary goal of this book is to inspire in students a sense of personal involvement with the subject of human services. To that end, the book contains a number of pedagogical features to help students personalize the chapter material via self-reflection (Critical Thinking/Self Reflection Corner, Suggested Applied Activities) and to actualize the material by seeing abstract concepts played out in a real-world context (True Stories from Human Service Workers, Case Presentation and Exit Quiz). Other special features, such as Chapter Review Questions and chapter Glossary of Terms, are provided to review and reinforce concepts presented in the chapters.

- **Critical Thinking/Self Reflection Corner:** Developing self-awareness is an important challenge for those entering the helping professions. As a result, each chapter contains Critical Thinking/Self-Reflection Corner boxes with questions aimed to catalyze students to explore their own values and emotional and cognitive reactions to topics discussed in the chapters. These boxes appear throughout each chapter, in close proximity to the topics to which they relate, and they can be answered outside of class as students read the chapters, opened up to small-group discussions in class, or both.

- **True Stories from Human Service Workers:** These boxed items feature real-life experiences of human services workers in the field. Placed in close proximity to the topics to which they relate, the boxes are intended to help students visualize the topics under consideration in a real-world context.

- **Suggested Applied Activities:** Following each chapter's summary, these activities bring chapter concepts to life and help students to personalize what they have read by asking them to reflect on their own lives, role play with other students, make observations outside of class, interview people, visit human services agencies, and so on.

- **Chapter Review Questions:** At the end of each chapter, students are presented with several open-ended, short essay questions related to key points from the chapter. These questions may be used as course exam questions or by students to help clarify which chapter points they understand and which they may need to re-visit.

- **Glossary of Terms:** These are key terms that have been bold-faced within each chapter and are listed in alphabetical order at the end of corresponding chapters, along with succinct definitions. Students should review these pivotal terms prior to moving on to subsequent chapters in which knowledge of these terms will be assumed. The terms may also be included on multiple-choice quizzes.

- **Case Presentation and Exit Quiz:** At the end of each chapter, a case presentation related to concepts covered in that particular chapter provides students with further opportunities to see chapter concepts played out in a real-world context. The 5 to 12 multiple-choice questions at the end of each case presentation relate directly to the case and reinforce chapter topics.

- **Appendix: Human Service Career Inventory:** This inventory consists of 15 questions designed to aid students in formulating their career goals. The questions help students narrow their career focus in terms of what types of agency they would like to work in, what types of clients they would like to deal with, what duties they want to perform, and what educational level they want to complete.

Instructor's Resources

The Instructor's Resources for *An Overview of the Human Services* provides teaching suggestions, numerous multiple-choice and true/false exam questions and answers, suggested answers to the student text's chapter review questions, and a sample course outline.

Acknowledgements

I would like to give my sincerest appreciation to my mother, Joyce Kanel, who spent much time and energy reading the rough draft of this text. She is proficient at expository English and helped ensure that the writing made sense.

I would also like to thank Ray Estrella, a former student of mine, who researched some of the material for the chapters.

In general, I thank my Human Services students, who have given me feedback about what they would like to see in an introductory text.

Also, I thank Glennda Gilmour, a Human Services instructor who has taught this course for many years. She gave me valuable ideas about what to include, especially the idea of creating exit quizzes.

Many, many thanks to the following manuscript reviewers who carefully assessed drafts of this book and provided detailed and thoughtful comments to help keep the book on track and in focus:

Paul Ancona, Edmonds Community College
Jackie Griswold, Holyoke Community College
Diane McMillen, Washburn University
Walter Swett, Quinsigamond Community College
Rick Thompson, Austin Community College

Kristi Kanel

CHAPTER 1

What Are Human Services?

Introduction

When someone hears the words **human services** for the first time, he or she might wonder, "Is this a college major or a department in the federal government?" The answer is "yes" to both questions. Or one might ask, "If it is a viable college major, why doesn't it end in 'ology' such as psychology, sociology, anthropology, biology, criminology, and other traditional majors?" The study of Human Services involves studying certain aspects of all those "ologies" and more. Human services uses a multidisciplinary (when several different human services workers trained in different areas of expertise work together for one consumer of service), **holistic** (viewing a person and his needs from many different perspectives such as physical, psychological, spiritual, and cultural), and **eclectic** (intervening with a person in need using a variety of theories and strategies based on those theories) approach to helping people with various needs.

President Franklin Roosevelt (FDR) established the Department of Human Services within the federal government in the 1930s, during the Great Depression, to assist people who were down on their luck. The Department of Human Services grew stronger throughout the 1960s and 1970s as U.S. residents began to assert their rights to be treated fairly and to have their basic needs met. Human needs and rights were given prominence over preconceived, government-dictated notions of the basic necessities people require to live a healthy, productive life.

Some might believe that those who study or work in human services are "Jacks of all trades but masters of none." This text, however, supports the view that the generalist human services **model** enables those who work in the human services to become "masters of all trades." In other words, successful human services workers must know a variety of psychological, biological, and sociological theories so they can understand the causes of human behavior and use a variety of intervention strategies that take into consideration all models available. Putting the knowledge of these many and varied approaches to use can help human services workers successfully help their **clients** deal with their various problems. Developing an open, nonjudgmental attitude helps human services workers to determine which approach will be the most effective in meeting a particular client's needs.

Defining Human Services

Generally, "human services" is a broad term that includes services and programs provided to meet the needs of a person, a family, or an entire community. These services and programs are varied and ever changing as the needs and demands of society change. Maslow (1968) developed his hierarchy of needs that human services workers often focus on when providing services. Based on Maslow's model, one might suggest that activities that aim to meet the physiological needs, safety needs, social needs, self-esteem needs and the need for self-actualization are human services. Alle-Corliss and Alle-Corliss (1998) present a simple definition of human services as "encompassing professional services provided to those in need."

People in the Human Services

Human services' multidisciplinary, holistic, and eclectic approach to helping people requires that it employ many different types of people whose skills, education, and experience differ widely. The following are some examples of the types of people who work in the human services professions.

What Is a Human Services Worker?

A **human services worker** can be anyone, from psychologists and social workers to data managers. Neukrug (1994) describes a human services worker as "a person who has an associate's or bachelor's degree in human services or a closely related field." Others use "helper and human services **professional** interchangeably to refer to a wide range of practitioners, including social workers, clinical and counseling psychologists, marriage and family therapists, pastoral counselors, community mental health workers, and rehabilitation counselors" (Corey and Corey, 1993). Alle-Corliss and Alle-Corliss consider "that people who have undergraduate or graduate degrees and who work in human services are indeed human services professionals." They support the idea that there is great variance among human services workers.

Human services workers might work in **nonprofit agencies,** such as the Red Cross, or in a psychiatric hospital. Any facility that focuses on helping its clients meet their needs will have human workers on staff.

For example, teachers, coaches, the clergy, guidance counselors, probation officers, gang-prevention specialists, outreach workers, advocates, social workers, and psychologists may all be considered human services workers.

What Is the Difference between a Professional and a Paraprofessional?

Many believe that human services workers attain professional standing when they have earned at least a master's degree. Some might say that only a person who is licensed or credentialed is a professional. Yet others use human service workers only when referring to those who do not have a master's or doctoral degree. **Paraprofessional** usually refers to community workers who have not completed a bachelor's degree but have completed some training or education at a community college, university, or human services agency (for example, at many clinics, rape counselors must undergo 60 hours of training to be considered paraprofessionals). Yet others would use the term human services worker instead of paraprofessional for those who have not earned an advanced degree. Both professionals and paraprofessionals in human services usually receive a salary rather than work as a volunteer. Many agencies could not provide the services needed without hiring paraprofessionals who often receive a lower salary than their professional counterparts. Paraprofessionals can be as competent and effective as professionals, although their responsibilities may be different.

What Do Volunteers Do in Human Services?

Anyone who works at an agency without pay is considered a **volunteer.** Volunteers often donate their time for altruistic reasons. They do not receive credit from a school and are not considered **interns.** Volunteers are integral to the operation of most nonprofit agencies. Professionals who have been working in the field for years may choose to volunteer to work alongside those with little or no experience in the human services. Services provided by agency volunteers aren't less effective or of poorer quality than paid workers. Volunteers often bring an enthusiasm to a situation that longtime employees may lose. Volunteers should be treated with the same respect as employees no matter what their education and abilities. The fact that they are helping clients and the agency because they truly care gives them a special place in an agency.

Volunteers may provide medical services at free clinics, serve food at homeless shelters, nurture babies at homes for abused children, and answer phone calls at crisis center hotlines.

What Is an Intern's Role?

Interns are usually enrolled in a college and work at an agency for course credit. Interns' experiences at agencies may be discussed in class or with an advisor and are essential to a student's overall education. Some internships are paid, whereas others are not. The purpose of an internship is to use the theories learned in class with the actual on-the-job experience. Interns are often encouraged to reflect on their personal reactions to working at the agency as well. Interns are also expected to gain awareness of how their agency experience fits into their career goals. For example, an intern might discover that after working with elderly people at a senior center, she definitely does not want to work with that population during her career as a case manager. She may, however, find that she is much more effective and therefore prefers working with children after interning at a home for abused and neglected children. An internship experience should match an intern's level of training. Students may be encouraged to begin their first internship by shadowing (following and observing) an agency employee with considerable experience. As interns gain confidence in their ability to work effectively with clients, they may seek out more direct client contact. Instead of merely observing a support group, they may choose to interact with clients and offer educational presentations. At some point, students feel confident enough to work with clients as if they were employees of the agency.

Participating in an internship is an invaluable opportunity. Not only does it provide experience, skills, and confidence, it may increase the chances of finding full-time work in the future. Interns must adhere to the same ethical standards and work ethic as the employees who work in the agency. Interns are often required to meet an agency's highest expectations, despite the behavior of the full-time staff. For example, some employees may show up late to work. An intern would not be given the same latitude but expected to display a strong work ethic. Internships may take place at daycare centers, at homes for abused children, at outreach programs that work with teenagers, at after-school programs, at centers for senior citizens, at shelters for battered women, and at state and local social service departments.

Key Terms Used in the Human Services

Clients

A client, or recipient, is any individual, family, group, or organization that seeks assistance from a human services worker. Some people refer to clients as consumers.

Patients in psychiatric hospitals, people on probation (probationers), abusive parents, students, children who have survived abuse, survivors of rape or domestic violence, the elderly attending a senior center, and people struggling with addiction who are attending 12-step programs are all considered clients.

Clients with Multiple Needs

While a client may only have one need and therefore require service from one human services worker (e.g., seeing a guidance counselor who recommends a class to take), other clients may come in with many different concerns and who would then need the assistance of a variety of workers. Some refer to clients who have many needs as **Multi-Needs Clients.**

For example, it is not rare for a client to have emotional issues, such as depression, to need housing and food stamps, to be involved in child custody disputes, and to struggle with substance abuse. Each issue requires the collaboration of different human services workers to meet this client's needs. While one human services worker may sometimes be designated as the case manager (this is true in cases where a child has been removed from the client or if the client is on probation), all the workers servicing the client must work together cooperatively for the benefit of a client. Difficulties that may arise include trying to separate out which need came first. Was the client depressed first and then did she abuse her child? Did the client lose her job, become poor, lose her home, and then become depressed? These questions become irrelevant at some point. The main goal is to assess for all the needs of the client and then to set up plans that can address them all.

Model

A **model** is a theory or approach that is used to understand a situation or to help work through a problem. It usually includes related terms that attempt to explain something.

Examples of models include the psychoanalytical model, the **generalist model,** the humanistic model, and the behavioral model all of which offer strategies to use to help clients and understand their needs.

Multidisciplinary Team Approach

The reason that a multidisciplinary team approach is needed is because many individuals and families have multiple problems and needs. In human services agencies, it is typical for several workers to provide services for one client, each with a different duty, all working collaboratively.

For example, a case manager might assess a family's financial eligibility for welfare, a psychiatrist might prescribe antidepressant medication for the mother's depression, a social worker might investigate a report of child abuse made on the father, and a probation officer might monitor compliance with terms of probation on the teenager in the family who sold drugs. Although each team member would focus on the family member who they are best qualified to assist, they all would communicate and coordinate care with one another.

Another typical example often occurs in a group home for abused and neglected children. A child will usually have an individual counselor (possibly a masters-level therapist) who provides ongoing counseling to deal with long-standing emotional and behavioral issues related to prior abuse and neglect and issues related to being separated from parents. Additionally, if a child demonstrates serious psychiatric symptoms or unmanageable behaviors, a psychiatrist may be called in to prescribe medication. On a daily basis, this child will interact with paraprofessional case workers and child-care workers who may lead groups and provide continuity of care and ongoing support and who may step in for crisis management situations. A child may also have an assigned social worker from the state department of social services who oversees the entire treatment plan and consults with all service providers. At times, the child may see a psychologist for more intense therapy or psychological testing.

The box below describes a current and very innovative example of how a multidisciplinary team approach is used in the area of child welfare to create more standardization of care. The approach ensures that families receive services based on collaboration among the various workers involved in the case and that all involved are informed about the essentials of the case and the case plan. It is hoped that misunderstandings and families slipping through the cracks will be minimized by this type of approach.

Encapsulated or Specialist Approach

Someone who practices from this perspective only views clients' problems from one theoretical model or from the helper's own belief system. The helper adhering to an **encapsulated approach** does not take into consideration cultural tradi-

In 2005, California's Department of Social Services along with the California Social Work Education Center, California's Regional Training Academies, and the Inter-University Consortium developed a program in an attempt to standardize case-management practice of the agencies' social workers. This **multidisciplinary approach** uses a team decision-making model. Team decision making takes place in a meeting that includes family members, foster parents (when children are in placement), service providers, community representatives, the caseworker of record, the supervisor, and other staff from the child welfare agency. In these meetings, the team shares all information about the family that relates to the protection of the children and functioning of the family. The goal is to reach a consensus on a plan that protects the children and, if advisable for the safety and health of a child, preserves or reunites a family (Annie E. Casey Foundation, 2005).

How a Multidisciplinary Team Approach Works

tions, economic status, religious beliefs, or issues regarding gender and race. This approach focuses on intervening from a limited set of strategies based on a narrow model for understanding client needs.

The Generalist Model

A generalist model takes a flexible, all-inclusive approach to helping clients deal with their problems. Rather than using one theoretical model or one duty or function, a generalist considers which theories and interventions are most appropriate to meet a client's needs. Rosenthal (2003) sees human services workers as functioning as "generalists, like general practitioners, who are the primary contact." Rosenthal also suggests that most human services workers view themselves as generalists with a multitude of skills, who can work with a vast range of difficulties and perform a variety of functions.

Rather than deny the usefulness of any theory of human personality or human development, the generalist model considers all theories as valid and useful when working with a client. The generalist human services worker uses a holistic approach that looks at the biological, psychological, and social aspects of a client. We refer to this approach as a **bio-psychosocial** model, which Chapters 5 and 6 will examine in detail. Zastrow (1995) stresses the importance of considering all systems within the social environment and the interactions between physical and social environments when trying to understand a client. An eclectic approach to intervention is used in which the worker selects methods of interactions and strategies for helping from a variety of theoretical modalities. In other words, the generalist approach views clients from a holistic perspective, understands their needs from a bio-psychosocial perspective, and intervenes with an eclectic attitude. What is most important to remember is that people have multiple needs. The attitude of a human services worker is one of openness regarding how to best help meet those needs. This often includes collaborating with other human services workers, performing a wide variety of duties, and encouraging the client to utilize various services in the community. The following scenario is cast using two providers, each of whom uses a different approach to treating a client's problems. Marilyn is a 38-year-old woman who is depressed. Her primary-care physician recommends her to a psychiatrist (a medical doctor who specializes in treating mental disorders). The first psychiatrist she sees is a generalist practitioner. He not only prescribes antidepressant medication, but he also spends time talking with her about her social, family, and work life. He discovers that she has a variety of needs. Not only has she been suffering from depression, which probably has a biological basis, but she is also having serious marital problems. The psychiatrist recommends that Marilyn and her husband see a marriage counselor. Additionally, her employer has been pressuring her to work overtime three days a week for the past two months. Marilyn has been unhappy at work for many years. The psychiatrist encourages her consider other job opportunities. Finally, Marilyn says that she doesn't participate in any activities that she finds pleasurable. The psychiatrist recommends that she try joining a health club or a church group. The psychiatrist consults with her marriage counselor to ensure continuity of care.

Although psychiatrists are sometimes considered specialists who only dole out medication, the human services mentality allows for a more encompassing and effective approach. The next scenario demonstrates what can happen if the generalist model is not utilized.

Here is the same scenario but with a psychiatrist who uses an encapsulated approach. Again, at her primary-care physician's suggestion, Marilyn goes to a psychiatrist for treatment of her depression. This psychiatrist thoroughly explores all her symptoms of depression and discovers she has been depressed for many years. She meets all the criteria for diagnosis of a major depression. He believes this is due to a biochemical imbalance, and so he treats her with medication. As he sees it, his responsibility is to determine whether the medication is effective in relieving Marilyn's depression. The psychiatrist schedules monthly visits to assess for side effects of the medication. Two months pass, and Marilyn feels no better than she did before beginning treatment. Meanwhile, her problems at home and at work persist. The psychiatrist tells her to stay on the medication and give it more time.

These may seem like dramatic examples. Unfortunately, they are not atypical. Many professionals and paraprofessionals alike do not adhere to a generalist approach. Instead, they limit their responsibilities to only certain functions.

Here is another scenario that shows how different approaches yield very different outcomes. An eligibility worker for the county welfare department conducts an intake interview with a new client. Esperanza is a 22-year-old, Spanish-speaking mother of three children, ages 3 months, 2 years, and 5 years. She is unmarried and the fathers of her children all live in Mexico. She doesn't work and needs help raising her children. She yells frequently and often feels overwhelmed. The generalist worker shows Esperanza how to apply for financial assistance, medical and dental coverage, and food stamps and also gives her information about classes for adults who want to learn English and that have free babysitting. She is also referred to free, Spanish-speaking daycare and parenting classes. This client needs some social support and is also encouraged to attend one of several churches in her community. The human services worker provides Esperanza with bus tickets for doctor visits and also suggests that she enroll her five-year-old in kindergarten and should consider participating in school activities.

This generalist worker realizes that the client needs more than welfare. If services are not provided now, Esperanza will be unable to provide her children with the parenting they need to develop into productive citizens. By encouraging her to use these various services now, Esperanza and her family have a better chance of leading a successful and happy life. The following shows the effects of an encapsulated approach: Esperanza visits the county welfare office to apply for financial assistance for her family. The eligibility worker decides she qualifies for basic financial assistance, food stamps, and medical care. The worker shows Esperanza how to complete forms and tells her that she will begin receiving assistance immediately. The worker suggests that Esperanza and her children may be better off moving back to Mexico and getting their fathers to take care of her kids.

This worker is culturally insensitive as well as insensitive to this family's variety of needs. This approach is devoid of caring and appears to present the stereotypical attitude of government workers (Chapter 12 includes a discussion of the bureaucratic technician).

CRITICAL THINKING / SELF-REFLECTION CORNER

Imagine that you are Esperanza.

- How would you feel about each of the different workers?

- How do you see yourself fitting in with other human services workers?

- In what areas do you need to improve to be able to collaborate effectively with other workers? Do you need to boost your self-confidence? to work on becoming more cooperative? to improve your decision-making skills?

- How would you describe your own work ethic?

- What do you need to do to prepare yourself to work as an intern in a human services agency?

- How would feel about working for no pay?

Where Do Human Services Workers Work?

Many different types of agencies and organizations employ human services workers. These range from community organizations, large and small nonprofits, and **public** and **private agencies.** Many operate using volunteers, interns, and salaried staff, all of whom have different backgrounds and levels of education.

Nonprofit Agencies

According to Kramer (1981), a nonprofit agency is a bureaucratic organization that is governed by an elected, volunteer board of directors, employing professional, paraprofessional, and volunteer staff to provide ongoing services to its clients. Funding for nonprofit agencies may come from private donations, fundraisers, and both private and government grants. There are two types of nonprofit agencies. The first type provides face-to-face service to various client populations. It is usually staffed primarily by volunteers and interns, with a few administrative paid workers and serves victims of domestic violence, child abuse, rape, seriously ill people with limited income, and people who are battling alcoholism and other addictions. The second type of nonprofit is more of an administrative organization whose main function is fundraising for a specific cause, such as the United Way, Easter Seals, and the American Heart Association. They provide community education and distribute money to direct-service organizations.

Public Agencies

These are agencies funded by government taxes at the city, county, state, or federal level. Sometimes consumers pay to receive services. Some public agencies don't provide direct services but are administrative or provide community education. Such city–level agencies include senior centers, park and recreation centers, and gang units in police departments. At the county level, human services agencies include the departments of social services and welfare, the department of mental and behavioral health, and the department of corrections. State- and federal-level human service agencies include the department of rehabilitation, state regional centers for developmentally disabled persons, and the department of social security.

Private Agencies

These agencies are funded by consumer fees and usually operate on a for-profit model, such as some hospitals or convalescent homes. Clinicians who engage in private practice as mental health counselors also fit into this category. Perhaps the most widely used types of **private agencies** are health maintenance organizations (HMOs). HMOs began to replace private medical and mental health insurance usage in 1980s. HMOs also provide educational information and treatment for substance abuse. HMOs tend to utilize more professional-level workers. Some may use volunteers, but their role is less vital to the daily operation of an HMO than they are to nonprofits and public agencies. Funding for HMOs comes partially from client co-payments and partially from insurance carriers, primarily acquired from clients' place of employment, and some may also receive third-party payments from Medicare and Medicaid.

Why Choose a Career in Human Services?

There are many reasons to seek a degree in human services and help others in need. This is an exciting field with much opportunity for professional enrichment, job promotion, and personal fulfillment. It is a chance to encounter people who are both different and the same as you. Human services workers can gain a sense of pride for contributing to the well-being of others. Human services jobs allow for autonomy and varied job duties. While some human services jobs conduct business during the traditional hours of 9 a.m. to 5 p.m., many offer flexible scheduling. There is constant growth—both personal and professional—for those who work in human services. Challenges abound, and this can be an intellectually rewarding occupation as well.

Reasons Not to Choose a Career in Human Services

If your goal is to make a million dollars and retire by age 55, human services may not be for you. Other motivations, such as a need to save others and take care of others or a need to be depended on or to control others may not be appropriate reasons to enter the helping field either. Sometimes a well-meaning helper may inadvertently use clients to meet his or her own personal emotional needs rather than focusing on the client's needs. If a person's motivation to enter the helping field is to feel good because someone else needs him or her or if the helper feels powerful when someone depends on him or her, the prospective human service worker should discuss these feelings with a counselor or an instructor. It isn't fair to clients to use them to meet our own emotional needs.

While one can make a decent living in this field, money is usually not the primary goal of those in human services. The field can be personally taxing, and dedication to helping others live better lives is key. Also, this is not just an easy degree that anyone can obtain. Many of the classes are both academically and emotionally difficult. Working on a daily basis with people who suffer from emotional and physical problems can be difficult. A person who works in human services must be committed to ongoing self-development and self-examination. These processes are part of the training for human services workers. For those who find these challenges appealing, human services may be a good career choice.

Chapter Summary

The field of human services includes a wide range of activities that focus on helping people meet a variety of needs. Human services workers perform many functions and are skilled to perform many duties. This generalist approach is one of the hallmarks in the field of human services and allows for an interdisciplinary approach to working with clients. Human services workers may use a variety of theories and interventions, may be volunteers or paid employees, and may be highly educated or have minimal formal education.

Suggested Applied Activities

1. Interview someone who works in human services in a nonprofit agency, a public agency, and a private agency. Ask this person to describe the types of other workers he or she deals with regularly. Inquire about the multineeds of the clients who come into the agency. See if you can determine whether this person uses a generalist approach.

_____

_____

_____

_____

_____

_____

2. Observe any differences among the workers you interview, based on the type of agency for which they work, whether they use a multidisciplinary team approach or a generalist model, and the types of needs of their clients have.

_____

_____

_____

_____

_____

_____

Chapter Review Questions

1. What is meant by a generalist approach?

_____

_____

2. Why is eclecticism considered necessary for being an effective human services practitioner?

_____

_____

3. What are the differences and similarities between an intern, a volunteer, and an employee?

_____

_____

4. Name two appropriate reasons to work in human services.

_____

_____

5. Name two inappropriate reasons to work in human services.

_____

_____

Glossary of Terms

Bio-psychosocial model is a theoretical model for understanding what causes deviance that includes physiological, psychological, and sociological theories.

Client is a person who receives human services.

Eclectic approach uses a variety of theoretical models and interventions to deal effectively with clients.

Encapsulated approach uses a narrow, theoretical model to understand and serve clients.

Generalist model uses a variety of theoretical models and interventions to assist client.

Holistic is an approach that considers the clients in their entirety, including their biological, psychological, and social needs.

Human services are services provided to help people with various needs live better lives.

Human services worker is any person employed by or volunteering in a human services agency.

Intern is a person who works in the field of human services as part of formal education.

Model is an approach that usually has a theoretical basis that helps workers understand clients and help them out with their problems.

Multidisciplinary team approach is an approach that requires collaboration and open communication among various workers to best meet the needs of clients with multiple problems.

Multineeds clients are individuals or families with a variety of needs who seek assistance from human services. Such clients require workers to be knowledgeable and competent in many areas and to practice a generalist approach.

Nonprofit agencies are community organizations funded by donations, fundraisers, and charity whose focus is providing service and effective programs rather than focusing on making a profit.

Paraprofessionals are human services workers who do not have a professional degree or license.

Private agencies are organizations that are not funded by municipal, state, or federal government programs.

Professional is a human services worker with a college degree or license.

Public agencies are agencies that are government run or funded.

Case Presentation and Exit Quiz

General Description and Demographics

Jenny is an unmarried 27-year-old woman with three children, all of whom have different fathers. She has never been married and is currently four months pregnant with a child from yet another man. Jenny has never worked nor graduated from high school. She survives through financial assistance from Aid to Families with Dependent Children (AFDC) but has recently been told that she must find a job or enroll in a vocational-training program. Jenny and her children live in a two-bedroom apartment in federally subsidized housing, receive monthly checks from AFDC, and are enrolled in state-funded medical programs. Two of her children go to public school where they get free breakfast and lunch. Jenny stays at home during the day to care for her two-year-old. She has yet to seek prenatal care for her current pregnancy.

Jenny was raised by her mother, had very little contact with her father, and has one brother, three years her senior who is in jail. Her mother works, lives close by, and often baby-sits for Jenny. Despite this help, Jenny and her mother are not close, but Jenny's children feel very close to their grandmother.

Problems That Need Assistance

Both of Jenny's school-aged children often show up at school improperly dressed and unwashed. But recently, Jenny's eight-year-old daughter, Rebecca, came to school with bruises on the backs of her legs. The teacher reported this to the child protective agency within the state department of social services.

Jenny has had drug problems for the past 10 years. She uses crystal methamphetamine at between three and five times a week, even when the children are home and hangs out regularly with other crystal-meth users. Despite this, she prepares dinner for her children every night and never leaves them alone.

First Human Services Worker Involved in the Case

When the report of child abuse came in to the department, the case was assigned to an emergency investigative social worker. He met with Rebecca at her school and spoke with Jenny at her home; he then referred the case to another social worker who began to develop a case plan.

Based on the details of this case, respond to the following questions. The concepts in this quiz have been discussed in this chapter.

Exit Quiz

1. Jenny is an example of
   a. a client with a very specialized need
   b. a multineed client
   c. a client who is undeserving of service because of her drug use
   d. none of the above

2. The most effective way for the social worker to deal with this case would be to
   a. conduct one-on-one counseling with Jenny
   b. focus on the children and let Jenny find her own case worker
   c. collaborate with several other human services workers to help the entire family
   d. all of the above

3. If the social worker sets up a case plan that requires Jenny to participate in her own therapy and drug treatment, undergo an assessment for depression, and to seek prenatal care, it would require
   a. a multidisciplinary team approach
   b. that each worker specialize in a specific task and let the others do their jobs as specialists
   c. that only the professionals be allowed to treat Jenny
   d. none of the above

4. If the social worker in this case understands Jenny and her children's various needs and is capable of coordinating all the necessary services, the social worker is considered
   a. a jack of all trades, but a master of none
   b. a generalist worker
   c. ambivalent
   d. all of the above

5. The most effective way to understand Jenny's problems would be from a
   a. a psychoanalytic view
   b. purely biological view
   c. bio-psychosocial view
   d. none of the above

Exit Quiz Answers

1. b   3. a   5. c
2. c   4. b

CHAPTER 2

A Brief History of the Human Services

Introduction

While the term "human services" is rather new, services provided to people in need by governments, religious organizations, and communities have been around since recorded time. There has always been a need to take care of people in the community, whether it be disabled members of the clans of caveman days, the lepers from the biblical times, the sick during the leech-sucking days of Aristotle, or the 'possessed witches' of the Middle Ages. Taking care of those around us was most likely a way to ensure survival of the species, which is an intrinsic drive in all species. It wasn't until Queen Elizabeth of England created the **Elizabethan Poor Laws** in 1547 that the government stepped in and officially declared its part in assisting those in need. Since then, programs have become more sophisticated and complex, but the type of individuals who receive assistance seem to stay the same. Let's go on a brief journey into the past to better understand the state of affairs in the twenty-first century.

Early Humans: Charity, Punishment, and Abandonment (Prehistory to circa 600 B.C.)

Charity, punishment, and **abandonment** are still integral aspects of human services. People who exhibit behaviors outside the boundaries of societal norms or who are lacking in the ability to survive as a human being, are treated with compassion (e.g. abused and neglected children), are sometimes punished (e.g. murderers), or are sometimes abandoned and rejected (e.g. homeless drug addicts). It can be conjectured that charity, punishment, and abandonment were the options in dealing with **deviance** and people with special needs in the days of early man. Picture yourself walking through jungles, deserts, and icy tundras with heavy loads of food and other survival gear such as hides for ensuring warmth and weapons. What would you do with a member of your clan who was physically disabled? How would you manage that cousin who suffered from mental retardation? Who would assist the elderly that were often too frail to travel? On the other hand, what should the clan do if someone steals food or items from another?

Worse, how would a murderer be handled? Would that oddly behaving uncle be given charity or would he be punished? The members of the clan had to decide whether to punish, take care of, or abandon these individuals. Although much change has occurred throughout time regarding how to manage deviance and assist those in need, modern day human services still operate under the same perspective of ancient man for the most part. Those in the human service field still approach those in need with charity and take care of them, or if deemed to be purposefully bad, punish them, and sadly sometimes, those in need are abandoned, neglected and excluded. Just as it was probably confusing back then as to who was deserving of charity and who deserved **punishment,** it is still sometimes confusing today who is entitled to services and who is not. Much of this confusion is due to the way in which human service workers attribute the causes of the problems.

One of the causal theories that anthropologists believe was adhered to by prehistoric civilizations is **animism,** in which spirits were believed to inhabit inanimate objects (Clodd, 1997). At times, evil spirits were thought to inhabit a person's brain and cause deviant behaviors, similar to what we now call psychotic delusions and hallucinations. A technique used to rid a person of evil spirits was called **trepanning** (see Figure 2.1), in which a hole was drilled into the skull of

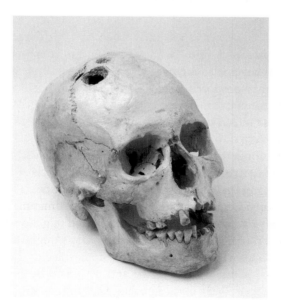

Figure 2.1 Trepanning, the procedure of boring a hole in the skull, is the earliest known medical operation. Some anthropologists believe that trepanning was performed on people with mental illnesses to drive out evil spirits from their heads. This skull dates from the Bronze Age, 2200–2000 B.C. © *SSPL / The Image Works*

the affected person to release evil spirits. This may have been one of the first attempts to treat mental illness, and it was certainly one of the first surgical procedures practiced. Trepanning, sometimes referred to as trephinning, might still be performed today on certain individuals. Sophisticated tools are used to relieve pressure from the brain caused by skull fracture or cerebral abscess.

While this sounds barbaric, when one compares it to a frontal-lobe **lobotomy** practiced in the 1930s and 1940s, it is not so unthinkable. Lobotomies were performed by using an ice pick through a slot above the eye into the brain to excise the frontal lobe—the part of the brain theorized to control aggressive and violent behaviors. The theory of causes may be different from our earliest ancestors, but the practice of trepanning may have been effective in the same way lobotomies were effective in managing psychotic behaviors. While modern-day psychiatry does not perform lobotomies with ice picks anymore (this was deemed too barbaric), some individuals suffering from severe mental disorders still undergo **psychosurgery,** in which parts of the brain are excised. History does repeat itself! But with the introduction of antipsychotic medications, the once widespread use of lobotomy in America was all but extinguished (El-Hai, 2004).

Ancient Civilizations: Scientific Inquiry Evolves (600 B.C. to the Common Era)

Enlightened Greeks, circa 600 B.C., such as **Hippocrates** (see Figure 2.2), Aristotle, Socrates, and Plato began exploring humans physically, mentally, and politically as their civilizations grew and became strong. Unlike their primitive predecessors, they proposed a scientific explanation for illness. Hippocrates, for whom the physicians' Hippocratic Oath was named (Miles, 2003), believed that human diseases, including deviant behaviors, resulted from an imbalance in four bodily fluids referred to as **humours.** This theory led to such practices as bloodletting and leeching, used to rid the body of excess fluids, therefore restoring the balance. An interesting point to consider is that many people in modern times use these methods on themselves when depressed (e.g., cutting oneself with razor blades to see blood, and inducing vomiting to be thin and feel purified). Use of leeches to extract disease is still used by modern physicians as well. Also, although modern-day psychiatrists and physicians might not believe that illness is due to imbalance in blood, phlegm, and stomach acids, beginning in the 1950s when psychiatrists began to prescribe anti-psychotic medications to mentally ill patients, the idea of biochemical imbalances as the cause of deviance has become strong and the predominate causal theory for twenty-first-century practice. The perception by psychiatrists that biochemical imbalances cause many mental health disorders dictates intervention by many psychiatrists and physicians work-

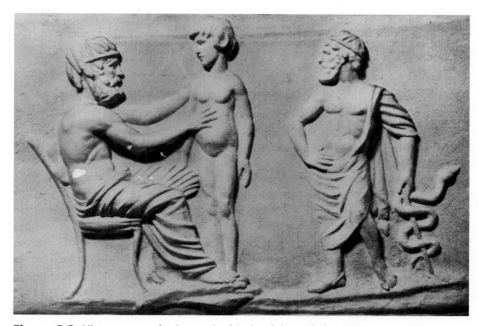

Figure 2.2 Hippocrates, who is seen in this Greek bas-relief watching as a doctor treats a young patient, believed most diseases were chiefly organic in origin. For example, Hippocrates believed that the brain was the center of intelligence, and mental disorders, therefore, were due specifically to the malfunctioning of the brain. *Hulton Archive / Getty Images*

ing in public and private agencies. Instead of having patients induce vomiting or release blood, modern-day human service workers prescribe medications to balance biochemistry.

Early Christianity and the Middle Ages: Punitive Approaches Prevail; Faith and Human Compassion Take Their Turns—and Back to Punishment (Eighteenth Century B.C. to Fifteenth Century A.D.)

Dealing with deviance, **poverty**, and human needs looks decidedly different from the perspective of the societies in which religious leaders ruled. Prior to Christianity, most deviant behavior was punished by putting the offender in stocks and gallows and having the public stone him or her for his or her misbehaviors.

The basis of criminal law in early civilizations was most likely based on the Semitic law of "an eye for an eye," and the earliest legal code known as the **Code of Hammurabi** (see Figure 2.3), in which equal retaliation was the basis for criminal justice (Harper, 2002).

In John 8:7, Jesus challenges a crowd, saying, "Let he who is without sin, cast the first stone" (Tyndale, 1611). Such renowned quotations may have reflected the changing attitudes of the time, from punishment to compassion. Jesus's stance toward the unfortunate may have lead to a trend toward forgiveness and empathy rather than the punitive stance that viewed people with struggles as being morally deficient.

As the Roman Empire lost its stronghold on the world by about 500 A.D., the era usually referred to as the Middle Ages began and continued until about 1500 A.D. The first couple hundred of years of the middle ages is often referred to as the dark ages because there was a lack of cultural achievements in contrast to the literary and scientific achievements during the Classic period of the Roman Empire (Mommsen, 1942). The dark ages most likely occurred due to the growing strength of Christianity and focus on faith rather than on science as

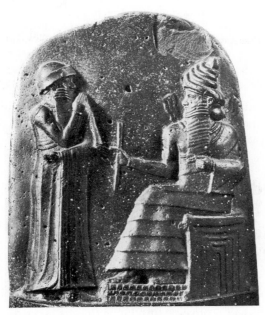

Figure 2.3 The Code of Hammurabi is engraved on the black basalt of this stele, which is 2.25 meters (7 feet, 5 inches) high and was made in the first half of the eighteenth century, B.C. *Time Life Pictures / Getty Images*

was seen in the classical era of the Greeks and Romans. The clergy was growing strong in terms of its influence on societal laws and norms. Lack of faith became the primary societal focus to explain deviance during these dark ages, and faith continued to be the primary explanatory model throughout the rest of the middle ages.

At times, prayer and faith healing were used to help those in need, along with compassion and charity. Later in the Middle Ages (during the time of the Spanish Inquisition between 1100 and 1300), the church dealt with perceived deviance by more punitive measures. Those who studied science or were associated with unexplained phenomena were considered heretics and in league with the devil, and the church often ordered them to be burned at the stake or to undergo exorcisms in which demons were ordered to leave the body of the person. Many women during this time were ordered to enter deep water after those in power filled their clothes with stones. If they drowned, it was proof they weren't heretics, and they would go to heaven. If they survived, they were witches and would be executed. The *Malleus Maleficarum* (a book written by clergy during the second half of the Middle Ages) was written to prove the existence of witches and warlocks and [to instruct] how to identify them and how to treat or help them (Summers, 1969).) The sick, the poor, and the needy were considered sinners and were left to die without any care. Only the very wealthy and most powerful were allowed to be educated.

It's interesting again to note how previous societal interventions with those suffering and in need can be observed today. For example, modern-day clergy still use prayer to heal a variety of ills. Also, the idea that deviance might be due to demonic possession sounds similar to prehistoric societal views that evil spirits possessed those who were suffering.

CRITICAL THINKING / SELF-REFLECTION CORNER

- What types of deviant behaviors do you think are caused by biochemical imbalances or other biological factors?

- Who do you think deserves punishment in today's society?

- Who deserves charity?

- Does any deviant group deserve to be abandoned, excluded, or neglected?

- Who is responsible for taking care of those in need?

- How would you respond to someone who believes that society should take a survival-of-the-fittest attitude and let people take care of themselves?

The Age of Reason: Scientific Discovery and Rational Politics (the Fifteenth Through the Eighteenth Centuries)

Fortunately, society made it through the Middle Ages, and science and rational politics returned, and at a more advanced level than of the ancient Greeks, Romans, and Egyptians. Monarchies ruled most countries, and the royals in power established civil governments that studied science systematically. Many commissioned explorers to travel the world and gather information and treasures, such as Queen Isabella of Spain who commissioned Christopher Columbus to find a trade route to the East. Human services were developing during this Renaissance in a very systematic way as well. Although average citizens had no access to education, and those accused of crimes were at the mercy of those in power, humanitarian philosophies influenced services established to aid poor, disabled, and infirmed people were being created. In 1601, Queen Elizabeth of England created the Elizabethan Poor Laws that authorized the British government to provide for the needs of people who were unable to care for themselves, such as children, the disabled, and the poor (Dean, Fletcher, Guy, and Morrill, eds., 1996). Shelters and workhouses provided for these populations. Modern-day social welfare is largely based on these same principles. Children and the disabled have priority in receiving governmental assistance. Although the shelters and services available in those days didn't focus on truly ameliorating the problems (they may have been a way to hide them), they do show that changes were being made in regard to these populations. At least they were being noticed by the governing class.

During that time, the mentally ill, mentally retarded, and criminals also received more humanitarian treatment than was given in the Middle Ages. In 1247, Bethlem Royal Hospital, popularly known as **Bedlam,** the first asylum for the insane was built in London to care for those with psychiatric illnesses (Hollingshead, 2004).

In France, institutions had been established to deal with members of its society who were insane and who broke the law by locking them in chains until they died. By the late 1700s, however, such institutions were being reformed, influenced largely by the work of **Philippe Pinel** (see Figure 2.4). Pinel was a physician who promoted the moral treatment of those who were institutionalized, not only by removing their chains but also by offering them food, shelter, and clothing (Weiner, 1979).

In colonial America, civil government was developing, and the country was governed administratively rather than by theocracy or monarchy during the 1700s. As the government became strong and independent, it developed public health and human services for children, the sick, and the poor largely because it

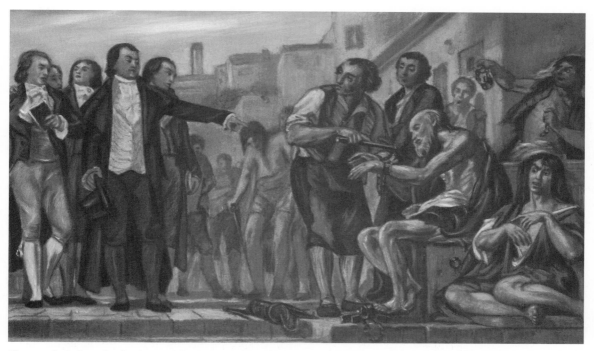

Figure 2.4 French physician Philippe Pinel supervises the unchaining of mentally ill patients in this painting by Charles Muller. © *Bettmann / Corbis*

was important to keep the streets clean from those afflicted with the plague and other public health nuisances. Although some people during this time period held punitive stances toward those exhibiting deviant behaviors (many people were called witches and burnt at the stakes such as during the Salem witch trials), it's possible that the Christian base of the growing nation allowed for humanitarian treatment of those in need. Also, the foundation of this new country was based on individual rights and pursuit of happiness. The government may have been compelled to take care of its citizenry in order to fulfill the dream of happiness and opportunity that was the foundation of the constitution.

Education in the United States was also undergoing major improvements. **Horace Mann,** known as the "great equalizer" (Compayri and Frost, 2002), worked with Thomas Jefferson to create mandatory education for everyone. Prior to that, only the wealthy and the powerful had access to education. Mann's reforms marked the beginning of government-funded school systems that would be regulated and would provide all U.S. residents access to literature and the fundamentals of learning that were the foundations of a prosperous standard of living.

The Nineteenth Century: Laying a Foundation for the Modern Human Services

Scientific interest in the causes of deviant behavior increased during the 1800s and led to different schools of thought about the causes of such problems as crime, mental illness, and poverty. For example, **Cesare Lombroso** began the systematic study of criminals, and scientists separated them from individuals thought to be mentally ill (Lombroso, Ferrero, Rafter, ed., Gibson, ed., 2004). **Emil Kraepelin's** practice of dividing mental illnesses into different categories set the stage for modern-day diagnoses. He is particularly well known for establishing the clinical pictures to diagnose schizophrenia and manic-depression (Columbia University Press, 2006).

Sigmund Freud developed his **psychoanalytic theory** which not only proposed a model for understanding abnormal and normal human behaviors, but introduced a systematic method for treating patients. His approach was novel in that he was the first physician to propose that mental health problems served a psychological function for the individual. He likened people to machines and suggested that failure in brain machinery may lead to mental illness. Rather than judge people or subject them to punishment or pity, Freud proposed that people could be helped by allowing them to speak freely about their problems and their thoughts to a doctor who would then interpret for the patients why they are suffering. His introduction of "talk" therapy was monumental in the field of mental health. Although many modern-day mental health workers use other approaches in their counseling practices, Freud must be credited with introducing the idea that a patient-therapist relationship can help people overcome emotional problems. For this, Freud probably deserves being considered the father of modern mental health.

Social welfare was also developing systematically during the 1800s. **Dorothea Dix** (see Figure 2.5) was well known for crusading on behalf of the insane, poor, and criminals (Grob, 1994).

In 1843, the New York association for improving conditions of the poor was created. Social workers of the time attributed poverty to "moral deficiency," and divided poor people into two categories: either unworthy or worthy. Sadly, many people today still adhere to this theory about the poor.

During the Industrial Revolution of the late 1800s, hundreds of thousands of people immigrated to the United States seeking a better quality of life. Another person interested in meeting the social welfare needs of people, **Jane Addams** (see Figure 2.6) founded **Hull House** as a settlement house to assist these immigrants in adjusting to their new homeland. Other similar houses were created in an initial attempt to provide housing assistance to the poor (Davis, K., 1990).

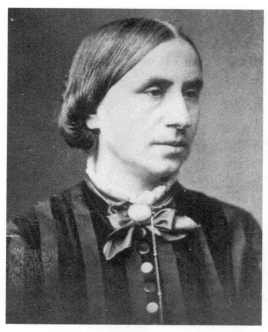

Figure 2.5 American reformer Dorothea Dix championed the causes of prison inmates, the mentally ill, and the destitute. *Photo by MPI / Getty Images*

Headway was being made in the criminal justice system during this century as well. Based on results of scientific studies, criminals who demonstrated signs of rehabilitation were being released from prison before the terms of their sentence were up. The **Elmira Reformatory** in Pennsylvania was the first U.S. prison to use the practice of "time off for good behavior." Past attempts at prisoner rehabilitation had failed, but prisoners given the chance of early release were more likely to reform their ways.

CRITICAL THINKING AND SELF-REFLECTION CORNER

Imagine what the United States would be like today if education was not government funded.

How do you think schooling would have progressed if the government had not intervened?

Consider both the pros and cons of the following statement:

Highly intelligent children should be exposed to a full education, whereas children of average and below-average intelligence should be taught only specific skills and certain trades.

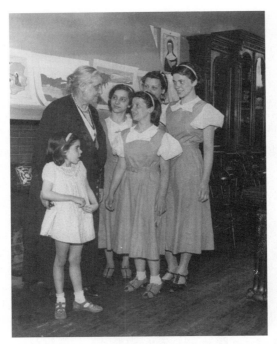

Figure 2.6   In 1889, Jane Addams, seen here greeting girls at Hull House, founded Hull House, a center for welfare work in Chicago. Fueled by Addams's exuberant personality, Hull House championed the causes of labor reform, public education, and immigrants' rights. Addams's book, *Twenty Years at Hull House,* details her service and social justice work in Chicago. *AP Images*

The Twentieth Century: Science Flourishes and Government Funds Human Services

Developments in Mental Health

Freud certainly set the stage for modern-day counseling with his **psychoanalytic approach** to treating emotionally troubled people. The idea that a practitioner would sit with a patient and talk about problems was unique. Of course now, we take this practice for granted, and various types of therapists and counselors abound in modern times. Psychoanalysis as a mental health theory and treatment model predominated until the 1940s when humanistic models such as Carl Rogers's nondirective approach (currently referred to as person-centered therapy, which is a form of humanistic counseling) became popular. Also, behavioral approaches (the use of rewards and restrictive methods to change behaviors) to treat certain problems were being used in schools, prisons and mental hospitals.

In the early 1940s, **Gerald Caplan** and **Eric Lindemann** developed crisis-intervention counseling through their work at the Wellesley Project in Boston (an institute involving research to learn about the reactions of survivors who had experienced serious trauma and grief). It also served as a training ground for people interested in providing crisis intervention. Their work was precipitated by the Coconut Grove nightclub fire in which almost 500 people died, and many more were injured (Lindemann, 1944). Using concepts and intervention strategies based on the psychoanalytic, humanistic, and behavioral models, Caplan and Lindemann developed ways in which individuals could benefit from short-term intervention. Caplan's preventive psychiatry, as it was first called, would ensure that individuals suffering from a life crisis wouldn't deteriorate and develop serious psychiatric illnesses. It promoted psychological and emotional growth and led to an acceptance of mental health consultation among the general public (Slaikeu, 1990). The practice of crisis intervention flourished over the next 50 years, and today's health maintenance organizations (HMOs) and many public and private agencies encourage its use. Besides being economically efficient, short-term therapy is effective in helping people return to a normal state of functioning and in preventing suicide and other dangerous behaviors.

In the 1950s, psychiatrists begin studying family therapy models. In the 1960s, other approaches to counseling were developed, such as gestalt therapy (that involves creating balance within an individual), and reality therapy (in which individuals are encouraged to take responsibility for their behaviors and to engage in more socially acceptable behaviors). Cognitive therapy (which focuses on how a person's perception of a situation can lead to emotional problems) became popular in the 1970s and 1980s. These approaches to counseling will be discussed in more detail in Chapter 5.

In the 1980s and 1990s, when health insurance companies began using **managed care** (which requires that treatment plans be preapproved before a person can receive care) **crisis intervention** (which focuses on coming to terms with a specific event that is keeping a person from functioning at a normal level) predominated, and still does in the twenty-first century. Specifics about crisis intervention and more details about managed care and HMOs will be discussed in Chapters 8 and 12.

The **deinstitutionalization of the mentally ill** during the late 1950s and early 1960s is considered monumental in the field of mental health services. When Thorazine, the first antipsychotic medication, was developed in 1955, many patients whose violent and unpredictable behaviors had made them unmanageable could be managed on medication and released from the mental hospitals. The advent of psychotropic medications set the stage for the **Community Mental Health Act of 1963,** which federally mandated communities to create mental health centers to provide crisis management and suicide prevention for formerly hospitalized patients. This created the need for workers to staff these centers. Initially, paraprofessionals, called mental health workers, were used. Later, licensed, **professional** therapists and psychiatrists staffed these centers.

During the antiestablishment era of the 1960s and 1970s, **grassroots** movements (programs and services that community activists started without government financing or a professional staff) established nonprofit agencies where people could go and talk about problems, often in support-group style. These were run by paraprofessionals and depended heavily on volunteers. These centers still exist today as viable alternatives for mental health treatment.

Social Welfare Development

In the twentieth century, social welfare has undergone many changes since the days of orphanages, settlement houses, and charity wards in hospitals. During the Great Depression of the late 1920s and 1930s, **Franklin Delano Roosevelt's New Deal** provided people in need with food, clothing, and other basic necessities of life and also created work programs so that people could earn a living wage (Davis, 1990). Under the leadership of President Roosevelt, government became strong in its focus on social problems, and the notion of **disparity** (inequality and differences) among **socioeconomic classes** (social class based on income per year; usually divided into upper, middle, and lower classes) was studied by social scientists. This disparity, especially between minorities and mainstream society, eventually led to the civil unrest of the 1960s in which minorities insisted on equality and reform.

In the 1960s, President Lyndon Johnson waged a **War on Poverty,** resulting in the passage of the 1964 Economic Opportunity Act, which created such programs as affirmative action, welfare, food stamps, low-cost housing, and federally funded medical insurance (Howard, 1972). While the welfare system has changed since the 1960s, the basic premise of government aid to those in need, still exists. The implementation of these welfare programs required the employment of thousands of social workers across the country. This catalyzed the formal study of social welfare in colleges, the increased usage of social workers in various agencies, and the sociopolitical premise that certain people are entitled to government charity.

Prison Reform

The twentieth century also brought reform to U.S. prison systems. In response to substantiated proof that there is a direct relationship between poverty, violence, and criminal behavior, the prison system has begun to focus on more humanistic approaches to rehabilitation. The proven connection between crime and poverty has made crime more of a social problem. Probation and parole programs were set

True Stories from Human Service Workers

Grassroots Movement Agencies

A Free Clinic for Women

The Anaheim Free Clinic, a community agency in California, was created in 1973 by two women interested in offering community residents, concerned about issues of confidentiality, an alternative to visiting a family doctor or a government-funded clinic. This clinic is a classic example of a grassroots agency. It was established during the time when women in America were beginning to assert their right to equal treatment. In particular, women wanted to be able to make decisions about their bodies. *Roe vs. Wade,* which gave women the constitutional right to terminate a pregnancy, had just been decided by the U.S. Supreme Court. The Free Clinic was developed to provide birth-control counseling, as well as birth control itself, and pregnancy testing and counseling. Participants didn't even have to give their real names or show identification.

I (the author) began interning at the Free Clinic in 1978, when I was a junior in college working toward my degree in human services. I chose that agency because I was interested in women's rights and in creating a safe place for women to learn and make choices about their bodies that could affect them for the rest of their lives. At the Free Clinic, I worked with physicians who volunteered because they also believed women needed to receive accurate information and testing so they could make informed decisions that would benefit them both physically and mentally.

In my role as an intern, I ran support groups, information groups, ran pregnancy tests, and counseled the woman about their options. Most of the clients were women and teenage girls who thought they might be pregnant or have a sexually transmitted disease or who wanted some form of birth control. Because sexuality was the primary issue at the clinic, it was vital to create a strong feeling of trust and confidentiality with the clients. All services were free. We did ask for donations from clients when possible. We held fundraisers in the community and sought donations from many companies to keep the clinic operating. I believe this clinic epitomizes a grassroots organization. Although I worked there more than 25 years ago, I still remember vividly my experiences there. It was a political as well as healing agency.

A Safe Place for Battered Women

Battered-women's shelters, another outgrowth of the women's rights movement of the 1970s, are also examples of grassroots agencies. The first such shelter was created in the mid-1970s to provide a safe haven for woman who were victims of domestic violence. At the same time that women were asserting their sexual rights, they were also realizing that putting up with physical and emotional abuse from a partner was unacceptable. This was and continues to be a political issue and to this day as various legislation dealing with domestic violence gets passed.

At first, these shelters were very small, involving women helping women. Over the years, they have become more elaborate agencies, with services ranging from employment counseling and legal advocacy to mental health treatment and child care. I also worked at a battered woman's shelter, and the following is a description of my experience there:

(continued)

(continued)

I remember immediately noticing the difference between this agency and the county mental health department, where I was a mental health worker for four years. At the shelter, clients were treated with more respect. The workers were motivated to make a difference in each of their client's life. Everyone talked about women's rights issues. Paperwork, while it existed, was not as extensive as it was at the county agency. The shelter focused on helping women feel empowered. Many of the advocates and counselors at the agency had survived abusive relationships themselves. The atmosphere was supportive, educational, and political. While furniture was somewhat old and dingy, it felt more homey than the county facility. Money was always a concern, but the autonomy gained from not having to abide by government regulations was worth the frantic, ongoing search for funding.

up to allow probationers and parolees to live in society under the supervision of human services workers who monitored their behaviors. Allowing certain individuals these freedoms seemed more economically efficient than sending all violators to prison. Many law-enforcement and correctional agency workers began to receive training in social and psychological theories so that they could better understand criminal behaviors. Even recent television dramas often have a character whose job it is to analyze the criminal mind.

Educational Reform

Education also progressed during the twentieth century. Although mandatory education had been around for a while, the quality of education was in no way the same for every child living in the United States. In the 1950s and 1960s, **Martin Luther King Jr.**, and other civil rights leaders, campaigned for an equal quality of education for minorities. Until the 1950s, and even into the 1960s and 1970s in some places, blacks and whites in the South were not allowed to attend the same schools. The **civil rights movement** of the 1960s focused national attention on the inequalities and abuses brought about by segregation and racism. Public schools throughout the country slowly became integrated.

Eventually, state governments began passing legislation that funded special programs in the public schools so that learning-disabled and developmentally delayed children, as well as children with physical limitations could be provided with the same educational opportunities as their peers. These growing programs required public school systems to hire human services workers to evaluate students' needs and to provide counseling to them and their families.

The Twenty-First Century: Conservatism, Volunteerism, and Political Correctness

Modern-Day Mental Health Programs

Today's human services exist amid a sociopolitical climate of conservative religious beliefs and conservative economic views. In the area of mental health, some states began using lottery monies and cigarette and gasoline taxes to increase state-funded services such as community mental health centers. In the private arena, HMOs provide mental health services which are low cost to clients, but which do not permit clinicians to provide long-term treatment for the most part. Also, HMOs have lowered the rates that clinicians receive for their services. For example, in 1984, the author was able to collect 90 percent of her fee from most private indemnity insurance companies for psychotherapy services. Twenty years later in 2004, most clinicians received a set rate made by the HMOs for their services, which is often half of what they would charge if they billed indemnity insurance or half of what they would charge a cash-paying client. Some clinicians still operate out of their own private practice collecting cash from clients, but in today's world where money is tight, not many people can afford to $100 to $200 an hour out of pocket for psychotherapy.

Nonprofit agencies still exist, but are more dependent on various government grants for funding. They still rely on volunteers and interns and the pay for employees is not comparable to those working for private agencies or public agencies. However, nonprofit agencies still maintain more autonomy from government regulations than other agencies and still operate from a strongly political perspective than other types of agencies.

Modern Social Welfare Programs

As for today's social welfare programs, government funding is fairly strong for child protection services and services that protect the elderly and the disabled. If someone does not happen to be an abused or needy child, a vulnerable and needy elder, or a person with a disability, most government run agencies will not provide social welfare. Nonprofit agencies do provide resources for the non-disabled adults and other needy people. There are many homeless shelters for families and adults. They are temporary and aim to help get people back on their feet. Many churches still provide food and clothes to the needy as well.

Modern Correctional Facilities

The correctional system is overwhelmed by inmates, and emphasis is placed on probation, counseling, and rehabilitation rather than incarceration when possible. Of course, when criminals pose a threat to society, they are still locked up and sometimes put to death. Because of the overwhelming numbers of criminals in society, private organizations and people have taken it upon themselves to intervene in some cases. For example, Oprah Winfrey, a national host of a talk show, has given large sums of money to people whose identification of child abusers leads to their arrest. Another television show, "America's Most Wanted" hosted by a man whose young son was abducted and murdered, presents case stories of criminals who are at large so that the American public might be able to identify these perpetrators. Such examples of enlisting the help of private citizens may be the beginnings of a trend in the human services to asking all members of society in intervening with deviance. The motivation behind private intervention is sometimes profit; often individuals receive rewards for their intervention.

Perhaps another future trend might be the privatization of rehabilitation services for the criminal population. It might be more cost effective for the government to pay private organizations to provide the necessary counseling and job training services for this population than to house them in prisons, especially if they are assessed to be non-violent and amenable to rehabilitation. Nonprofit agencies that rely on volunteers wouldn't have the overhead and other expenses that typical correctional facilities have.

Modern Educational System

The traditional public educational system is another area of human services that may be in trouble. Recently, the Bush administration (2000 to 2008) has backed up a program referred to as "no child left behind." The program is intended to expose all children to the same level of education and therefore increase literacy in our country. While it is true that public educational institutions have been studying the effects of racism and discrimination on academic achievement for many years, efficient change in the educational system has not been markedly demonstrated.

Over the past 20 years, dissatisfaction in public schools has spurred interest in privatizing education. Many Americans (especially those in the middle and upper economic classes) enroll their children in private, for-profit schools because they do not believe their children will receive a rigorous and safe educational experience in the public school system. Because these schools operate on a for-profit basis and often offer more luxurious work environments, they may be enticing teachers and other human services workers away from public educational institutions. The effect of this might be a return, at some level, to segregation. Private schools may also attract the most qualified and experienced teachers and counselors, leaving the public schools with a staff of inexperienced teachers and administrators. Wealthy citizens who can afford private schools might then receive better education while the more poor (and often minority) students would receive inferior instruction and services.

Of course, this may only be an ominous hypothetical scenario, but a serious possibility nonetheless. Human services workers in the future must focus on understanding low achievement scores and how they relate to poverty and racial discrimination. Interventions should be aimed at motivating students to achieve higher standards. Human services workers, such as school counselors and counselors and social workers, could run educational groups for families and students explaining how success in school is related to adult success and economic opportunity. Unless this type of service is encouraged, the public educational system might remain deficient.

Before concluding this chapter, please reflect on two more questions.

CRITICAL THINKING / SELF-REFLECTION CORNER

What is the role of human services in a for-profit environment?
Do clients receive better services when human service workers receive more pay?

Chapter Summary

Deviant behaviors have been documented throughout history. This has necessitated that methods of managing deviance be implemented. Although these methods have changed dramatically over the millenniums, certain patterns for dealing with fellow humans with special needs appear to still exist. Over the years, society has placed differing emphasis on whether to be charitable to those in need, to be punitive or to provide some form of healing to those suffering from maladies. The type of intervention has been related to the theoretical explanation accepted by society about why individuals engage in deviant behaviors or have special needs. Current human services focus on providing all of the above-mentioned types of interventions; some people in need receive charity, some are punished, and others receive various healing interventions, while some receive a mixture of interventions. These services are provided by family, charitable organizations, religious groups, and the government.

Suggested Applied Activities

1. Create a chart that compares the human services models used today to the societal interventions of previous eras.

_____

_____

_____

_____

_____

_____

_____

2. Note how views about human nature have changed permanently, changed and then reverted back to previous ways of thinking, or stayed the same over time. For example, the Elizabethan Poor laws set up a standard for social welfare that suggests that children, the disabled, and the deserving poor should receive government-sponsored social services. These same populations remain the typical recipients of modern day social welfare assistance.

_____

_____

_____

_____

_____

_____

_____

Review Questions

1. What is trephining and why was it used?

   _____

   _____

2. How does trephining relate to modern day mental health treatment?

   _____

   _____

3. How did the ancient Greeks view physical and mental health problems, and how did they treat them?

   _____

   _____

4. How did the clergy tend to view deviance, and how did they provide help to those in need?

   _____

   _____

5. When did modernized human service first begin?

   _____

   _____

6. Which populations tend to be considered deserving of human services?

   _____

   _____

7. What was the War on Poverty?

   _____

   _____

8. How did modern-day psychotherapy practice begin?

_____

_____

9. What was an important outcome of Caplan's and Lindemann's Wellesley project?

_____

_____

10. What are the current trends in social welfare?

_____

_____

11. Name five people who created reforms in social welfare and corrections.

_____

_____

Glossary of Terms

Abandonment refers to individuals who, during primitive times, displayed deviant behavior and were merely left behind when they became a burden to the clan.

Addams, Jane was a nineteenth-century social worker who founded Hull House.

Animism was a belief held by early civilizations that spirits inhabited inanimate objects and sometimes a person's brain.

Bedlam was an institution in London built in the thirteenth century that provided humanitarian care to the mentally ill and others who demonstrated deviant behavior.

Caplan, Gerald was considered the "father of crisis intervention" because he developed preventive psychiatry, a new approach to coun-

seling that he used to treat victims of the Coconut Grove nightclub fire in 1942.

Charity is giving services, money, or care to someone in need who is deemed worthy. This has been a practice since early times and was strengthened during the period of Jesus.

Civil rights movement began in the 1950s and 1960s. Many Americans worked to end racism and the inequities endured by the majority of black people in the United States. Many people engaged in protests and marches in support of these causes.

Code of Hammurabi is the earliest criminal justice code, which stated that equality of retaliation should be used when someone breaks the law.

Community Mental Health Act of 1963 is federal legislation that provided government funding for treating severely mentally ill patients throughout the country.

Deinstitutionalization of the mentally ill refers to the release of thousands of mentally ill patients who were hospitalized in government-funded mental hospitals during the 1950s and 1960s, after development of the antipsychotic medication Thorazine, which enabled many psychotic patients to live outside of the confines of a hospital.

Deviance is any social behavior that does not fit the normally expected way of behaving. It is the focus of human services workers.

Disparity is when things are not equal.

Dix, Dorothea was a nineteenth-century crusader for the rights of criminals, the mentally ill, and the poor.

Elizabethan Poor Laws were laws set up by Queen Elizabeth as a system of assistance for the worthy poor in England during the sixteenth century.

Elmira Reformatory was an eighteenth-century prison in Pennsylvania known for its reforms that included giving prisoners time off for good behavior.

Freud, Sigmund was a nineteenth-century physician who developed the psychoanalytic approach to understanding and treating individuals with mental disorders.

Grassroots is a movement started in the 1960s during times of civil unrest and lack of faith in the government to take care of the public's needs.

Hippocrates was an ancient Greek physician who proposed a biological basis for human illness and set ethical standards for doctors.

Hull House was a settlement house founded by Jane Addams in 1889.

Humours refers to Hippocrates' Proposition that an imbalance of four bodily fluids could cause mental and physical disturbances. This theory led to the practice of bloodletting and the use of leeches.

King, Martin Luther Jr. was an African-American minister who was a prominent civil rights leader during the 1950s and 1960s and used passive resistance to protest racial segregation and inequalities. He was assassinated in 1968.

Kraepelin, Emil was a social scientist of the late 1800s who categorized human deviance into separate illnesses such as schizophrenia and manic-depressive psychosis

Lindemann, Eric was one of the pioneers in the development of crisis intervention who worked extensively with Caplan on the Wellesley project. Lindemann worked extensively with many forms of loss including working with women grieving over the loss of infants through miscarriages and stillborn births.

Lobotomies is the practice of removing brain tissue in the frontal lobe to rid the patient of aggressive tendencies. It first began in the 1930s with the use of ice picks into the eyeball sockets.

Lombroso, Cesare was a social scientist of the late 1800s who began to understand the psychology and social needs of criminals.

Mann, Horace was the great equalizer who worked with Thomas Jefferson to create mandatory education in the United States.

New Deal was a program created by Franklin Roosevelt in the 1930s during the Great Depression that provided some basic needs and set up work programs to help destitute people.

Pinel, Philipe was a physician who humanized institutions not only by removing chains but also by offering food, shelter, and clothing to inmates.

Poverty is an economic state in which people have little or no income and are unable to their basic needs of survival.

Professional is a human service worker with a college degree or license.

Psychoanalytic approach is Freud's model of personality development based primarily on conflicts between instincts that focus on the unconscious processes as the major determinant of behaviors.

Psychosurgery is modern-day surgery that involves removing areas of the brain.

Psychotropic is a psychiatric medication given to people to control their behaviors, moods, and thought processes.

Punishment is an approach to dealing with deviance and emotional problems in which people with power impose negative consequences on the troubled person.

Roosevelt, Franklin Delano was President of the United States during the Great Depression who established the New Deal and began formal governmental funding of many social welfare programs.

Socioeconomic class is often referred to as SES and is a person's financial situation that usually determines a person's standard of living.

Trephaning/trepanning is a primitive method used to release evil spirits from the head by drilling holes in the skull.

War on Poverty Lyndon Johnson created the Economic Opportunity Act in 1964 aimed at reducing the amount of people living in poverty due to racism and other social factors.

Case Presentation and Exit Quiz

General Description and Demographics

Ann is a 39-year-old woman who has a four-year-old child and a seven-year-old child. She was divorced from her children's father a year ago and awarded primary custody. She receives $400 monthly for child support. Ann works full time for the phone company and makes $35,000 a year. Her seven-year-old attends public school, and her 4-year-old goes to daycare while Ann works. The 7-year-old get a ride to the day care center after school by the day care workers until Ann arrives at 6 P.M. to pick up both her children. She and the children live in a two-bedroom apartment, with the daughter sleeping in the same room as Ann. The apartment rent is $1,400 a month. Ann has $100 per month disposable income after all bills are paid. After the divorce, she was ordered to pay half of the liabilities incurred during the marriage even though her ex-husband earns twice what she earns. Ann couldn't afford a lawyer, so she was not represented during the divorce.

Although Ann has benefits from her company for mental health services, the health maintenance organization (HMO) provided by her employer pays for only 20 visits a year, for which she must pay a $20 copayment for each session as well.

While married, Ann was able afford $70 a month for ongoing therapy with a private therapist. Now that she is divorced, she cannot afford a private therapist.

Problems that Need Assistance

Ann has been depressed on and off for more than 20 years. She has attempted suicide twice, was hospitalized once, and has seen five different therapists in the past 20 years. Her depression has been managed through antidepressant medications and therapy. Her family doctor has always prescribed the antidepressants, but he is retiring this year.

Ann must change therapists for financial reasons. When she doesn't see a therapist, her anxiety increases so much that she often feels unable to go to work. She must keep her job and wants to work. When she called her HMO to get a referral for a new therapist, she was told that there was a three-week waiting list. She then called a few county-funded mental health services, but they told her that she makes too much money to be eligible for services. Ann also called a nonprofit agency and was told that because of her income level, she would have to make a $35 co-payment for services.

Ann is getting more and more depressed and anxious.

Based on this case, respond to the following questions. The concepts in this quiz have been presented throughout the preceding chapter.

Exit Quiz

1. Why might the nonprofit agency need to charge this middle-class client a $35 co-pay?
   a. the workers at the agency are usually highly trained professionals
   b. they have many paid staff that must be paid
   c. many nonprofits have been receiving less funding from government grants
   d. the client can easily afford the co-pay and must take responsibility for her problems

2. What treatment would a doctor in Ancient Greece, circa 600 B.C., use to treat Ann?
   a. lobotomy
   b. blood letting
   c. psychoanalysis
   d. prayer

3. What treatment would a doctor during the 1940s have treated Ann?
   a. leeches
   b. exorcism
   c. lobotomy
   d. public humiliation

4. What treatment would Ann receive in the Middle Ages?
   a. lobotomy
   b. blood letting
   c. exorcism
   d. person-centered therapy

5. Ann's HMO benefits her in all but one of the following ways:
   a. it permits her to receive the exact type of treatment she and her therapist think is best
   b. it permits her to receive medical benefits at a reduced rate
   c. it allows her to pay less per treatment session
   d. none of the above

Exit Quiz Answers

1. c	3. c	5. a
2. b	4. c	

CHAPTER 3

Human Service Workers

Introduction

Listing every possible human services job title would be difficult. Jobs in human services vary by city, county, and state. Even educational requirements change depending on the supply of and demand for human services workers and the specific needs of a community. For example, in 1997 the Los Angeles Mental Health Association conducted a study of the needs of clients with mental health problems in Los Angeles, a city that's home to millions of people of various cultural and ethnic backgrounds (Mental Health Association of Los Angeles, 1997). The study found that there were simply not enough mental health workers, social workers, and case managers to handle the needs of the population, especially those of the large Spanish-speaking and Vietnamese-speaking communities. To help meet those communities' needs, the city created a high-school program that trained students of various ethnic backgrounds interested in careers in human services to meet the needs of people in their communities. A contrasting example might be the use of psychiatrists to provide counseling services (a function not typically provided by that profession) in rural areas where there are few if any licensed master's-level **therapists.**

This chapter details some of the careers in human services and their educational requirements. You will get a fairly good idea about types of job opportunities and specific duties associated with each position. I've tried to showcase people who work in public and nonprofit agencies and deal with social welfare issues such as financial needs, child abuse issues, housing, criminal justice needs, mental health, and educational needs.

A few general job functions in human services are defined below to assist you in understanding the vast array of actual duties performed by human service workers in a variety of positions. It's not uncommon for human service workers to engage in many of these duties at one point in their careers. Because of the generalist approach used by human service workers, many of the functions listed below will be performed as part of one job title. In other words, human service workers wear many hats while servicing clients. The **Southern Regional Education Board** (SREB, 1969), a consortium of community colleges in 14 southeastern states, first proposed some of the positions and responsibilities discussed throughout this chapter. I've also added other functions to supplement SREB's list.

Job Functions of Human Services Workers

Administrators and Assistants

Someone must run an agency. These people are usually interested in the field of human services, but they don't want to work directly with clients. Agency **administrators** and **assistants** focus on program development, fundraising, grant writing, scheduling, and community representation.

Advocates

Human services workers who speak on behalf of clients to ensure that other agencies and people treat them appropriately are **advocates.**

Examples of advocates include a staff member at a battered women's shelter who helps a client file a restraining order in court and a family therapist who writes a letter to a school department for a Spanish-speaking family whose child needs an evaluation for a learning disability.

Behavior Changer

Clients who have debilitating behavioral problems may best be helped by receiving a very direct approach from human services workers. These clients can either be children or adults and may have a variety of issues, including those who are disabled, mentally ill, residents in treatment programs, in school settings, or in **correctional facilities. Behavior changer specialists** focus on eliminating, decreasing, or increasing certain behaviors and use such approaches as positive reinforcement and response cost or extinction (Kazdin, 2001) to work with clients to change a behavior.

For example, a hyperactive first-grader wins a happy face sticker every time she stays seated for an entire five minutes.

Another example of reinforcing desired behavior might involve a hospitalized, mentally ill patient who believes he is unable to care for himself. Every time he brushes his teeth, takes a shower, or puts his clothes on in the morning he receives a point that he can trade in for privileges, such as buying sodas or candy.

The following example demonstrates a method used to discourage unwanted behavior: a teenager in juvenile detention earns a two-day pass to visit her parents after going two months without receiving any warnings or violations.

True Stories from Human Service Workers

Administration in Human Services Agencies

Most nonprofit agencies employ administrative workers who engage in a variety of tasks. Four examples will be given of specific duties performed. The first agency is a center that helps individuals struggling with issues related to their sexual orientation identity, the second agency helps victims who have been sexually assaulted, the third agency provides shelter and other services for homeless families and individuals, and the fourth agency provides a variety of services to individuals struggling to overcome substance abuse.

Example 1: David Hart, the program manager at the Center of Orange County, describes his duties: "There are administration tasks such as evaluations, follow-up with staff, a lot of writing for grants, newsletters, and the press. I also see individual clients and run groups, and I go out to the community and do workshops and network. It really varies." One can clearly see that David epitomizes the generalist worker attitude.

Example 2: Brandi Titis of the Sexual Assault Victim Services in Santa Ana, CA, shares that her job as the Supervisor of Client Services includes "grant writing, agency reporting, writing reports for the human resources department, and keeping track of services for clients in order to provide three reports to the state every year. These reports consist of the age groups, gender, ethnicity, cities served, and services provided to each client."

Example 3: Cindy Snelling describes her duties as the assistant to the director at an agency in Santa Ana, CA, that serves individuals and families who are homeless. "There's daily administration support and little tasks such as making sure the newsletter is ready and out for delivery. There are also the tasks that are more relational such as checking with the case manager, the bookkeeper, and the community."

Example 4: Jan Tyler describes her duties as the program director at Heritage House, a drug and alcohol program in Costa Mesa, CA. "The program director is responsible for overseeing the running of the program and conducting and attending meetings. She is also in charge of hiring, training, monitoring, and in some cases terminating staff. The director monitors the residents and makes sure all the regulations are followed. I verify that things are flowing, and I write letters of recommendation, evaluations, and grants. Every day is different, and it all depends on what needs to be done, whether it is driving the women, conducting some of the sessions, or simply filling in wherever there is a need." This worker also shows the generalist attitude.

Brokers

Often, a human services worker cannot provide the exact service that a client needs. Brokering allows workers to connect clients with someone who can better meet their needs. A **broker** serves as a go-between, connecting a client to

True Stories from Human Service Workers

Advocates' Responsibilities

Those who work in human services have long been acting as advocates on behalf of their clients. Many political issues have encouraged agencies to help clients fight for their rights in a world in which people in certain situations, such as those who have been raped or who are dealing with unwanted pregnancies, can be stigmatized and treated insensitively by society.

Brandi Titis from Sexual Assault Victim Services describes what advocates do at her agency: "Volunteer advocates may accompany clients to hospitals, law enforcement agencies, district attorneys' offices, court proceedings or other agencies. There are also three paid advocates that work for the district attorney's office that help with these duties."

According to Kathryn Treachler, a client advocate at the Whittier Pregnancy Care Clinic in Whittier, CA, says that client advocates at her agency have a variety of responsibilities: "Staff and volunteers counsel women regarding pregnancy options, offer emotional support, and assess for community referrals."

another human services worker. **Brokers** must know a community's resources thoroughly.

A therapist acts as a broker when, in treating a woman for depression, discovers that his client is being beaten by her husband and provides names of shelters for battered women to her client.

True Stories from Human Service Workers

Focus on Changing Behaviors

Those who work with clients to change their behaviors often have a captive audience—that is, clients in residential facilities or students in a classroom. Patients in mental hospitals, inmates in prison, students in school, and residents of a **diversion program** or other 24-hour live-in facility are often involved in behavior modification programs.

Elizabeth Exell, a counselor at a home for abused children shares some of the ways she works with children to change their behavior. "I try to give them consequences that communicate that they did something wrong without replicating the shame and rejection experiences they had with their parents, because for these kids, it is easy to perceive anything as more abuse, deprivation, or rejection. I will have the child practice positive behaviors or have the child make amends to a person he or she has hurt; we usually do these things together so the shared activity will strengthen our relationship. This has the added benefit of giving the child an accomplishment to be proud of. The agency uses a philosophy called 'love and logic' when it comes to working with kids' behaviors."

A probation officer takes on the role of a broker when she notices that one of her probationers suffers from panic attacks at job interviews, and refers him to a therapist.

A teacher who hears that the father of one of his students wants to learn English, and he tells him about English-as-a-second-language classes at a local adult-education center is also being a broker.

Caregivers

At times, human services workers provide clients with direct care. **Caregivers** often provide transportation, food, shelter, medical assistance, or attention.

Examples of caregiver responsibilities include a worker at a senior center who serves clients their lunch, a case manager at a welfare office who provides a client with bus tickets and food stamps, and a worker at an HIV/AIDS clinic who makes home visits to provide critically ill patients with nurturance and support.

Caseworkers

This function epitomizes the generalist role of human services workers. **Caseworkers** manage all of the various needs of their clients and perform a multitude of duties.

Child protective workers are one example of caseworkers. They contact clients to verify that parenting and drug-awareness classes are being attended, that their homes are clean and have appropriate and sufficient food and heat, that they're working and that visitations with their children who are in temporary foster care are taking place.

Probation officers, another type of caseworker, meet with clients to make sure they are working, that their drug tests are coming back negative, and that they're not involved with people who will get them into trouble. If a client is in crisis because of a failed relationship, a probation officer may offer support and refer the client to a counselor.

Consultants

Some human services workers may have specialized expertise and might work as an independent contractor on specific issues with an agency. **Consultants** who are specialists in a certain area might work at an agency that provides services to other agencies that need a consultant's special knowledge.

A nonprofit agency that needs to submit a grant proposal to receive money may hire a consultant who has grant-writing skills to teach the agency's administrative staff how to write grants by working with them closely on the current proposal.

A consultant who specializes in gang prevention may be called in to an elementary school that's having trouble with gang membership among its sixth grade students. The consultant may set up a program aimed at diverting these children from gang affiliation before they enter junior high school.

A counselor at a local clinic may call on a consultant when a new client seems to have multiple personality disorder. No one at the clinic has treated this disorder so a therapist from the private sector is asked to consult with the supervisors and the counselor about how to proceed.

Crisis Workers

Many agencies deal with clients who have problems that need immediate attention. Without some resolution, these problems could lead to serious impairment in functioning. The **crisis worker** attempts to calm the client down, assesses the problem and needs; offers a different perspective on the situation, and connects the client to appropriate resources.

Crisis workers may work for suicide hotlines, conducting telephone interviews and attempting to get callers to calm down and to promise to get professional therapy.

A case manager at a drug rehabilitation center becomes a crisis worker when a client is struggling to stay sober. The case manager provides emotional support and allows the client to vent, then offers a new perspective on the issues.

In a very different example, an academic advisor at a local community college assists a student in crisis after receiving a failing grade on a test. The advisor offers suggestions about how to retake the course so that the "F" is replaced on the transcripts.

Data Managers

Most agencies have one or more people who collect data on how many people use the agency, costs, and other statistics. Often, surveys are conducted by **data managers** with former clients to gather information that can be used during an agency evaluation.

For example, an adult re-entry program on a college campus needs to keep track of how many students visit the center and what their needs are. The data manager develops a form that advisors and counselors complete after each visit

True Stories from Human Service Workers

Providing Crisis Intervention

People who have experienced a trauma are susceptible to entering into a crisis state. If a victim is not helped immediately, post-traumatic stress disorder (PTSD) may result. It is paramount to provide counseling and other services as soon after the trauma as possible.

Kara Hay, a counselor at the Orange County Sexual Assault Center, describes her duties. "Crisis intervention is a large part of what happens. The ABC model (a specific way of conducting crisis intervention to be described in Chapter 8) is taught to all volunteers because when a call comes into the hotline or a victim is taken to the hospital, it is very possible that the victim is in crisis. They need to get back to decent coping skills in order to handle what has just occurred."

with a student. These forms are given to the data manager and input into a computer program. In this way, the data manager has ongoing information about where the agency stands in terms of usage and needs.

Evaluators

Since most human services agencies are funded through grants, there is a need to assess the effectiveness of the program in order for the funding agency to continue the funding. **Evaluators** are trained to make a thorough assessment of the continuing need for a nonprofit agency and whether the program has been utilized effectively.

For example, the United Way has given a $25,000 grant to a community drug-education program for first-time teenage offenders. An evaluator visits the agency and studies the data collected over the past year. The evaluator looks at how many teens attended the groups, what the rates of success have been after attending the groups, and what is being done to increase the success rate. This process requires that agencies maintain detailed records and statistics.

Educators

Most human services workers who deal directly with clients perform educational functions. **Educators** disseminate information that will assist clients in making better choices, understand how clients' problems developed, or how to manage stress.

For instance, an educator will conduct a Parenting class for pregnant teens to help them prepare for the birth of their baby and how to succeed as a new mother.

Another example of an educator is a worker at a clinic for HIV-positive patients who provides a client with information on how HIV/AIDS is spread after that client's blood test came back negative.

A client advocate at the battered women's shelter becomes an educator when she holds discussions with shelter residents about the battering cycle and how women develop battered women's syndrome.

Fundraisers

In large, nonprofit agencies, staff may be hired to raise money by holding various events, such as charity balls and donation drives. **Fundraisers** may work for an agency full time or be hired periodically for fund-raising campaigns.

For example, a battered women's shelter may send invitations to former employees, local law enforcement, judges, and physicians to attend a charity gala where there will be dancing, food, and raffles. All the financial proceeds will go directly to the shelter.

Grant Writers

Although executive directors often write grants for their agencies, sometimes specialists are hired to prepare documents aimed at acquiring funds from various institutions to provide money to the agency for a specified period of time. **Grant writers** are in high demand because it is essential for the funding of nonprofit agencies.

For example, at the end of Chapter 12, a call for a proposal is presented. A grant writer would follow the instructions of this document and submit it to the funding source.

Outreach Workers

Outreach workers conduct presentations to community groups or make visits to people's homes rather than having them come into their office or agency. This is done because some people are resistant to visiting an agency, especially a government agency. Other reasons for outreach are that some people don't have transportation or time to go to an agency for services. At other times, it is more convenient for the agency because one outreach worker can reach multiple clients at one time.

One example of outreach work is done by community organizations that offer various services such as counseling, education, or medical care that are invited by a local factory to set up booths in its parking lot. The factory workers are given an extra 30 minutes from work to visit some of the booths. Each agency can talk to the people and assess any needs, explain what services are available at its agency, or make referrals to appropriate agencies.

Another example involves an outreach coordinator from a community college who visits high school seniors to tell them about various majors, careers, and how to enroll in that particular school.

A final example of outreach work is done by a community worker at a free clinic who visits tenth-grade health classes to talk about birth control and sexually transmitted diseases.

Therapists

Therapist is a broad term that can include a number of functions. It usually involves some type of intensive work to help an individual resolve a serious impairment in functioning. A therapist may help with physical or psychological problems.

For instance, an occupational therapist works in a convalescent home to help stroke patients relearn how to use their hands by getting them work on projects, such as ceramics, painting, or knitting.

A recreational therapist at a psychiatric facility teaches schizophrenic patients how to play card games, billiards, and ping pong.

A psychotherapist provides long-term counseling to a client who has difficulty functioning at work because of panic attacks that are related to being sexually abused as a child.

CRITICAL THINKING / SELF-REFLECTION CORNER

- Do you think it is more efficient for workers to be trained in one duty and then perform that duty exclusively, or for workers to be trained in many duties and perform them all when necessary?

- What types of duties could you see yourself performing on the job?

- Which of the previously mentioned duties would you be least interested in performing and why?

Educational Requirements
for Human Services Workers

Human services workers may be employed at a variety of levels, often depending on the extent of formal education, experience, and other forms of training. The higher the education level, the more responsibility one has, and the more money one makes. Below, a brief summary of what defines various educational levels is provided. Specific careers for each level will then be described.

High-School Diploma

This is the least educated human services worker. It does not mean that this type of worker is insignificant or useless. In fact, due to economic efficiency, many programs employ this level of worker and train the person on the job. Jobs for this person are considered entry level, and these workers are considered to be para-professionals.

Associate's Degree

Most community colleges offer courses that lead to an associate's degree of arts (an A.A.) or science (an A.S.). Students receive this type of degree when they complete a two-year course at a community or junior college. Community and junior colleges frequently offer associates degrees in human services such as drug and alcohol counseling, domestic violence advocacy, and gerontology.

Bachelor's Degree

To earn a bachelor's degree, students must fulfill course requirements of the college or university they attend. Students typically choose a specific major, such as human services, psychology, sociology, or history, and then take courses specific to that major. The time it takes to complete a bachelor's degree usually takes at least three or four years, depending on how heavy a course load a student takes on each semester. Students can earn a bachelor of science (B.S.) or a bachelor of arts (B.A.) degree, depending on their major. Both are considered equivalent in terms of hiring potential for most jobs. Some bachelor's degrees may allow a person to receive certification by various professional associations. For example, to qualify as a certified social work case manager, a human services worker must be an active member of the National Association of Social Work (NASW), hold a bachelor of social work degree (B.S.W.), have one year post-graduate, paid supervised work experience and hold one of the following: NASW ACBSW (National Association of Social Work Accredited Bachelor of Social Work) credential or a current state B.S.W.-level license (NASW website, 2/23/2006). In addition to certified social work case manager, human services workers with a B.S.W. may also be eligible for certification in the areas of children, youth and family; health care; alcohol, tobacco and other drugs; and school social work.

Master's Degree

Earning a bachelor's or an associate's degree is referred to as undergraduate education attainment. When students earn a master's degree, they have moved to graduate-level education. To enter a master's degree program, students must have already earned a bachelor's degree. Many graduate programs also require students to take graduate record exams, complete a thorough autobiography, and supply letters of reference. In human services, the most common master's degrees are a master of science (M.S.) or master of arts (M.A.) in counseling, which would qualify you to become a licensed marital and family therapist or professional counselor, a master of social work (M.S.W.), which could lead to licensure as a licensed clinical social worker, a master of arts or science in psychology, and a master of science or arts in sociology. These graduate-level programs can take from two to four years to complete. Students who earn a master's degree are usually considered professionals and are eligible for more challenging and responsible positions than with only associate's or bachelor's degrees.

Students often wonder about the difference between an M.S.W. and an M.S. in counseling. Both degrees allow people to be licensed counselors and practice on their own or in a variety of agencies. Licensed clinical social workers, licensed marital and family therapists, and licensed professional counselors may be employed as psychotherapists or as social workers. Some agencies may prefer one over the other. The coursework differs in the various programs. M.S.W. programs usually have courses that focus on program development and community assessment, whereas counseling programs usually focus primarily on mental health counseling issues. Because licensing requirements differ from state to state, students should investigate the specific requirements for licensure in their state of interest.

Doctoral Degree

When students earn a doctoral degree, they usually receive a doctor of philosophy (Ph.D.) in Psychology, Counseling, Sociology, etc., or a doctor of psychology (Psy.D.), or a doctor of social work (D.S.W.). These degrees may allow students to become licensed psychologists in some states. Many people who hold doctoral degrees also teach at colleges and universities. Doctoral programs may take from three to six years to complete. Students usually select a specific area of study that interests them and must either complete a dissertation (a thorough research study in written form) or a thorough clinical paper. Both of these papers may be as long as 100 pages. They may officially be called "doctor."

Some people earn an Ed.D., which is a doctor of education. These programs vary from university to university. After completing an Ed.D. program, students may gravitate toward the field of psychology or education. In some states, a person may sit for the psychologist licensing exam with an Ed.D. Persons interested in pursuing careers as school principles and other school administrative positions may opt for the Ed.D. as well.

Medical Degree

Human services workers with medical degrees are psychiatrists. Psychiatrists attend medical school and then specialize in psychiatry. They must become certified medical doctors before they can practice psychiatry. Medical school may take from 6 to 10 years. Psychiatry focuses on learning about the physiological causes of mental disorders and various treatments to minimize symptoms of these disorders. Typically, psychiatrists emphasize the use of medications to assist people in leading better lives. Sometimes, psychiatrists engage in more drastic forms of treatment such as brain surgery or electroconvulsive therapy (sometimes referred to as electric shock therapy).

CRITICAL THINKING / SELF-REFLECTION CORNER

- How do you feel about continuing your formal education at a college or university?

- Are there any specializations or certifications that you are interested in obtaining?

- What are your concerns about applying for graduate school?

- Can you see yourself working as a licensed professional?

- How much responsibility do you see yourself accepting in your career?

- At what level of education do you think you will feel the most satisfaction?

Human services workers no matter what their education may work in a variety of settings. The arena of human services may be categorized into four separate but interrelated settings. When individuals are trained to be generalists, they are usually competent to work in any of the following types of agencies, depending on their interests. Of course, some human services workers take courses and participate in training that provides specialized knowledge and skills that have proven to be helpful in serving at one of the types of agencies over the other types of agencies.

Four Types of Human Services Agencies

Social Welfare Agencies

Social welfare agencies usually provide services to families and individuals who need financial assistance and housing and may also have child-abuse or neglect issues. The elderly and disabled might also receive public welfare assistance. Federal and state governments fund social welfare programs to protect vulnerable populations and ensure that the deserving needy have basic needs taken care of such as food, shelter, and medical care. Private, nonprofit agencies offer services to people who do not qualify for government-assisted programs, such as able-bodied men and women who have no children. Homeless shelters and churches are examples of such agencies. Private institutions may also fund programs for those in need.

Mental Health Agencies

The workers in mental health programs usually focus on the emotional, psychological, behavioral, and social world of the client. These human services workers function as counselors and psychotherapists. The counseling might be done in groups, with families, with couples, or with individuals. There are many approaches to counseling, ranging from psychoanalysis to humanistic approaches to cognitive behavioral and family approaches. It may be crisis intervention or long-term counseling. However, most nonprofit and public agencies, and to some extent private mental health insurers, prefer short-term approaches that cut down on the cost of the mental health treatment. The Community Mental Health Act of 1963, passed during the Kennedy administration, ensured that federal funding would be available to all communities nationwide to provide mental health treatment to at least the most seriously mentally ill. Since most mental health clients do not qualify as seriously mentally ill, nonprofit mental health centers and private practitioners are invaluable in serving those in need of mental health treatment. As is the case in the medical field, managed care and HMOs have played prominent roles in controlling the extent and type of mental health treatment people receive.

Correctional Facilities

Programs and agencies that provide services for individuals who violate laws and rules range from punitive to rehabilitative. Some agencies are 24-hour-a-day residential facilities, while others employ workers that provide services at an office or conduct home visits. Sometimes the workers at these agencies do not receive training as human services workers. They tend to focus on punishment and enforcement. Others have an educational background in counseling, social work, sociology, psychology, or criminal justice, and emphasize helping the perpetrator. In reality, working with this population requires focus on both law enforcement and rehabilitation. Too much emphasis on one without acknowledging the need for the other does not usually allow for effective service.

Government-funded correctional agencies include the court system, prisons, juvenile detention centers, and departments of probation. These agencies are involved in the investigating, trying, sentencing, and incarcerating of criminals and other violators of laws. Nonprofit facilities, such as halfway houses and diversion programs, are designed to facilitate the transition from prison life to life as a productive member of society. These agencies focus on counseling and rehabilitation rather than punishment. Human services workers often run groups and coordinate programs.

Specialized Education Programs

Specialized education programs are geared for students who need additional attention in academics and emotional guidance. These programs have special services for students with learning disabilities, development delays, and behavioral problems. Other programs provide tutoring and after-school activities for children whose parents may work or are otherwise unavailable.

These **specialized education programs** are found in public and private schools, from primary through high school. In addition to classroom teachers, these programs have a variety of academic and guidance counselors and program administrators.

Careers in the Human Services

Specific career opportunities will now be described based on educational level and type of agency. Additionally, specific responsibilities frequently performed by workers in these careers will be described.

Opportunities for People with Associate's Degrees

SOCIAL WELFARE AGENCIES

Positions in social welfare agencies that require some education beyond high school include social workers in group homes for abused and neglected children or for disabled people and in nursing homes for elderly people and those unable to live independently. These workers are often caretakers, supervisors, and crisis managers. They may take clients on outings, prepare food with clients, or provide an understanding ear for someone who's lonely. They usually work with professionals in a multidisciplinary-team approach.

In addition to social service agencies, there are many nonprofit agencies, such as shelters for the homeless, sanctuaries for battered women, hospices for the terminally ill, and rehab facilities for alcoholics and drug users. These shelters often have a staff of people who do not necessarily have impressive academic credentials but who do have a lot of life experience and possibly have been in similar situations to the people they are now working with and therefore are effective in gathering intake information, conducting phone interviews, managing cases, and providing data management.

Organizations, such as Easter Seals, the United Way, the American Heart Association, and the Ronald McDonald House, also use workers to greet people who enter a facility, to work on pamphlets and outreach programs, or to collect data. Some organizations use minimally trained workers to supervise field trips and other outings for children, developmentally disabled people, or the elderly. The worker may also help serve food at senior centers or assist Alzheimer's patients at daycare centers. While this is not an exhaustive list of possible job opportunities, this may give you an idea of what is available for people who, at most, have an associate's degree.

MENTAL HEALTH AGENCIES

Although the community mental health centers of the 1960s employed nonprofessionals to provide crisis management services, current hiring practices in government-funded **mental health agencies** tend to emphasize the employment of workers with at least a master's degree. In facilities that work with people dealing with substance abuse and chemical dependency, certified chemical dependency workers may be hired. This certification can be achieved at the "paraprofessional" level after two years of college. These positions can pay well and offer the worker the opportunity for challenging duties such as group counseling, educational group presentations, and individual counseling. Many community colleges offer courses that will qualify students to apply for certification not only in chemical dependency but also in gerontology and domestic violence.

These human services workers are often employed at nonprofit agencies, where they provide group and residential counseling and do intake work. They may provide guidance, problem solve, and help with everyday crises. Some agencies that typically hire such workers include juvenile halls, battered women's shelters, and group homes for developmentally disabled people.

CORRECTIONAL FACILITIES

A good example of this type of position would be the counselors at juvenile detention facilities. These workers generally do not need advanced degrees. They conduct group counseling and crisis management for the inmates at these correctional facilities for youth.

Many interns and paraprofessionals work as group counselors in halfway houses. They may also provide drug-awareness classes if they are certified chemical-dependency counselors. Sometimes they provide case management services at diversion programs and residential homes as well.

SPECIALIZED EDUCATION PROGRAMS

Workers at this level might serve as a classroom aide, perhaps a bilingual aide in a variety of specialized education programs. There may also be positions at this educational level for workers to assist with data management at community colleges and state universities. Some outreach duties might also be available. Tutoring opportunities might be available in some school systems as well.

Many human services workers enjoy working in recreational, after-school programs, such as the Boys and Girls Clubs, the YMCA, and other organizations for children and teens. These are viable careers and require some human services generalist skills. While the pay may not be great, these are worthwhile programs.

Some programs are designed to assist youth considered to be "at risk" such as those involved in gangs, drugs, or at risk for pregnancy. These agencies may be funded through public monies or may be nonprofit. Positions may be available for those with, at most, community college-level education, depending on the function of the agency. Some agencies may provide residential living for pregnant teens and need counselors, case managers, and caretakers. Others need outreach workers that can educate the at-risk populations.

Opportunities for People with Bachelor's Degrees

SOCIAL WELFARE AGENCIES

Having a bachelor's degree makes it easier to find better-paying jobs in social welfare agencies. Most communities have county- or state-run agencies for families and single parents with children, as well as for elderly and disabled people who need financial and social services.

In some social service departments throughout the nation, having a bachelor's degree might permit someone to work in the area of child protection. These workers provide case management, advocacy, crisis management, and they may be asked to testify in court. Their first priority is to act in a child's best interests, which may or may not be to reunite parents with their children who might have been taken from their home because of abuse and neglect. The social worker may make referrals to other agencies and professionals if a family or an individual has a need that can be met through counseling, parenting classes, and drug-education classes.

Adult protective services also offer bachelor's-level positions that involve working with elderly and disabled adults. In addition to being a case manager, adult protective workers might also act as an **ombudsman** who visits nursing homes to ensure the residents are receiving appropriate services. This worker might also serve as a **conservator** for individuals who are disabled when families cannot do so. Social welfare programs might employ someone at this level who would conduct financial need assessment and provide general case management to assist families in finding work, enroll in college, and find housing and child care.

Generalist skills are definitely needed to deal with issues related to child abuse, poverty, drug addiction, spousal abuse, and criminal activities. These workers must be able to communicate effectively with different types of people from a variety of backgrounds.

Nonprofit social welfare agencies often employ bachelor's-level workers to perform functions that public agencies might not deem appropriate. Using paraprofessionals in nonprofit agencies is cost effective and is more widely accepted than in county or state facilities where money is not as big an issue as it is for nonprofit agencies. The bachelor's-level worker might serve as client advocate, case manager, intake worker, or group counselor. They often conduct educational groups. For example, in a home for teen mothers, a bachelor's-level worker might conduct groups for the teens about parenting, nutrition and how to utilize community resources. At a battered women's shelter, this level of worker might run groups related to childcare, how to re-enter the workforce, and how to access legal assistance or financial assistance.

MENTAL HEALTH AGENCIES

There are probably not many positions available for counselors with only a bachelor's degree in county facilities. Some agencies may still employ this level of worker if there is a great need for counselors and not enough master's-level therapists available to handle the case load. Some agencies may employ a bachelor's-level worker if he or she is working toward a master's degree. Typically, bachelor's-level counselors are employed more in nonprofit agencies than in government funded mental health institutions.

Because nonprofit agencies must function with very little money, it is not uncommon for counselors at these agencies to conduct individual and group counseling especially for people in crisis. Often, these workers are working toward a master's degree, but not always. Sometimes, they attend special training programs to become certified in a specialty such as domestic violence or sexual assault intervention. The focus of these counseling sessions is to resolve immediate crises and receive education. Sometimes, this level worker may serve as a coordinator of a program within the agency and provide outreach and informational services.

True Stories from Human Service Workers

Career Opportunities for Workers with Bachelor's Degrees

Some agencies might even hire someone who has not even quite earned a bachelor's degree based on the person's experience at the agency. The following human services worker served one of her required internships at a group home for abused children and was hired as a paid employee while still working on her bachelor's degree. She describes some of her job responsibilities below.

For example, Elizabeth Exell, a residential support counselor at a home for abused children, recalls, "I was hired even before I graduated with my bachelor's degree in human services. I pick children up from school, hang out with them, help them with homework, and do something fun with them. I may spend time with the children and their parents or talk with the parents alone. Sometimes crisis situations arise. I don't do therapy but instead try to empower the children and focus on making better choices. I use Reality therapy and stay in the here and now."

The next example is a personal one that illustrates how an internship turned into a full-time job, which then led to a position with a county mental health center, where I worked while pursuing a master's degree in counseling.

My third internship was at a nonprofit organization called the Free Clinic, where I conducted support and educational groups on birth control and sexually transmitted diseases. When a job opening for a counseling services coordinator became available, I applied. Although other applicants held master's degrees, I was hired because of the experience and training I received at the clinic while completing my bachelor's degree in human services and because of the good rapport I had with the director.

As I recall, the pay wasn't very much, but the experience was invaluable. It allowed me to transition from my college job as a clerk at the department of motor vehicles to a real human services job. This job gave me experience beyond that of an intern. In addition to running groups, I learned how to coordinate volunteer schedules and responsibilities, how to manage data, how to write grants, and how to provide outreach services. This job was an entry-level position that gave me more credibility when I applied for my next human services position as a mental-health worker with County Mental Health. Although I only had a bachelor's degree, I was hired because of my experience at the Free Clinic, and also because I was working toward a master's degree and I could speak Spanish—a definite advantage, especially in Santa Ana, CA.

My duties at County Mental Health included running groups at a day-treatment program for severely mentally ill patients, conducting intake interviews, and providing case management for the patients. While there, I learned how to diagnose and make treatment plans.

CORRECTIONAL FACILITIES

In many probation departments, workers with bachelor's degrees may be hired as deputy probation officers. They may supervise inmates who are working out in the field (cleaning up the highways). They may also assist probation officers in monitoring cases. Some probation departments may even hire a worker at this level as a probation officer. These duties include case management, counseling, and crisis management for the probationer.

In addition to probation work, this level worker may also work at Juvenile Hall as a counselor, case manager, or supervisor. Some police departments have positions available at this level in gang prevention and drug education. Outreach work and field crisis management may be duties in these positions.

As with the entry-level worker, this worker may provide case management and crisis management for residents at halfway houses. They may also conduct outreach educational services for diversion programs. Counseling would most likely be limited to group counseling at diversion programs with teens or with residents in the halfway house. They may also be involved in grant writing, fundraising and data management.

EDUCATIONAL PROGRAMS

It is possible for workers at this level to work as kindergarten through twelfth-grade (K–12) classroom teachers, preschool teachers and as special-education teachers and resources specialists. However, many schools require a graduate degree for a resource teacher who works with learning-challenged students K–12. Community colleges and state universities often hire this level worker to provide guidance counseling to at-risk students, to work as resident advisers in dorms, or to provide orientation for new students. Administrative positions, such as data management and program coordination, might also be available.

Opportunities for People with Master's Degrees

SOCIAL WELFARE AGENCIES

Once a human services worker attains a master's degree or above, duties and responsibilities increase. More job opportunities exist, more money can be made, and more autonomy on the job is available.

These people might serve as supervisors in financial assistance programs and work as administrative personnel in the federal, state, or county welfare systems. They often work in group homes for abused children as therapists, they conduct investigations into child abuse and elderly abuse, and maintain caseloads of families who may be trying to adopt. Sometimes they work in hospitals and provide crisis management and counseling to medical patients.

The M.S.W. is a flexible degree that is recognized nationwide. It allows the worker to perform a variety of duties and work in many settings.

People who hold master's degrees may sometimes serve as an executive director at a nonprofit agency where the functions include administration of the program, grant writing, fundraising, and meeting with community board members and other community representatives who may have an interest in the agency.

The master's-level social worker may also provide supervision for interns at shelters and develop new programs and policies. They may also serve as mental health counselors (this will be discussed below in the section on mental health).

Some master's-level social workers are employed in nonprofit programs in hospitals and serve as a link between the patients and their families. They also assist with referrals and discharge plans. Much of a social worker's function has to do with connecting people with community resources to meet a variety of needs.

MENTAL HEALTH AGENCIES

Community and county mental health and behavioral health services often hire therapists who hold master's degrees in counseling or social work. Whether a license is required would vary from state to state. These counselors provide all basic counseling, psychotherapy, and crisis management services to the clients who utilize county services. These clients are often very emotionally disturbed individuals who also need the services of a psychiatrist who prescribes the medication.

While students are working toward a master of science or master of arts degree in counseling, psychology, social work or some other related field, they often work in nonprofit settings as part of their licensing internship. Here, they have an opportunity to provide in-depth counseling and psychotherapy and receive supervision from a licensed therapist as a way of earning hours toward their own license. The benefit for the worker is gaining experience and hours. The benefit for the clients is receiving therapy at reduced fees in comparison to what it might cost to see a licensed therapist in a private setting. However, many nonprofit agencies hire licensed therapists to provide counseling as well. Also, these agencies often use these licensed therapists as supervisors and administrators. Of course, some of the supervisors might also hold doctoral degrees, and they may be the directors of the agencies. Individuals who don't wish to obtain a clinical license may choose to merely coordinate and administer programs. Across the nation there are several types of master's-level licenses. As discussed previously in this chapter, some typical ones include licensed clinical social worker, licensed marital and family therapist, and licensed marriage counselor. In addition to acquiring a master's degree, these counselors usually need to complete 3000 hours of supervised experience and pass a written and sometimes oral exam through the state's licensing board.

CORRECTIONAL FACILITIES

The department of probation may employ master's-level workers some of whom may be licensed therapists or social workers, while others may have master's degrees in sociology or criminal justice. These workers often serve as probation officers and supervisors. They provide case management services, crisis intervention, and some law-enforcement activities when the probationer violates the

True Stories from Human Service Workers

Master of Science in Counseling Leads to More Challenges, Pay, and Status in Mental Health

"I'm going to continue to share my chronology of employment beginning at county mental health, where I worked for four years. During the first two years, I was working toward the 3,000 required hours to become a licensed marital and family therapist (MFT). Once I completed my master of science in counseling and completed 3,000 hours of counseling required to sit for a licensing exam, I became a licensed MFT. I was then promoted to mental health specialist. In addition to earning more money, I also performed slightly different duties. I now provided individual psychotherapy to all types of clients. I was qualified to diagnose and conduct emergency evaluations in the community. I could also supervise MFT interns as well.

I was offered a position as a therapist at a managed-care facility where my salary increased considerably. At this HMO, I provided individual, family, marital, and group therapy for a variety of clients. My hours were more flexible, and the pay was good. During this time, I returned to school to work on my doctoral degree in counseling psychology. Once I earned the doctorate, I opened a private practice as an MFT but was able to increase my fees because of my advanced degree. I also contracted with many managed-care insurance providers at that time, and I earned more money for my services than I had received at either the private HMO or the public county mental health facility.

terms of probation. At this level of education, administration and management duties are frequent as well.

As with most of the nonprofit agencies that have been discussed, the worker at this level often serves as a primary counselor, psychotherapist, case manager, supervisor, and manager. He or she may be the executive director of a program as well. Depending on a person's desire, he or she may conduct fundraisers, write grants, provide outreach, and serve as a liaison with other programs. This person may testify in court at times. The worker at this level might run a Batterers Treatment Program and be involved in all aspects.

SPECIALIZED EDUCATION PROGRAMS

With a master's degree, a person might provide counseling, either personal or academic to students. This worker might be a school psychologist or a guidance counselor. Many schools employ master's-level social workers to be on campus to aid in the detection and resolution of child abuse issues. As stated earlier, many schools require a graduate degree for employment as a resource specialist.

There are a variety of programs on college campuses that utilize master's-level workers. These range from psychological counseling to coordination of programs, to student retention management. Some universities offer specific master's-degree programs in student assistance at the college level.

Table 3.1 provides a sampling of available jobs in the human services that were posted on the web during May 2005. Job descriptions and salaries are included. The jobs are listed in order of level of education required (master's first, then bachelor's, and so forth).

Table 3.1 A Sampling of U.S. Job Openings in the Human Services (posted online in May 2005)

Job Title	Requirements	Salary	Duties	Agency Name and Location
counselor (part-time, 20 hours a week)	master's degree, three years' experience	$18,000 yearly, no health insurance	offer short-term counseling, respond to hotline calls, manage cases, provide advocacy	Deaf, Abused Women and Children Advocacy Services, Austin, Texas
domestic violence counselor	master's degree, must be Spanish-speaking	$32,000–$34,000 yearly	provide empowerment-oriented individual and group counseling, advocacy, intake, and assessment	SafePlace, Austin, Texas
child and adolescent counselor	master's degree/ Spanish-speaking strongly preferred	$32,000–$34,000 yearly	assess children and adolescents and their accompanying guardians, provide crisis intervention, counseling to children and teens who have been abused or witnessed domestic violence	SafePlace Supportive Housing Community, Austin, TX
child welfare specialist	master's or bachelor's degree with one year experience	$3144–$4645 monthly	manage casework and cases of at-risk families whose children are in foster care or at home	Department of Child and Family Services, Chicago, IL
child protection specialist	master's degree and two years experience or bachelor's degree with four years experience	$3,144–$4,645 monthly	investigate reports of child abuse and neglect, including conducting interviews and assessments, preparing for and testifying in court	Department of Child and Family Services, Chicago, IL

(continued)

Table 3.1 *(continued)*

Job Title	Requirements	Salary	Duties	Agency Name and Location
assistant director of family investment and child support	master's degree and eight years experience	$48,405–$75,389 yearly	establish and sustain a customer-focused practice in the delivery and supervision of core services	St. Mary's County Department of Social Services, Maryland
support groups coordinator	master's degree/ five years experience	not available	evaluate effectiveness of support groups, develop and manage program budgets, provide ongoing education and support for volunteer group facilitators	Alzheimer's Association, San Diego chapter, San Diego, CA
public outreach associate	master's degree/ five years experience	$55,000–$60,000 yearly	provide trainings, set organization's mental healthcare priorities, advance systemic reform	Stop Prisoner Rape, Los Angeles, CA
volunteer advocate coordinator (part-time, 20 hours a week)	bachelor's degree or equivalent experience	$12,000 yearly	recruit and coordinate training of volunteer advocates, provide ongoing training and support and networking to volunteers, write reports	Deaf Abused Women & Children Advocacy Services, Austin, TX
executive director	bachelor's degree or five years experience	depends on experience	develop programs, write grants, raise funds, administer budgets, working with board of directors and public relations staff	Montana Coalition against Domestic and Sexual Violence, Helena, MT
children's advocate	bachelor's degree or equivalent experience	$9.50–$19.00 an hour	work with children with histories of domestic violence and homelessness, implement therapeutic activities	SafePlace, Austin, TX
social worker supervisor/ program manager	bachelor's degree, three years experience	$54,433–$64,997 yearly	plan, supervise, coordinate and monitor the work of team leaders, social workers, and support staff	Child Protective Services, Green Bay, WI
chief of administration	bachelor's degree and experience	$60,530–$75,663 yearly	oversee budget and financial management activities and manage staff development and training	Department of Health and Social Services, New Castle, DE

(continued)

Table 3.1 *(continued)*

Job Title	Requirements	Salary	Duties	Agency Name and Location
sexual assault coordinator	bachelor's degree, five years experience	not available	coordinate sexual assault program, provide direct services, make community presentations, write grants	The Crisis Center, Sherman, TX
resident adviser	no degree required, must be bilingual	$10.00 an hour	respond to domestic violence and sexual assault hotline calls, gather intake information, monitor shelter security, and assist shelter clients	SafePlace, Austin, TX
sexual assault advocate	no degree required	not available	not available	Women's Center of East Texas
coordinator, professional training and continuing education	two years of college and three years experience	$24,000–$29,000 yearly	coordinate speaker logistics, process registrations, prepare planning schedule, maintain database, generate marketing reports, prepare brochures	Family Violence and Sexual Assault Institute, Longview, TX

Opportunities for People with Doctoral Degrees

PUBLIC WELFARE AGENCIES

People with a doctoral degree, have more choices in occupations and typically have greater earning potential than those with lesser degrees. In the field of social welfare, those with doctoral degrees may work as psychologists for group homes, serve as expert psychological evaluators in regard to custody disputes, and may serve as managers and directors of various programs. Some choose to serve as lobbyists to help change legislation. Others may choose to spend their time in grant writing and other community activities.

MENTAL HEALTH AGENCIES

Workers who hold a doctoral degree may choose to work in public mental health clinics, private practice, HMOs, or nonprofit agencies. They often acquire a license as a psychologist. Whatever the setting, they typically engage in the provision of psychotherapy, group and family counseling, and psychological testing. They are qualified to treat almost any client population and are usually paid more than a master's-level therapist. Some doctoral-level workers prefer to serve as supervisors and administrators at clinics and hospitals. They may be more likely to work for facilities such as the Veteran's hospital or prisons because these are often used as internships in doctoral programs. Although they can't prescribe medication, they often consult with physicians about appropriate medical treatment for their clients.

CORRECTIONAL FACILITIES

Psychologists hold a special place in the court system. The courts often require that people undergo psychological evaluations in order to stand trial, to gain custody of children, or to be deemed disabled. They are qualified to conduct a variety of tests such as the MMPI (Minnesota Multiphasic Personality Inventory) in their evaluation of people. Some psychologists provide counseling services in correctional facilities as well. No doubt, some doctoral-level workers serve as probation workers, probation supervisors, and administer nonprofit diversion programs.

SPECIALIZED EDUCATION PROGRAMS

With a doctoral degree, people are able to become professors at community colleges and most universities. They may choose to work as deans, coordinate various student programs, and serve as counselors at a college as well. In the K–12 system, many people with doctoral degrees become school principals. Some may serve as school psychologists, too.

Chapter Summary

Careers in the human services are varied and include positions that require minimal college education to graduate degrees. Human services workers often work in social welfare agencies, mental health agencies, correctional facilities, and in the educational system. The duties performed by human services workers may be specialized such as performing data collection or general such as performing case management functions. While most human services workers deal with similar types of populations and work in similar settings, those with higher education usually perform the most challenging jobs and earn higher pay than those with lower educational attainment.

Suggested Applied Activities

After learning about various careers and their duties, you may be feeling overwhelmed regarding deciding on a career. To help clear up any confusion, you might want to take a few minutes to answer the questions below to see where you stand at this point. These reactions may change once the text and course are completed. As you respond to the questions, you may want to organize your career options using the SREB's 1979 model that sorts various roles and functions into four classifications (see Table 3.2).

BRIEF CAREER-DECISION INVENTORY

1. Do I want to work directly with people?

   _____

   _____

2. Do I prefer to create and design programs?

   _____

   _____

3. Do I want to organize fundraisers, write grants, and manage data?

   _____

   _____

Table 3.2 Southern Region Education Board Career-Classification Model

Linkage/ Advocacy	Treatment/ Planning	Administration/ Management	Therapeutic Environment Control
outreach worker	behavior changer	consultant	teacher-educator
broker	caregiver	community planner	
advocate	specialist's assistant	data manager	
mobilizer		administrator	

4. Do I want more than an associate's degree?

_____

_____

5. Do I want more than a bachelor's degree?

_____

_____

6. Do I want to work toward a master's degree?

_____

_____

7. Do I want to work in a government-funded agency or a nonprofit agency?

_____

_____

8. Do I want to provide counseling-type services?

_____

_____

9. Do I want to provide more general case management?

_____

_____

10. Do I want to educate others?

_____

_____

Chapter Review Questions

1. What are some of the differences in responsibilities between human services workers who hold associate's or bachelor's degrees and those who hold master's

or doctoral degrees in the field of social welfare, mental health, corrections, and education?

_____

_____

2. What is the function of social welfare agencies?

_____

_____

3. What is the function of mental health agencies?

_____

_____

4. What is the function of correctional agencies?

_____

_____

5. What is the function of educational agencies?

_____

_____

6. What duties would a social worker typically be engaged in on a regular basis?

_____

_____

7. What types of duties are a large part of a mental health worker's day?

_____

_____

8. What skills and duties do teachers often perform?

_____

_____

Glossary of Terms

Administrators focus on management, policy-making, and budgeting.

Advocates intercede for clients to help them receive fair treatment and access to programs.

Assistants provide a variety of services ranging from grant writing, to bookkeeping, to serving as the executive director's right-hand person.

Behavior changers focus on systematic interventions designed to help clients change specific behaviors and improve functioning.

Brokers refer clients to other human services workers who are better equipped to handle a client's specific issues.

Caregivers provide direct daily care to clients such as shelter, transportation, or food.

Caseworkers manage different activities and services for a client or a family that may involve networking with other workers as well as providing direct services, such as crisis management.

Conservator A person designated by the county department of social services to make financial and personal decisions for someone who has been assessed by the courts as incompetent to care for himself.

Consultants specialize in a certain function that contributes to an agency, such as grant writing, program evaluation, or treatment of certain populations.

Correctional facilities are residences that provide shelter, punishment, and rehabilitation for criminal populations.

Crisis workers focus on assisting clients through immediate, serious problems to help their clients maintain functioning and prevent dangerous behaviors such as suicide.

Data managers input information into computer systems, analyze it, and create effective data management at an agency for purposes of statistical collection and accountability for program evaluation.

Diversion program A program that typically includes some form of education (e.g. about alcohol and drugs), group counseling, and family counseling. The purpose is to provide an alternative to incarceration.

Educators provide information to clients to increase awareness and greater choices.

Evaluators monitor the effectiveness of programs and offer suggestions on how to better meet clients' needs and work more cost effectively.

Fundraisers focus on raising money through various events, such as charity balls and donation drives.

Grant writers prepare documents for submission to organizations that may provide funding to an agency for a specified period of time.

Mental health agencies provide therapy, crisis management, and case management to clients with psychological and behavioral disorders.

Outreach workers disseminate information to groups of at-risk populations or visit people where they live in an effort to assist them in making changes to enhance their lives.

Ombudsman A person whose primary function is to monitor the conditions of residential facilities where the elderly and the disabled reside. They work with county and state officials to ensure proper treatment is provided.

Social welfare agencies are government-run programs that provide money, housing, child care, and protection to people in need.

Southern Regional Education Board is a consortium of community colleges in 14 southeastern states.

Specialized Education Programs are programs within public and private school systems that provide education for students (from kindergarten through twelfth grade) with needs that cannot be met in a regular classroom environment.

Therapists help clients learn new life skills, become aware of behavior patterns that have caused them difficulties, or work on physical rehabilitation. It may be psychological or physical.

Case Presentation and Exit Quiz

General Description and Demographics

Glen, age 52, and his wife of 20 years, Karen, age 50, have a daughter Jenna, age 18, and two sons Jacob, who's 15 and Eric, who is 10. The family lives in a very nice neighborhood, and both parents work full time in administrative positions. Both parents have medical insurance and pay very little out-of-pocket expenses for medical, dental, and eye care.

Recently, Glen's father died, leaving his 75-year-old mother, Emma, a widow. Glen's siblings live in another state but do visit their mother occasionally. Both of Karen's parents have died several years ago. Emma lives in the house she raised her children in still and lives off of her and her late husband's social security checks.

Jenna was supposed to graduate from high school this year but has been ditching classes recently and may have to go to summer school if she doesn't graduate in the spring. Jenna is quite popular and has always been an average student.

Jacob started high school this year and seems to have adjusted well. He is involved in sports and hangs out with his friends most of the time at an internet cafe.

Eric is doing well in school but has recently gained about 20 pounds. He likes to play video games most of the time rather than play outside with friends.

Problems that Need Assistance

Emma has been showing symptoms of Alzheimer's disease for the past 10 years. She cannot remember her grandchildren's names and at times forgets her son's name. Her husband used to take care of her when he was alive, but now she lives alone and her children are worried about her. She sometimes forgets to eat and bathe. She is often found sitting alone in her living room, smelling of body odor. Her son pays her bills and takes her to doctors' appointments

Glen and Karen have begun to have arguments about Emma's care. Karen thinks the other siblings should put more effort into Emma's care, but Glen believes that since he lives locally that he should shoulder the bulk of the responsibility, especially since his brothers and sister have been uninterested in their mother's care. Glen has always been very attentive to his mother's needs, which has created resentment between Emma and Karen for many years. Karen and Glen have been growing apart since his father's death and can barely speak without arguing.

Jenna has been using crystal methamphetamine for the past five months and has been hanging around with friends who do the same, instead of her former friends who don't use drugs. Her parents just found out about her drug use after she stayed away from home for two days straight without calling them. When her parents confronted her and threatened to take away her car, cell phone, and all other privileges, Jenna said she needed help to stop using drugs. This was the reason she was ditching school and not passing her classes.

Jacob has also gotten into trouble. He and his friends stole a car to go joy riding. Although the car belonged to one of his friend's parents, they were all arrested.

Eric has been feeling depressed lately. He says he eats because he's sad and has had thoughts of suicide but has not tried to kill himself.

Services Provided for Each Family Member

Glen took his mother to her family doctor and explained her worsening symptoms. The doctor referred Glen to an Alzheimer's Association and prescribed his mother medication to attempt to slow down the progression of the disease. Glen called the Alzheimer's Association and spoke with someone about his mother's behaviors and about the family's lifestyle. The worker recommended that Glen explore the possibility of having his mother attend a special daycare program and live with him at night. A worker was assigned to visit his mother's home to assess her level of functioning. Another worker came to visit Glen and Karen to talk about caretaking responsibilities. They gave Glen and Karen information about the progression of Alzheimer's disease as well as information about respite care that provides workers who can stay with an Alzheimer's patient when caretakers need a break.

Karen doesn't want Emma to stay with them, but Glen does. Karen sets up an appointment with a licensed marital and family counselor to help them deal with this major difference of opinion and potentially life-altering decision. At their first session the counselor recommends to Karen and Glen that he should urge his siblings to get involved with their mother's life and perhaps share caretaking responsibilities. Glen is resistant, but the counselor points out that at a time when their children are getting into trouble, he and Karen need all the support and help they can get.

After hearing about Jenna's drug problem, the counselor refers all of them to a facility that offers drug-education classes and group counseling for Jenna and her parents. The counselor also gives them a list of appropriate 12-step programs and then schedules regular marital counseling sessions for Karen and Glen.

Jenna and her parents enter an outpatient drug-treatment program paid for by the family's medical insurance. Jenna attends groups five days a week, and her parents will be going to group and family therapy once a week for the next 12 weeks. A psychiatrist evaluates Jenna and prescribes antidepressants for her. The program emphasizes changing behaviors through parental reinforcement of appropriate behaviors and parental removal of privileges after negative behaviors.

Jacob and his parents go to court where he is put on probation and must attend a diversion program if he wants to stay out of jail. Jacob must also meet with his probation officer once a month and stay away from other criminal offenders. Jacob's probation officer monitors his progress in school and makes sure Jacob doesn't associate with anyone who has had problems with the law. Jacob must also attend group counseling and classes at a community services agency.

Eric visits his pediatrician who sets him up with some nutritional guidelines and an exercise program. He doesn't feel the need to see a counselor yet. Karen and Glen's counselor has suggested that they keep a close eye on his suicidal feelings and encouraged them to bring him in to her if he doesn't feel better soon.

Exit Quiz

1. Which service provider has the highest level of education?
   a. Glen and Karen's counselor
   b. Jenna's group counselor
   c. Eric's pediatrician
   d. Jacob's probation officer

2. Jacob's probation officer is serving as
   a. a data manager
   b. a caseworker
   c. an advocate
   d. an educator

3. The model at Jenna's substance-abuse program encourages workers and parents to serve as
   a. outreach workers
   b. therapists
   c. behavior changers
   d. brokers

4. Karen and Glen's counselor most likely holds a
   a. Ph.D.
   b. M.S.
   c. B.S.
   d. M.D.

5. What function does Emma's family doctor serve when he referred Glen to an Alzheimer's association?
   a. broker
   b. administrator
   c. evaluator
   d. grant writer

6. Which organization is most likely to use volunteers and paraprofessionals primarily?
   a. pediatric clinic
   b. probation department
   c. Alzheimer's association
   d. Jenna's psychiatrist's office

Exit Quiz Answers

1. c   4. b
2. b   5. a
3. c   6. c

CHAPTER 4

Communication Skills and Personal Characteristics of Human Service Workers

Introduction

All people undoubtedly benefit from clear and sensitive communication styles. In the field of human services, the need for effective communication skills is more important than it is for most other fields because clear communication between a worker and a client do more to benefit the client. Even if a human services worker does not work directly with clients, he or she will be interacting with workers who do, as well as other colleagues at an agency. Learning how to present one's point of view clearly to others is helpful to anyone, and we'll take time now to address communication styles that can lead to effective interventions with clients and good working relationships with coworkers.

In addition to acquiring effective communication skills, human services workers must also develop and strengthen certain personal qualities. The person-hood (the overall way in which a person relates to others and to himself including personal characteristics such as warmth, sensitivity, and so on) of a human services worker can be that worker's best resource when dealing with people in need.

This chapter presents specific communication skills that are essential to being an effective human services worker. The suggested applied activities at the end of the chapter offer suggestions on using role-play to practice these skills. Following the discussion on communication skills are some personal characteristics that are considered vital for human services workers to possess.

Effective Communication Skills of Human Service Workers

The idea that there are certain methods of interacting with others that enhance trust and promoted open sharing has been supported by many. Books entitled *Effective Helping* (Okun, 1992), Basic Attending Skills (Ivey, Gluckstern, and Ivey,

1997), and *Helping Relationships and Strategies* (Hutchins and Cole, 1992) all indicate that professionals in the field of helping others have formulated ideas about how to proceed in an organized, effective manner. Of course caring about people and wanting to help them fix problems is important; however, providing intuitive **feedback** and advice are not effective in actually helping people. If that were all that was needed, you could simply find a caring and intuitive friend or family member to talk with. Often, talking to family and friends is not enough to solve people's problems. Also, many people do not have the support of family and friends and need outside intervention when facing problems.

General Goals of Effective Communication

Certain communication methods and interaction strategies have been shown to be effective in helping people work through their problems. To successfully work with people in overcoming their problems, a sense of trust must be developed that allows clients to open up and speak honestly about the problems. If clients do not feel comfortable sharing their problems with a counselor, then their problems will remain unresolved. Effective strategies (that may also be helpful in dealing with your own family and friends) for establishing trust between a counselors and clients and for helping clients work through problems will be covered later on in this chapter. But first, let's briefly review the goals of effective communication.

GOAL ONE: CREATE A SENSE OF TRUST

A human services worker must help people talk about their problems to assess their needs and create appropriate interventions. Because people often feel that their problems are personal and are perhaps ashamed of them, human services workers must work to establish a relationship in which the client can openly speak about their problems.

First steps to creating trust: When speaking with a client for the first time, maintain a calm demeanor and comfortable eye contact, nod your head to let the client know you are listening carefully, and remain nonjudgmental, no matter what the client is saying.

GOAL TWO: CREATE A SENSE OF EMPATHIC UNDERSTANDING

In addition to developing trust, clients must believe that their worker understands their problems and therefore is able to help them. If workers do not seem to "get" their clients' problems, how could the worker do anything to solve it?

Some examples of empathic statements include, "I can see how this is painful for you." "I hear that since your husband left you, finances have been difficult." "Your fears about relapsing are understandable since you had been using for over 10 years."

GOAL THREE: ALLOW CLIENTS TO EXPLORE AND CLARIFY THEIR THOUGHTS

Clients don't always express themselves in an organized manner. Human services workers must often help clients verbalize what they're trying to say to better assess their clients' needs. Certain communication strategies provide an arena for **clarifying** and exploring a problem.

Examples of comments and questions that can help that process along include: "How does that make you feel as you think about losing your job?" "So I hear you saying that after your son tore your book in front of you, you became so angry that you hit him with your belt." "What do you feel about your husband giving you a black eye?"

GOAL FOUR: INSTILL CONFIDENCE IN YOUR ABILITY TO HELP YOUR CLIENTS

Clients also need to believe that their worker is knowledgeable and confident so that when clients get feedback, suggestions, and information about other resources they will accept and put all that information to use. Certain comments and observations help establish a confidence building rapport: "I have recently attended a seminar about marital infidelity and the speaker provided many examples of couples who have been successful in reuniting." "I know of a great support group for women who have survived date rape. Let me give you the phone number." "Perhaps you could contact the district attorney's office about getting a restraining order."

Specific Effective Communication Skills

The skills detailed below are presented in order from basic to advanced; however, they are not necessarily used in this order with a client. Beginning workers will probably be most comfortable with the first few skills, and as workers become more experienced, they will be comfortable incorporating other skills in their client interactions.

Active listening is the basis for all effective communication between a helper and a client. The difference between simply hearing and listening to what someone says is considerable. Active listening requires a listener to concentrate solely and without distraction on what someone is saying to you at the moment; that means putting aside personal problems and daydreams. It also means hearing beyond what the person is saying—trying to understand deeper levels of meaning when appropriate, and encouraging the person to say more. In our everyday conversations with family and friends, this is not how we usually listen. Often, people are so wrapped up in their own problems and concerns that when someone is talking to them, they barely let the other person get out a statement and are ready to add something about themselves.

True Stories from Human Service Workers

Building Trust in the Real World

The following comments are from two human services workers who share their views about building trust with clients. Although they do not consider their primary role as being a therapist, they still emphasize the goals previously discussed.

Elizabeth Exell, who works at a group home for abused children, shares her communication methods: "My focus in working with these kids is on building relationships. I am not a therapist, and I do not do therapy with the kids. However, I believe it is therapeutic just to establish a relationship with the kids and be someone they can trust. Showing **empathy** for these kids helps them learn to soothe themselves when they are overwhelmed or upset. It helps the kids feel safer with their own feelings."

Kathryn Treachler, a nurse manager and client advocate at a pregnancy care clinic, says that "no deep psychological counseling is done here. Emotional support is given when the clients are in crisis, and appropriate feedback and education is given for each client's unique situation."

These examples illustrate how basic counseling skills are used by various human services workers.

Because people are unaccustomed to listening in this manner, active listening may seem odd or unnatural at first. In an average conversation, one person says something, the other either gives a suggestion, discloses something that may be related to what the first person said, or tells the other person not to worry because everything will be all right. The result may be feelings of frustration and lack of validation. Human services workers must learn to interact in a way that assures clients that they are being heard, understood, and are allowed to explore problems or needs thoroughly. The personal concerns of a human services worker should not be part of these interactions.

Active listening includes a variety of skills that have been studied by many professionals in the field. When Rogers (1970) was first conducting his research on the therapeutic effects of encounter groups, he found many therapeutic benefits resulted when group facilitators used active listening techniques. Additionally, he discovered that certain qualities (discussed later on in this chapter) of group facilitators influenced therapeutic outcomes.

Some active listening skills that contribute to effective communication are discussed below.

USING MINIMAL ENCOURAGERS

Using **minimal encouragers,** though simple, is the foundation of active listening in all interactions. Minimal encouragers are both verbal and nonverbal signals that indicate the listener is interested. When you feel that the person you are talking to is really interested in the conversation, you are motivated to keep talking. Likewise, when you feel that your words aren't being heard, you're more apt to quit talking. Being interrupted, having a completely new topic brought up, or simply being ignored does not usually make people feel good about themselves, nor does it encourage them to keep talking. Effective communication encourages clients to keep talking and makes them feel that what they are saying is important.

One technique that encourages conversation is head nodding. When people are truly interested in what you are saying, they tend to unconsciously nod their heads. In addition, maintaining good eye contact says, "Go on, I'm with you, and want you to continue." Of course, adding a few "uh-huhs," "I sees" or "ohs," along with attentive body language, also lets clients know you're involved in what they are saying. In American culture, the "basic listening posture is a slight forward trunk lean with a relaxed easy posture" (Ivey et al., 1997).

CRITICAL THINKING / SELF-REFLECTION CORNER

- Have you ever been bored while someone was talking, having no interest in what the person is talking about?
- How easy is it to drift off and stare into space?
- How often have you drifted off during class, or while reading this text?
- What did you do to bring yourself back to listening and paying attention?
- Have you ever felt someone shut you out? How did that make you feel?
- Can you think of someone in your life who makes you feel listened to? What does that person do to make you feel like truly heard and understood?

VERBAL FOLLOWING

The next level of active listening is to focus on what clients have already said instead of "topic jumping" (Ivey et al., 1997). One way to let the clients know that you are listening and understanding them is to paraphrase, reflect on, or question what a client has just said. There is usually no need to bring up new topics or issues. Following a client's lead will get you to the relevant problems. This will create a climate of understanding and empathy that assures clients that their experiences are understood, both emotionally and intellectually. Here are two examples of **verbal following.** In each example, two possible responses are given to show poor and effective verbal following.

Scenario 1 client: "I'm pretty bummed out because I didn't study hard enough and I got a D on my exam. My parents are going to be mad, and I'm not gong to be able to go out this weekend."

Poor response: "Who's your favorite teacher?"

Better response: "It sounds like you understand why you didn't do well on the exam and are concerned about your parent's reaction to your grade."

Scenario 2 client: "I forgot to bring in the paperwork to verify my income level. I really need the food stamps today. How are my kids going to eat?"

Poor response: "When is the last time your kids have seen a doctor?"

Better response: "I can see it's really important for you to make sure your kids eat today."

PARAPHRASING

This can be done either by restating in your own words what you heard your client say or by clarifying what was said in the form of a question. This technique can clear up confusion or ambiguity and thus avoid misunderstanding and confirm the accuracy of what was heard. It is not parroting or repeating exactly what the client says, but the goal is to share with the client what you heard (Kanel, 2007). This allows clients to either correct any misunderstandings or to confirm that both of you are on the same page. As you become more sophisticated and skilled, try to develop this skill and paraphrase at deeper levels. When Carl Rogers was first developing his theory about empathic understanding, he expressed a desire to understand the exact meaning of what a person is communicating. He believed that this could clarify a speaker's message and helps others understand some complicated details that are often missed (Rogers, 1970).

The following example of **paraphrasing** and clarifying statements contains a poor response and an effective one.

Client: "My son upsets me so much. He stays out too late and refuses to do his homework. I don't know how to get him to cooperate."

Poor response: "Your son upsets you so much. He stays out too late and refuses to do his homework and you don't know how to get him to cooperate." (This is merely parroting the client verbatim).

Better response: "It sounds like you just can't find a way to get your son to adhere to your curfew rules and schoolwork which makes you upset" (puts client's comments into own words).

REFLECTING EMOTIONS

Listeners use **reflection** to reflect the affective part or emotional tone of a client's message. It is a powerful tool that can create an empathic environment (Kanel, 2007). Reflection says to the client, "Your feelings are understood and it is ok to continue talking about them and feeling them." Expressing feelings openly has been considered a characteristic of effective coping people and should be encouraged when possible (Caplan, 1964). Reflection is most effective when it simply emphasizes the emotional aspect of a client's spoken and unspoken emotions. Below are examples of reflection. One is too wordy while the other is simple and more effective in keeping the client in touch with his feelings.

Client: "My wife left me this past weekend, and I can't stop crying. I can't eat, sleep, and don't feel like going out at all."

Poor response: "I hear that you've been crying since your wife left you and don't feel like doing anything" (doesn't encourage client to focus on his feelings and may distract him from his feelings).

Better response: "It sounds like you are hurting a lot" (encourages client to focus only on feelings of sadness).

ASKING OPEN-ENDED QUESTIONS

Sometimes you can guide the flow of a conversation by asking questions based on information already given by a client. As with paraphrasing, you should not topic jump but instead ask questions to help clients explore more of what they have already said. The key here is asking pertinent questions to which the client will relate. "**Open-ended questions** provide room for clients to express their real selves without categories imposed by the interviewer. They allow clients an opportunity to explore themselves with the support of the interviewer" (Kanel, 2007). It is useful to ask questions that begin with "what" or "how" because these types of questions allow clients to explore their ideas and feelings without being defensive. Asking too many close-ended questions might make clients feel that they are in a police interrogation, and so questions that begin with "do," "did," "why" are often avoided in client interviews. It is a good idea to communicate by combining paraphrases, reflections, and open-ended questions. This will reduce defensiveness and increase trust and **openness** on the part of the client. Below are examples of effective and ineffective questions.

Client: "I'm scared to apply for graduate school. Where should I go? How do I know if I can make it?"

Helpful response: "What would you like to go to graduate school to learn?" (allows client to explore her motivation).

Helpful response : "What are you scared of exactly?" (allows client to explore her fears).

Poor response: "Do you want to make more money?" (might have the effect of client answering "yes" or "no." How is this even relevant?).

Poor response: "Why do you want to go to graduate school?" (This almost sounds like the worker doesn't believe the client should go to graduate school and may make the client feel like she must justify herself. It might create a less defensive response by the client to ask, "What are some reasons you would consider going to graduate school?).

PROVIDING FEEDBACK

Once you clarify and understand a client's needs, you need to provide your client with feedback that is based on objective observation and thoughts about the client's needs. During the verbal-following stage of communication, you are formulating ideas about the problem. This is often referred to as assessment. Once you believe you have something to offer your client in terms of help or assistance, you can begin to communicate various ideas in a nonjudgmental manner. Sometimes this feedback is very supportive and easy for a client to accept. At other times, feedback must include candid appraisal of certain behaviors' consequences, for both the client and others who may also be affected (Hutchins and Cole, 1992). This can be more difficult for some clients to accept, and so it must be presented in a way that allows clients to maintain dignity and save face.

Feedback can range from validation of a client's behaviors to confrontation of discrepancies in a client's behaviors and words. Some feedback is educational and provides information about which a client was misinformed or ignorant. An effective form of feedback is to try to help a client perceive a situation in a new way that may make the situation seem more solvable. Cognitive approaches to counseling emphasize this type of feedback (Kanel, 2007).

Sometimes, feedback comes in the form of direct suggestions about how to solve a problem or meet a need. This may be a referral to another agency, an assignment that encourages a client to try a new behavior, or that highlights the benefits of reconnecting with family or friends. The key to all forms of feedback is to offer it without judgment. The focus should be on creating a climate that lets a client hear the feedback as being helpful and in the person's best interest. The following provide examples of appropriate feedback.

Client: "I know I should quit drinking so much, but my life is so stressful that I need the wine to fall asleep. I'm not happy, but I just don't know how to reduce stress but still keep my job and manage my kids' social world."

Helpful feedback: "Perhaps you could make a list and prioritize your activities. Maybe some days you could put off one of the least important activities until the next day."

Helpful feedback: "Many people drink as a way to medicate depression and reduce stress. In fact, alcohol is a biochemical depressant and can actually worsen depression. Although it seems to work at first, at some point, too much alcohol consumption often has the effect of increasing stress because it affects the body negatively. Also, it's probably not good to depend on alcohol to sleep. Would you consider seeing a physician about your depression and stress?"

Personal Characteristics of Human Services Workers

Perhaps more than in any other profession, the personhood of human services workers is integral to becoming a competent practitioner because the nature of the work demands close interaction with others. As human beings, we are all full of emotions and needs. These emotions can, however, become overwhelming and needs can go unmet. When people find themselves in such difficulties, extensive research (Gibb, 1970) has shown that they tend to respond more openly to practitioners who interact appropriately and possess certain traits.

Rogers (1970) also studied the effectiveness of various client-counselor interactions. Additionally, he examined the ways in which clients respond to various personal qualities of a counselor. Based on his findings, Rogers proposed that there are certain qualities—genuineness, acceptance, and empathy—in order for therapeutic change to occur. What follows are descriptions and examples of each of Rogers's conditions for positive, therapeutic change.

Congruence or Genuineness

Congruence and **genuineness** both mean that interactions with clients must be sincere, allowing both you and your client to openly express feelings, thoughts, reactions, and attitudes that are present and relevant to the relationship. Displaying authenticity also serves as a model of a real human being who also struggles with life (Corey, 2005). Of course, no one is expected to be authentic 100 percent of the time, but it is a quality worth developing. On the other hand, authenticity does not mean sharing your every thought and feeling, but only those that are relevant for the situation, as the following example illustrates.

Client: "I am so sad. I'll never get over my father dying."

Appropriate response: "I was sad too when my father died and never thought I'd get through it. Thankfully, I did though, and I think you can too" (response is relevant to client's experience, validates feelings, and comforts feelings of hopelessness).

Unconditional Positive Regard and Acceptance

Both **unconditional positive regard** and **acceptance** mean that interactions are "not contaminated by evaluation or judgment of the client's feelings, thoughts, and behavior as good or bad" (Corey, 2005). When clients feel accepted and worthy of being understood, they may be more inclined to speak honestly and reveal the real issues and problems. As a result, they have a better chance of being helped, and receiving the most appropriate interventions, as exemplified below.

Client: "I am so ashamed to tell people that I'm HIV-positive and that I got it because I use heroin. If I got it through a blood transfusion, people wouldn't be so weird about it."

Appropriate response: "No matter how you got the virus, you are deserving of the same respectful service and treatment as anyone with a serious disease" (response shows no judgment of the client or the disease).

Empathy

Rogers (1958) also found that clients must be assured that their frame of reference is understood from their own point of view—viewing a situation from their perspective. Empathy assures clients that their problems are really understood. Consider the following interaction:

Client: "I didn't really do anything that bad, my parents are just overreacting. I just smoked pot once, and now everyone's making a big deal out of it. Like no one else has smoked a joint before. I don't need counseling."

Empathic response: "Sounds like everyone else thinks smoking pot is a big deal, but for you, it's just not that horrible. After all, a lot of kids smoke pot." (Response lets client know the situation is being viewed as the client sees it, even if it is a big deal.)

Concreteness

Carkhuff and Berenson (1967) have identified four basic traits that seem to facilitate effective client-practitioner relationships. The first three, like Rogers's, are empathy, respect and positive regard, and genuineness. To those, they have added **concreteness** that, in essence, refers to the ability to respond accurately, clearly, specifically, and immediately to your clients. Carkhuff and Berenson made significant contributions to the field of human services by conducting their studies using applied research, which demonstrated that the quality of client-practitioner interactions had a greater effect on the outcome than the educational level of the practitioner. Therefore paraprofessionals can be just as effective as professionals if trained to develop these traits and communicate them to clients, as the following scenario reveals.

Client: "I am so overwhelmed. I need to go to court, apply for welfare, enroll my kids in a new school, get the restraining order, and now I find out I have to help clean the shelter and cook too. How am I going to do all of this?"

Appropriate response: "There is much to do, so let's prioritize the tasks. Since you are safe for now, the restraining order can wait until later. It would be good to ensure your kids are enrolled in school, so why don't we go to the school, get that done and then while we are out, we can stop off at the welfare office. When we return to the shelter, we can set up your cleaning and cooking schedule and have you start some groups. Tomorrow, we'll go to court and file all necessary documents."

Developed Sense of Well-Being

Bugental, a proponent of the **existential-humanistic counseling approach,** addressed the need for therapists to have a **developed sense of well-being** when he asked, "How can someone who's messed up himself help someone else get unmessed up?" (1978). This does not mean you must be problem-free, but you are expected to seek help with your problems to be able to maintain emotional stability while working with others, as illustrated in the scenario that follows.

Janice has been feeling increasingly tired. When she arrives at her office, she feels angry and resents having to talk to her clients. She realizes that something is wrong. At lunch, she goes to the gym to try to work out her feelings. Since she still feels very negative, she phones her health-insurance to get a referral for a counselor. Janice sets up an appointment and discovers during the first session that her anger stems from her mother-in-law's interference with the raising of Janice's child. Her husband hasn't helped the situation, so Janice discusses this with her husband, who talks to his mother, which leads to an honest conversation between Janice and her mother-in-law. Janice feels better and returns to work with a refreshed outlook.

Self-Awareness

Self-awareness can help you recognize whether you need help yourself. That means paying close attention to who you are, what values you have, what your emotional needs are, and how you interact with others. Self-awareness makes the helping profession unique in comparison to other fields in which this quality is not necessarily encouraged. Besides being aware of your own values and needs, you must also be aware of cultural biases and other values and attitudes that influence your thinking so as not to inappropriately impose these biases on your clients. Human services workers should be able to recognize "the strong set of Western assumptions underlying helping theories and techniques, and realize that helpees from non-Western cultures may have altogether different perceptions of their problems and what to do about them" (Okun, 1992).

For example, John has been interning at the YMCA. In a session the other day, a girl confided that she was pregnant. John became enraged and told her to quit having sex, she was too young. John was brought up to believe that people, especially teenagers, should not have sex unless they're married. Obviously, John was not being aware of his own values when he spoke with the girl. Since he has such strong beliefs, he should be very careful when working with clients who might believe it is all right to have sex, whether or not you're married. He must also try to understand why he gets so angry about this issue or he may take out his own feelings on his clients, which would be inappropriate and irresponsible.

Presence of Mind

Another quality somewhat unique to human services workers is the importance of having **presence of mind.** Presence means "being in a situation in which one intends to be as aware and as participative as one is able to be at that time and in those circumstances. It is being totally in the situation" (Bugental, 1978). This means developing the ability to leave your own personal problems or plans behind when working with clients and give your undivided attention to your client. This is not as easy as it sounds, as the follow example illustrates.

Before leaving for work, Penny had a horrible fight with her 16-year-old daughter, Amanda. Penny feels badly about yelling at Amanda and realizes now that the situation was blown out of proportion. When Penny's first client arrives, she makes sure to write down her feelings and her decision to talk to a co-worker about her daughter after her client session is over. This clears Penny's head and can now focus on her client's needs instead of her own.

Flexibility

Generally speaking, all people have multiple needs and can be unpredictable, even more so for those who seek out human services. Therefore, human services workers must learn **flexibility** and allow for modifications in assistance plans when appropriate. While structure is helpful, and in many circumstances necessary, you should not rigidly implement your intervention plans or expectations. Things happen to people that make changing the rules at times necessary. For example, many people who use human services must rely on public transportation to get them to their appointments. Someone might be late for an appointment because the bus was running late. The worker might need to allow the person to still be seen despite his being tardy. Flexibility simply means to learn how to "roll with the punches" by keeping in mind that people are not always consistent and by being realistic about an intervention's results, which might not turn out as you expected. Preparing alternative plans and keeping an open mind about new methods or ideas are imperative for working effectively with clients.

For example, Maria's friend Claudia gets called into work unexpectedly, just 10 minutes before Maria's social work appointment. Maria doesn't drive and was depending on Claudia to drive her to her social worker's office. Maria now has to take a bus, which doesn't leave for 45 minutes. Since she realizes that there's no way she can get to her appointment on time, Maria called her social worker to tell her about what happened. Her social worker makes another appointment for the next day and suggests that Maria always have available an alternate plan, such as various bus route schedules, in case this happens again. The social worker also says that she'll allow this to happen once but doesn't want last-minute calls about appointments to become a habit.

Openness

Closely related to flexibility is openness, which means having an open mind to different views and behaviors, to learning something from and about clients from the clients themselves, and to making mistakes and learning from them. Having a nondefensive attitude when getting feedback from clients and coworkers is also part of this openness. Human services workers must freely admit when they are wrong or need to improve. Making mistakes is inevitable, and making an effort to learn from your mistakes sometimes even makes them worthwhile. The field of helping is ever changing, and therefore human services workers must remain open to changing and learning. The need to be perpetually learning is acknowledged by most human services agencies and professions. Most agencies and licensing boards require ongoing, continuing education and in-service training for workers. This is what makes the field dynamic and interesting.

The following interaction is an example of a worker's open attitude:

Client: "Last week you told me that you would have a hard time taking back your husband if he had cheated on you. That made me feel really bad, like I was doing something wrong by getting back together with my husband."

Appropriate response: "I'm sorry. I sure didn't mean to make you feel that way. I was trying to impress on you how much I admire your strength for being able to cope with something very difficult."

Knowledgeable and Resourceful

Although it is important to care and be genuinely concerned about your clients, it is also necessary to be **knowledgeable and resourceful** so that you have the best information on how to work with your clients and about other places for them to get help. Some of this information is usually based on research studies or anecdotes from workers who have many years experience serving people. Recipients of human services are entitled to be served by workers who put thought into interventions rather than merely offering intuitive and spontaneous advice. In addition to acquiring knowledge about client needs and interventions, human services workers should develop a list of resources by actively seeking connections with the rest of the human services world. This involves using a collaborative approach. Human services workers should want to give their clients access to as many resources as are available to assist them with whatever problems they may have. Human services workers should use all available resources and knowledge to meet as many of a client's needs as possible. This is part of the eclectic and integrative, generalist attitude discussed in Chapter 1.

Here is an example of such an attitude. Client: "I tried going to the grief group at the hospital, but I can't relate to anyone. They are all old and all their spouses died of heart attacks and cancer. My son was five when he got run over. No one there understands what I'm going through."

Resourceful response: "I can see why that group may not work for you. Your loss is very devastating, and you need a very special group. I have read about a group called, Compassionate Friends. They only take members who have lost a child. I think you might do better in that group."

Caring Professionalism

Another quality that human services workers should develop is **caring professionalism** in which they demonstrate both their knowledge and their humanity to their clients. This attitude allows workers to present information and give feedback to their clients in a way that doesn't make their clients feel like they are just another case.

Helping people based on research and the experiences of others is part of being a professional. Human services workers must be both professional and real. This can take years to develop. Beginning human services workers often feel awkward when first trying to be professional. Many times these workers approach clients as they would their own friends and family. Learning to set boundaries as a professional may initially seem as if you're being uncaring, however, clients deserve to receive services from a professional who can objectively help them with their needs.

For example, I conducted a research study of Latinos in Southern California that revealed that the vast majority prefer counselors who are very professional and give a lot of advice. The study participants didn't want their counselors to get too personal (Kanel, 2002). These results are particularly interesting because Latinos are known for having very warm and personal relationships. There is even a word for it in Spanish: *personalismo.* This suggests that while people want friendly and personal disclosures from family and friends, they might not want this from people whose professional services they need.

Desire for Self-Preservation

Finally, is the important quality of **self-preservation,** which involves finding a balance between work and a satisfying personal life outside of work. Human services workers deal with people on a regular basis who have severe problems. It is not easy to listen to these problems daily, and stress and even burnout are not unusual. Hearing about trauma and injustices may cause human services workers to feel traumatized themselves. Therefore it is vital for human services workers to take care of themselves emotionally and physically so they can handle the stress that comes with the job. Having a life outside of work that is healthy and active can help you reenergize you for work. Self-preservation involves leaving your clients' problems at work and seeking help when you need it. Overusing alcohol and drugs are not optimal ways to handle stress. Burnout can be avoided by seeking out personal relationships that are fulfilling and healthy and by exercising and doing fun things.

Self-preservation is so important that Chapter 10 is devoted to ways that people can handle stress and avoid job burnout. By taking care of yourself, you can better take care of others.

The following example profiles a human services worker who has found a healthy balance between work and play. Judy regularly jogs and rides her bike after work and on weekends. She also reads novels for fun. When she goes out to dinner, she may have a glass of wine, or might just have water. Judy is not perfect, but she does try to eat nutritious food when possible. Although she cares for her clients, she does not think about them after work hours. Someone asked her if she feels guilty about having fun when she knows her clients are suffering. She said, "Absolutely not! I would feel more guilty if I thought about them all day and didn't take care of myself. I wouldn't be worth anything to them if I was depressed."

CRITICAL THINKING / SELF-REFLECTION CORNER

- Do you think people who work in human services should be held to a different standard of self-development than those in other professions, such as doctors, lawyers, and businesspeople? Why?

- What are some ways in which you take care of yourself to ensure that you don't burn out and deplete your energy?

- Should human services workers be required to work through their own problems with a professional therapist? Why?

Chapter Summary

Because the primary role of human services workers involves human interaction, certain skills are considered vital for effective job performance. Table 4.1 summarizes the qualities and communication skills that human services workers need to develop over the years.

Most of these communication skills emphasize communicating genuine empathy and acceptance of clients' feelings and views about their situation. Skills such as active listening, feedback, and reflection help show clients such empathy. In addition to various communication skills, human services workers must also possess certain personal qualities that can increase their effectiveness. Some of these qualities include warmth, self-awareness, flexibility, openness, and self-confidence. Human services workers are encouraged to develop both effective communication skills and their own personhood as they begin helping others.

Table 4.1 Qualities and Effective Communication Skills

Personal Characteristics	Effective Communication Skills
congruence/genuineness	
unconditional positive regard/acceptance	using minimal encouragers
empathy	verbal following
concreteness	paraphrasing
developed sense of well-being	reflecting emotions
self-awareness	asking open-ended questions
presence of mind	providing feedback
flexibility	
openness	
resourcefulness and knowledgeable	
caring professionalism	
desire for self-preservation	

Suggested Applied Activities

1. Find a partner to play the role of a client or simply ask someone to talk with you. Let the person know you are interested in listening to whatever he or she wants to talk about for about five minutes. As the person talks, maintain good eye contact, nod your head, and say "uh-huh" every half minute or so. After the five minutes, ask the person if he or she felt heard and did it seem that you were paying attention to the conversation.

_____

_____

_____

_____

_____

_____

2. Find a partner to role-play an interaction between a counselor and a client. As the client talks, try to restate what you heard. Try to reflect feelings or information. Remember, the goal is to understand your client's experience. Do not try to solve any problems. Don't give advice. Just try to understand the problem or the client's needs.

_____

_____

_____

_____

_____

_____

3. In another client-counselor role-playing exercise, ask five close-ended questions in a row. For example, "Do you feel angry?" "Do you want to cry?" "Did you tell anyone?" "Why did you do it?" or "Does it make you want to get back at him?" Ask your role-playing partner for feedback about what it feels like to be asked those types of questions. Next, try asking open-ended questions. A simple trick is to reword the first set of questions by beginning each with the words "what" or "how." For example, "How do you feel"? "What does it make you want to do?" "What did you do?" "What made you decide to do it?" "How do you feel toward him?" Then find out if these questions make your partner feel any different.

_____

_____

_____

_____

_____

_____

_____

4. During your everyday social interactions, pay attention to how people listen to each other. Can you observe people interrupting each other in the middle of a thought or sentence? Do people ask questions that allow the speaker to continue with his or her thoughts? Make a list of the types of things people actually say to each other. Are any of these things similar to the types of communication skills presented in this chapter?

_____

_____

_____

_____

_____

_____

Chapter Review Questions

1. What are 3 active listening skills?

   _____

   _____

2. In what way are open-ended questions more effective in helping clients open up than close-ended questions?

   _____

   _____

3. What personal characteristics are human services workers encouraged to develop that differentiate them from other professions?

   _____

   _____

4. What is meant by "being there"?

   _____

   _____

5. What is empathy?

   _____

   _____

6. What do the concepts of authenticity and genuineness mean when referring to qualities of human services workers?

   _____

   _____

7. How might you show someone that you are verbally following them?

   _____

   _____

Glossary of Terms

Active listening involves not only hearing what clients say but offering feedback and helping them explore more about what they are saying.

Caring professionalism says to clients, "I care about you and your needs, but I am a professional and the nature of our relationship is professional. I will be friendly but not your friend."

Clarifying is paraphrasing in a questioning tone what a practitioner thinks a client is saying to make sure that what the client said was accurate. Concreteness is an accurate, clear, specific, and immediate response to clients.

Congruence and genuineness involve being real and genuine in the moment.

Developed sense of well-being requires human services workers to take care of their own emotional needs and actively deal with any life struggles so that they may be fully available to their clients.

Empathy involves being able to put yourself in another person's shoes and understand that person's emotional and cognitive experience of a situation.

Existential-humanistic counseling approach A philosophical approach to counseling in which the client is invited to examine his or her values and human needs and is encouraged to grow and expand his or her existence. Choice and growth are the foundations of this approach.

Feedback provides clients with an assessment of their problems. It can be both supportive and confrontational but should always be based on an objective assessment and presented in nonjudgmental terms.

Flexibility is being open to adopting and modifying new ideas and behaviors and to learning new ideas.

Minimal encouragers are verbal and nonverbal cues that let clients know that their human services worker is interested in hearing what they are talking about. Head nodding and a forward-leaning posture are two examples.

Open-ended questions begin with *what* and *how* and allow for further exploration of what a client is saying. Clients feel less defensive answering these types of questions.

Openness is a nondefensive approach that actively seeks new information with the realization that there is always something new to learn.

Paraphrasing is used to restate what a client is saying to make sure that the practitioner and the client are understanding each other.

Presence of mind keeps practitioners in the moment and participating with a client during a session rather than being focused on other things.

Reflection is the use of verbal and nonverbal cues to reflect back a client's emotions.

Resourcefulness is the ability to work collaboratively to learn about all the agencies and services that are available to help out and meet the needs of clients and requires the use of active problem-solving methods.

Self-awareness is the recognition of your own feelings, thoughts, values, and behaviors, and how they affect people around you, as well as the awareness of your strengths and the areas in your life that need improvement.

Self-preservation gives you the ability to protect yourself from harm (and job burnout) by regularly monitoring your emotional well-being and doing what is necessary to stay healthy.

Unconditional positive regard and acceptance of clients allows them to believe that feelings, thoughts, or behaviors are not being judged.

Verbal following keeps the focus of a conversation on what a client is saying rather than jumping from topic to topic.

Case Presentation and Exit Quiz

General Description and Demographics

The client presented in this counseling session is a 23-year-old woman, named Gloria, who entered a battered women's shelter last night. Gloria has been married for six years. She has two children, a three-month-old baby girl, and a 4–year-old son, both of whom are with her at the shelter because she has no relatives living in the area. Her family lives in Mexico, and she rarely communicates with them since she's been married. Gloria married a U. S. citizen whom she met in Mexico. He brought her to the United States and began beating her two months into their marriage.

The abuse escalates when he is drinking. Gloria has had bruises around her eyes and on her ribs. He even beat her while she was pregnant, and yesterday he attempted to choke her. She is so afraid that he might kill her that she finally told a neighbor what's been happening. The neighbor gave her the number of a battered women's shelter. Gloria called the shelter, and an intake worker made arrangements to get her and her kids to the shelter while her husband was at a bar. Gloria speaks English, but not fluently. Her client advocate speaks some Spanish. The following conversation takes place the next morning, and is the first that Gloria and her advocate have had.

Interview between Gloria (G) and her client advocate (A.)

A: What happened yesterday that made you call our hotline, Gloria?

G: My husband, he choked me bad.

A: How are you feeling now?

G: I am scared.

A: What scares you?

G: He might try to find me and kill me.

A: That does sound scary.

G: Yes, he told me he will kill me if I leave.

A. Uh-huh.

G: He gets drunk and is very mean. I hope he doesn't find me here.

A: It sounds like you believe he might look for you and hurt you.

G: Yes, he told me many times that I am his now, and that I won't be allowed to stay in the U.S. if I leave him.

A: I can see why you would be afraid then. I am not sure if that is true, but we have an attorney who comes here weekly and we could find out about that if you like.

G: That would be good.

A: Are you saying that you want to leave your husband?

G: I want our family together so the children can have a father, but I . . .

A: This seems like a difficult decision for you.

G: Yes, my family told me not to marry him because he would be a bad father. He was known to have a bad temper in our town in Mexico. My mother told me I should stay in Mexico.

A: So even before you got married, your family didn't really think he was right for you.

G: I am ashamed to tell anyone that he beat me. They will think it is my fault.

A: Unfortunately, many people don't understand these types of situations. I don't think it was your fault at all. Nobody deserves to be mistreated. It is a crime to beat your wife.

G: But I don't keep my children quiet enough, and sometimes I don't want to be close with my husband.

A: It is hard to keep children quiet all the time, especially a baby.

G: My husband says he will take the children from me. I cannot live without them. I love them so much.

A: You sound like a good mother.

G: My husband says I am a bad mother and that the children love him the most.

A: What do you think about that?

G: I don't think so. My son is afraid of his father.

A: How do you mean, afraid?

G: He told me he is scared when Papa comes home.

A: Has your husband ever beat your son?

G: He yells at him, but has not hit him yet. He hits me instead because I don't raise our son right.

A: I am sure glad he hasn't hurt your son. But I am scared that your husband could get violent with your children. Your husband might have a serious problem with his anger and with the need to be in control.

G: I think you are right, but my husband, he does love us. Sometimes he is nice and brings us to the park, and we eat McDonalds. My son loves that.

A: That is good that your son has some good times with his father. It is important that children have a father and a mother in their lives. It is not good for children to watch their father hurt their mother. It could affect them later on in life. Many children who see violence in the home repeat it as adults.

G: Of course, I saw my father beat my mother, and I was afraid. But I thought it was normal.

A: It is very common. About one woman out of three lives with a man who mistreats her. But it is not normal, and it is against the law. Your husband needs professional help to stop doing it.

G: But I don't want him in trouble with the law. He needs to work.

A: It is your choice to decide whether you want to report it to the police. If you do, the court will most likely make your husband go to group counseling and get educated about his problems. Here at the shelter, you will have a chance to learn more about this problem and how you want to handle it. I am so glad you are here with your children. You will all be safe from violence while you are here. You can talk to an attorney and other women who have gone through this. Try to focus on getting help for your family while you are here. We will take it one day at a time. You have at least 45 days to make decisions.

G: Thank you. I need to go feed my baby now, but I will see you later. You have been so much help.

A: Good, I'll see you in group at 10 a.m.

Exit Quiz

1. When the advocate says words like "seems" and "sounds," she is
   a. providing direct feedback
   b. asking open-ended questions
   c. clarifying and paraphrasing
   d. unsure of what to say

2. When the advocate tells Gloria that she is glad that her son hasn't been hurt, the advocate is
   a. showing professional caring
   b. crossing the line between being a professional and being a friend
   c. lacking empathy
   d. all of the above

3. An example of a reflective statement is
   a. uh-huh
   b. Are you saying that you want to leave your husband?
   c. How are you feeling?
   d. That does sound scary.

4. When the advocate tells Gloria that it is good that her son has some good times with his father, the advocate is demonstrating
   a. lack of empathy
   b. lack of congruence
   c. unconditional positive regard
   d. lack of flexibility

5. Including an attorney to help this client is an example of the advocate being
   a. lazy
   b. resourceful
   c. uncaring
   d. incongruent

6. When the advocate asked questions related only to what Gloria said in the session, this is an example of
   a. the advocate's inability to develop empathy
   b. lack of trust between Gloria and the advocate
   c. verbal following
   d. lack of creativity

Exit Quiz Answers

1. c	3. d	5. b
2. a	4. c	6. c

CHAPTER 5

Biological and Psychological Theories of Causality

Introduction

We will be discussing in this chapter biological and psychological theories that have been developed that explain **social problems** and **deviant behaviors** that people who use human services may have. Some of these theories explain problems as being due to physical factors. While human services workers deal with many problems that seem to be caused by physical factors, this text only deals with problems that effect an individual's emotional and behavioral functioning. Most medical diseases are not dealt with by human services workers. Instead, medical doctors and nurses generally deal with purely medical disorders. That is not to say that medical disorders do not impact a person's overall well-being. Human services workers are often needed to assist people in dealing with medical disorders. It is just beyond the realm of human services workers to provide medical treatment, except in the case of psychiatrists, who usually prescribe medications.

The majority of this chapter focuses on psychological factors that often cause emotional, social, and psychological problems. Throughout the twentieth century, a variety of **psychological theories** were developed that offered strategies for helping people with deviant behaviors and other emotional disorders. Human services workers at all levels should be familiar with the best-known of these theories and strategies so they can be used in a client's best interest. Familiarizing yourself with these various approaches and implementing them when appropriate is largely the basis of the generalist approach and an eclectic point of view.

Sociological theories also attempt to explain social problems. These theories include looking at the effects of societal norms, social roles, cultural expectations, and social inequities such as racism, sexism, ageism, and socioeconomic status (SES) on a person's behaviors and emotional needs. Also included in this category are political factors such as the administration's tendency either toward social programs or away from social programs. More recently, many human services workers have been looking at the effect that spirituality and religion have on creating or maintaining various problems. Many of the problems that human services workers deal with have strong social factors that maintain the problem. These social theories are essential in understanding the issues facing many recipients of human services. Chapter 6 is devoted to exploring the social, cultural, spiritual, and political factors that influence human services delivery and that may explain certain problems faced by various populations. Because human services workers are generalists who use an eclectic, holistic, and multidisciplinary model, their knowledge of various theories lets them understand and serve their clients best. Some theoretical models may be more appropriate for certain clients than for others. Determining the suitable model for a client will be examined in subsequent sections of this chapter and in Chapter 7. A **bio-psychosocial model** takes into account the ways in which biological, psychological, and social factors affect clients and gives workers a multitheoretical foundation for working with clients. It is all-inclusive and permits a multitude of interventions.

Biological and psychological theories are discussed throughout this chapter. Chapter 6 goes on to examine how human behavior is affected by social factors, including those that focus on religion, gender, ethnicity, politics, and economic class.

The Biological Model

The **biological model**—sometimes referred to as the **medical model**—uses medical, genetic, neurological, or biochemical factors to attempt to understand emotional, behavioral, and social problems. Many studies have been conducted to pinpoint how biological factors affect various problems. Although proving that biological factors definitely cause certain behaviors, attitudes, and emotions is extremely difficult due to the difficulty in pinpointing which parts of the brain cause specific behaviors and emotions, such theories are widely accepted by many human services workers. Physicians and psychiatrists who deal with severe deviance and mental illness often adhere exclusively to this approach when understanding and treating their patients. Not only do psychiatrists use this model, but non-medical human services workers do as well. In fact, the fourth edition of the Diagnostic and Statistical Manual of Mental Disorders (DSM-IV) lists a multitude of mental disorders whose primary cause is believed to be biological because they include impairments in functioning and are frequently related to emotional suffering such as bipolar disorders, schizophrenia, and dementia. The DSM-IV contains the universal codes for diagnosing clients used by most mental health practitioners nationwide. Although human services workers do not typically treat mental disorders that have a primarily biological basis, they do offer help by providing information about the disorder and by supporting and helping the person who is ill, as well as family members affected by the illness, lead as normal and productive a life as possible. The disorders commonly seen and dealt with by human services workers are mentioned in the section

"Implications of the Biological Model in the Human Services" along with services typically provided for these disorders.

Because we are all physiological beings, it is hard to claim that there is no biological component to a person's problems. Some problems, however, seem to be more influenced by sociological, political, or psychological factors. Poverty is one such example that is easy to grasp. Chapter 7, in its discussion of various client populations also looks at what, if any, biological factors contribute to the needs of these populations. If biological factors have been determined to be an important aspect of a client's problem, interventions are usually tailored to include biological treatments, such as medication.

Biological Factors

Since this is neither a physiology nor a biology book, this chapter will provide only a basic discussion of the most common biological factors that can affect psychological, emotional, and social functioning. Specific disorders encountered frequently by human services workers will be linked to these factors.

NEUROTRANSMITTERS

Neurotransmitters are chemicals released from one neuron in the brain that travel through a small gap called the synapse until they reach the receptor site neuron. Communication of information between neurons is accomplished by movement of these neurotransmitters. When a receptor site is activated, the result may be either an excitatory potential or an inhibitory potential. Most emotions and behaviors, it is believed, are triggered by the release of these chemicals, and that some people are born with a tendency to release an imbalance in certain neurotransmitters that may lead to abnormal behaviors, emotions, and thoughts ("Neuroscience for Kids" website, 6/17/2006).

Some of the most common neurotransmitters that affect clients seen by workers in the human services include dopamine, serotonin, norepinephrine, and epinephrine. Dopamine is essential to a normally functioning central nervous system, and a reduction within the brain is associated with Parkinson's disease. Norepinephrine reduction has also been linked with other such disorders as schizophrenia. Serotonin, which has been linked with norepinephrine, affects mood, as well as levels of anxiety and pain. "Implications of the Biological Model," which is farther along in this chapter, discusses medications that have been developed to balance the transmission of these neurotransmitters.

GENETIC AND HEREDITARY FACTORS

Genetic disorders are caused, at least in part, by the genes of the person with the disease. These are congenital (present at birth) and are often referred to as **hereditary disorders.** There are a number of possible causes for genetic defects. They may be caused by random mutation or by the accidental duplication of a chromosome, as in Down syndrome, or by repeated duplication of part of a chromosome (wikipedia.org website, June 2006). In essence, genetic disorders are caused by an anomaly in a person's genetic structure, manifest themselves by limiting a person mentally and physically as determined by a person's genetic structure (at http://en.wikipedia.org/wiki/List_of genetic_disorders 6-17-06).

Some of the more widely known genetic disorders are cystic fibrosis, sickle cell anemia, spina bifida, Huntington's chorea, Alzheimer's disease, Down syndrome, Rett syndrome, dwarfism, and hemophilia.

BRAIN TRAUMA

Brain damage from either an accident or a disease is another biological factor that may cause emotional, behavioral, social, and psychological impairments. People suffering from **brain trauma** often need the ongoing assistance of human services workers to help them live as fully and as independently as possible. Others can be rehabilitated through occupational and recreational therapy.

TOXIC SUBSTANCES

Some people's mental and behavioral disorders result from exposure to various poisons, radiation, alcohol, drugs, and other **toxic substances,** all of which can impair a person's functioning and even cause permanent brain damage. In some instances, people choose to intoxicate themselves, such as when people abuse drugs and alcohol. Others are victims of those choices, such as babies born with fetal alcohol syndrome, which results from women who drink while they are pregnant.

Implications of Biological Theory for the Human Services

All of us are biochemical beings, and therefore one can argue that all of our actions have a biological basis. In human services, certain problems lend themselves most appropriately to biological theory and corresponding treatment approaches. Many disorders found in the DSM-IV are usually treated as medical disorders. In fact, medical insurance covers treatment for a variety of these mental disorders because they are thought to be caused by physiological factors. The most common disorders in the DSM-IV that are thought to stem from biological factors include delirium, dementia, amnesia, and other cognitive disorders; substance-related disorders; schizophrenia and other forms of psychosis, major depression, bipolar disorders, panic disorders, anorexia nervosa; mental retardation; learning disabilities; obsessive-compulsive disorder; and hyperactivity attention-deficit disorder.

Human services workers may provide services for individuals suffering from these disorders and their families in residential facilities such as hospitals, board and care homes (private homes where patients reside and are monitored by board and care operators and often receive medication by psychiatrists who frequently visit at the home), outpatient clinics, and group homes in conjunction with physicians and psychiatrists. Some human services workers provide supportive and educational counseling, others serve as behavior managers with these populations. Psychiatrists usually prescribe medications, and neurosurgeons may sometimes operate.

Many times, families of impaired clients need assistance in taking care of their loved ones. Human services workers may offer **respite care** (which gives family members a break from their caretaking responsibilities). The overall goal in working with people suffering from biologically based illnesses is to provide them with the highest possible standard of living that their disorder allows. Total cure is not typically the focus of intervention.

CRITICAL THINKING / SELF-REFLECTION CORNER

What aspects of your psychological, emotional, or social functioning are influenced by your physiological makeup?

The Psychological Model

Many different theories have been devised in an attempt to understand our psychological makeup. Some are fairly well known, such as Freud's psychoanalytic theory. Others are new approaches or modifications to more traditional methods, such as current trends in family and cognitive therapies. Psychological theories try to explain a person's behaviors and emotional states by looking at childhood interactions with family and friends, traumatic events in the person's life, and choices that a person makes.

Psychoanalytic Theories

THE PIONEER: SIGMUND FREUD

Sigmund Freud is credited with having developed the first of the **psychoanalytic theories** in an attempt to understanding how symptoms and deviant behaviors serve a psychological function for individuals. Freud proposed that all humans are born with certain instincts that need to be expressed. These instincts reside in the part of the psyche that Freud called the **id.** The instincts, often called **libido** or eros (sexual and pleasure drives) and **thanatos** (aggression and death drives) are considered primitive drives and include all the impulses, fantasies, wishes, and feelings all people have (Brenner, 1974; Guntrip, 1973; Strachey, 1966). Freud suggested that as we grow, we develop another aspect to our personality structure, the **ego,** which is our sense of self. As children's egos develop, they begin to understand that a separate reality exists outside of their own drives, needs, and feelings. While the id operates under the pleasure principle, the ego operates under the reality principle and is vital for healthy functioning. A weak ego may hinder an individual's ability to approach the world realistically and thereby hamper that person's ability to manage daily stress and problems. By about four years of age, children begin to develop another part of their personality, the **superego,** commonly known as a conscience. At that point, children begin to internalize the demands and societal boundaries that their parents, teachers, religious leaders, and other authority figures have placed on them (Guntrip, 1973).

Freud postulated that problems may occur when the demands of the id are in conflict with the internalized boundaries of the superego. A person may have impulses (the id) to assault someone but if that person has internalized the parameters of appropriate behavior (the superego) such aggressive urges will not be acted on. Conflicts between the id and the superego can make people feel threatened and anxious. To abate those negative feelings, Freud suggested that the mind represses these conflicts. This concept of **repression** relates to another concept that Freud postulated, the **unconscious.** Freud believed that the bulk of our mental lives resided in a part of our mind not readily available to conscious scrutiny. To manage our daily lives, Freud believed that we bar from consciousness (in other words, repress) psychological and emotional knowledge and experiences that would cause us overwhelming anxiety and shame, and prevent us from functioning normally. In addition to basic repression, Freud theorized that we engage in other behaviors—**ego defense mechanisms**—that help us cope with unmanageable feelings of threat and conflict, and that are believed to operate outside of conscious awareness. These behaviors allow the ego to manage reality without the burden of anxiety (Brenner, 1974; Strachey, 1966).

Some of the ego defense mechanisms that we humans use are defined below.

- **Projection** is used to attribute to others qualities and actions that are considered unacceptable to yourself. For example, a husband might accuse his wife of having an affair when in fact he is the one who has been unfaithful.

- **Denial** is used when a problem is too threatening to acknowledge. Refusing to recognize and get treatment for a health problem is one example of denial that can have serious consequences.

- **Minimization** is used to turn a serious problem into a minor one, such as the battered wife who says that her husband isn't being abusive since he hasn't broken any of her bones.

- **Reaction formation** is denial of a certain desire or impulse while responding vehemently to an opposite impulse or desire. For example, a new mother who has thoughts of drowning her baby instead overindulges the baby in front of other people.

- **Regression** is used to cope with an intolerable situation by returning to an earlier and safer level of functioning. For instance, a five-year-old who's been toilet trained for three years starts wetting herself after her baby brother is born. Unconsciously she feels threatened by the attention her parents are giving to the baby and reverts to an earlier stage of development to get the attention and comfort she feels she has lost.

- **Intellectualization** is used to distance yourself emotionally from a difficult situation. A rape victim who calmly and unemotionally describes the attack in full detail is using this defense.

- **Compensation** uses strengths to make up for difficulty or an inability to do something, such as an athlete who becomes paraplegic and gets actively involved in wheelchair sports.

- People use **displacement** to direct feelings away from the threatening object that's causing the emotions and toward a safe one instead. For instance, a husband who's angry with his boss comes home and yells at his children and his wife instead.

- **Sublimation** is a healthy, socially acceptable way to express psychological energy and drives. For instance, when a woman takes out her frustration with rush-hour traffic by playing a rigorous game of tennis (Brenner, 1974; Corey, 2005).

CRITICAL THINKING / SELF-REFLECTION CORNER

What are some examples of ego defense mechanisms that you use or that you observe others using? When have you used them?

How do these defenses help you or others cope with difficult situations?

Freud also proposed that people develop through certain stages that he called, **psychosexual stages.** He believed that if children are overindulged or deprived during these stages of development they could become **fixated** at that stage and develop personality problems in adulthood.

Oral Stage This is Freud's first stage of psychosexual development. In infancy, the basic source of pleasure is the mouth. All needs should be met during infancy. When infants are appropriately nurtured, they will feel safe and develop a sense of trust in the world. When basic needs during this phase are not met adequately, individuals may grow up to have issues with dependency and trust.

Examples of appropriate behavior at the **oral stage** are babies who, as soon as they learn to crawl and walk, begin sticking everything—even inedible things like dirt—in their mouths. Also, when babies cry, they are given a bottle or pacifier to quickly stop their crying.

Anal Stage As toddlers, children need to learn how to be independent and empowered, but they also need boundaries. While infants don't usually have boundaries placed on them, children at this age begin to hear and understand the meaning of "no." Freud believed that at this stage, much of the instinctual and psychological energy revolves around toilet training. Parents of two- and three-year-olds can verify that this is a truly difficult time because toddlers are learning to assert their independence. If needs are not met adequately at this stage, children may grow up burdened by shame and doubt. Freud claimed that those who are fixated at the **anal stage** often develop obsessive-compulsive personality disorders.

Normal behaviors at this stage are toddlers who fly into a tantrum when they can't have a toy that they want. They often insist on feeding themselves and refuse to hold their parents' hands when walking up stairs.

Phallic Stage At the **phallic stage**, development moves from biological to social. Preschoolers learn to engage in relationships and begin to develop a sexual identity. This is accomplished primarily by interacting with their parents. Primitive sexual and aggressive drives need to be repressed, and children need to internalize socially appropriate behaviors. Problems during this stage might lead to faulty superego formation, difficulties with sexual identity, and primitive sexual longings.

Appropriate behaviors observed at this stage may be a four-year-old girl who asks a boy in her class to play house, where she's the mother, he's the father, and a third classmate is the baby. A three-year-old sees his mother and father sitting close together on the sofa and sits between them.

Latent Stage During the elementary school years, if repression of a child's primitive drives was accomplished in the previous stage, children are basically free from mental conflict and engage in the process of learning new skills and social behaviors.

Examples of typical behaviors during the **latent stage** may include a fourth-grade boy who feels proud when he learns how to do long division or a third-grade girl asks if she can sharpen pencils for her teacher.

Genital Stage In adolescence, teenagers should be developing mature ways of relating to others and turning primitive energy and instincts into socially acceptable behaviors, such as being responsible sexually and having a mature work ethic.

Appropriate behaviors at the **genital stage** are seen when an eighth-grade girl asks a boy to dance at a school prom or a 17-year-old boy kisses his girlfriend at the end of a date (Brenner, 1974; Corey, 2005; Guntrip, 1973; Strachey, 1966).

OBJECT-RELATIONS THEORY

Object-relations theorists, while still proponents of Freud, focus more on the impact the relationship between a mother or primary caretaker **(object)** and her baby has on a child's psychological development. **Object-relations theory** proposes that, rather than being controlled by instincts, a person develops a self-concept and a procedural code about how to have relationships. When children are traumatized or endure unhealthy parenting practices during the first three years of life, they may become deficient in relational skills and develop inappropriate or unrealistic self-concepts (Gabbard, 2000; Guntrip, 1973).

Margaret Mahler's (1975) emphasis in object-relations theory was on the stages during a baby's first three years of life. She proposed that the inability to move from one stage to another may develop into **personality disorders** in adulthood. Mahler's stages of development are described below. Notice that both this theory and Freud's model do not contradict each other. Object-relations theorists use these stages to determine when people begin to develop their own self-concepts and to learn to relate to other people.

Autistic Stage　Infants live in their own world of feelings, impulses, and drives. For them, life is about survival. **Normal (infantile) autism** occurs during a baby's first three or so months of life. If infants are not nurtured sufficiently so that they can move on to the next stage, deficits may develop in emotional relationships with others. They may be distrustful and may have difficulty receiving realistic feedback about their self-identity. This may lead to a schizoid, paranoid, or antisocial personality disorder.

Appropriate behavior for babies at this stage is, for instance, not crying when strangers hold and kiss them.

Symbiosis　During **symbiosis**, an infant (at about three months) begins relating to others, primarily the mother or primary caretaker. All of an infant's needs are met by the mother, and a sense of total relatedness to the **object** (mother) develops. It is as if the two are connected and live as one. This phase should last until children are about two years old, when, as toddlers, they begin the process of becoming independent.

Children who do not move on from this stage may, as adults, feel incomplete when not involved in an emotionally intense relationship and even may worry about being abandoned. Fixation at this stage might also result in borderline personality disorder. Adults with this disorder have great difficulty managing relationships, emotions, and impulses. They often feel empty, have intense fears of abandonment, and may have suicidal thoughts.

A 14-month-old who cries when her mother leaves for work or a 9-month-old who will only calm down and go to sleep when his mother puts him to bed are both examples of normal behavior at this stage.

Separation/Individuation   From ages two through four, children learn how to experience themselves as separate individuals who must get along with other separate individuals. At this stage, children need to receive validation and empathy for who they are. Children who do not receive proper validation may become fixated at this stage. As a result, they may continue searching for validation and empathic response throughout their lives. Individuals who don't receive appropriate validation during the **separation/individuation** stage may lack of a sense of a cohesive self-identity, which can develop into narcissistic personality disorder. Those with this disorder are, typically, obsessed with self-acceptance and self-affirmation and appear self-involved and to lack empathy. They often have difficulty developing intimate relationships and may use others only to meet their own needs (Gabbard, 2000).

CRITICAL THINKING / SELF-REFLECTION CORNER

- Do you believe that people can be fixated in an early stage of development, and that this fixation can determine their personality in adulthood?

- Have you noticed any of your own or anyone else's personality traits described in Freud's or Mahler's stages?

THE NEO-FREUDIANS

Neo-Freudians, most of whom were students of Freud, offered another theory to explain internal conflicts that can lead to psychological problems. Alfred Adler, Karen Horney, Harry Stack Sullivan, and Erich Fromm proposed that children, rather than being instinct-powered and preprogrammed, are instead beings who, aside from such innate neutral qualities as temperament, are entirely shaped by their cultural and interpersonal environment. A child's basic need is for security, acceptance, and approval from significant adults. The quality of interaction with these adults determines adult character structure (Yalom, 1980).

Adler emphasized that the ways in which people perceive their interactions with others greatly influence how they feel and behave. He proposed that every person has a unique, **individual psychology** that is determined by mistaken beliefs and faulty logic. Adult behavior that is considered deviant may result from distorted perceptions developed in childhood. Adults with mental health problems may be discouraged because they can't find ways to feel secure and accepted in childhood. Adler believed that understanding each person's own frame of reference is vital to understanding that person's unique lifestyle and choices. He used a **phenomenological** approach to understanding people and a cognitive approach to affecting change in their behavioral patterns. Adler introduced a more integrative way of dealing with people that continues to be practiced today by human services workers.

IMPLICATIONS OF PSYCHOANALYTIC THEORIES FOR HUMAN SERVICES DELIVERY

The psychoanalytic models offer human services workers a theoretical basis for understanding clients. Many of these concepts can be used in counseling or providing other service. In terms of a typical human services worker practicing psychoanalytic therapy, there are some limitations. This type of therapy usually involves a long-term commitment, is costly, and should be limited to clients who have enough ego strength to handle the stress of uncovering painful emotions and to those who have enough money to pay an analyst for several years. This is not to say that counselors, social workers, probation officers, and other human services workers cannot successfully put to use some of these models' ideas and techniques. If these methods are used, workers will most likely modify their interventions to fit the needs of their clients. The idea of gaining **insight** into a person's unconscious is the main goal of psychoanalysis, and this is done is by having the client talk freely about whatever comes to mind during a session. Many human services workers provide an opportunity for their clients to talk openly and freely about their problems. Although the goal may not be to uncover unconscious conflicts, the idea of a client talking to a human services worker was introduced by the psychoanalytic theorists.

Adler's model of providing encouragement and focusing on a client's strengths is probably used more often by typical human services workers. His model can be modified to benefit clients who are in short-term treatment because, unlike Freudian and object-relations psychoanalysts, Adler focused on the conscious mind and conscious goals. This focus is more amenable to short-term interventions.

The Existential-Humanistic Theories

While Freud was developing his psychoanalytic model for understanding people, a group of philosophers and novelists were establishing their views about the human condition. Existentialism is a philosophy that examines the meaning of being human. It examines the basic core of the human condition and how that condition influences behavior and emotions. **Existential-humanistic theories** focus on conflicts that flow from an individual's confrontation with certain **givens** of existence. These "givens are the intrinsic properties that are a part, and an inescapable part, of the human being's existence in the world" (Yalom, 1980, p. 8).

IRVIN YALOM'S THEORY

Yalom, a well-known existential therapist focused on four ultimate givens: death, freedom, isolation, and meaninglessness. He believed these concerns create conflicts within humans. In *Existential Psychotherapy* (1980, p. 10), Yalom states that awareness of these concerns leads to anxiety when an individual realizes he or she is alone to make choices and then must accept responsibility for the consequences of those choices. To cope with this existential anxiety, many people use psychological defense mechanisms that can create dysfunction and unhealthy behaviors and restrict a full existence in which people can realize their full potential. Instead of facing anxiety and making choices based on will, people may instead seek an ultimate rescuer to make those decisions for them. Although anxiety may be reduced, the cost, according to Yalom, is an inauthentic existence, depression, and a feeling of psychological deadness.

In Yalom's *The Theory and Practice of Group Psychotherapy,* he describes how to assist clients by having them engage in **group therapy** that focuses on the existential givens (Yalom, 1985). His work has long been considered the standard text for group therapists and is also included among the decade's 10 most influential publications in its field. Yalom's group therapy model also provides a detailed understanding of the group therapy process as experienced by individual group members and by the group as a whole. Group therapy is used frequently in many human services settings, and many use Yalom's model. Rather than talking to clients one at a time in private sessions, Yalom's approach has group members talking directly to one another while the therapist serves as a relationship-building facilitator among members. Of course, the therapist also speaks to clients about what they are talking about but is encouraged to disclose more than typical therapists might in individual therapy.

CARL ROGERS'S PERSON-CENTERED APPROACH

Rogers's **person-centered model** followed existential theory more closely than it did the psychoanalytic theories, and heavily emphasized the concepts of self-awareness and human growth and potential. Rogers believed that humans behave in symptomatic ways because they suffer from blocks to this growth. He also believed that people would be able to actualize their potential by forming a relationship with a genuine, nonjudgmental, and empathic person. Chapter 4 presents many of Rogers's ideas about how workers should relate to their clients and what characteristics typically lead to being most effective in their job.

Rogers also considered group participation to be very beneficial for many clients. He described the values of groups in *Carl Rogers on Encounter Groups*

(1970), in which he shows how his original ideas about the necessary and sufficient conditions of therapeutic change can be used in a group therapy setting.

Although Rogers is known for these conditions of change, he has also written about the humanistic basis of becoming a person in *On Becoming a Person* (1961). Rogers's works all focus on the positive elements of humans and encourage all of humanity to communicate respectfully with one another. In his later years, Rogers's writings and presentations focused on world peace and race relations (1987). He believed that his approach to counseling could be implemented in a variety of situations, not just therapy.

FREDERIC PERLS AND GESTALT THERAPY

Gestalt therapy is a type of existential therapy that focuses on the maturation process of individuals. Perls claimed that for people to relate to the world maturely they must integrate all aspects of themselves and own all of those parts. Additionally, he believed people must resolve interpersonal conflict to feel whole and complete. According to Perls, **unfinished business** and **fragmentation** of the self can lead to phony and phobic living. Perls recommended that people engage in the process of self-awareness at an emotional and experiential level instead of the intellectual level recommended by psychoanalysts. Symptoms, he said, resolve themselves once a person moves from dependence on others for emotional support to self-reliance. Mental health problems result from immaturity and the inability to face yourself and others honestly (Perls, 1969).

In *Gestalt Therapy Verbatim* (1969), Perls catalyzed a movement during the late 1960s and 1970s that encouraged full expression of the self. The rebellious political climate of the time provided fertile ground for growth of a nontraditional approach to therapy. Perls's charismatic leadership spurred development of many gestalt therapy institutes, one of the best-known, the Esalen Sensitivity Training Institute was located in Big Sur, CA.

REALITY THERAPY: WILLIAM GLASSER'S APPROACH TO WORKING WITH JUVENILE OFFENDERS

Glasser developed his approach in the 1960s when he was involved in treating teenage girls in the Ventura, California, correctional facility. He found that the long-term psychoanalytic models and the humanistic self-examination models weren't effective for this population. Rather than examining anxiety derived from being aware of core human conditions, Glasser focused on changing deviant behavior into responsible behavior. However, his model did incorporate many of the existential and humanistic concepts such as stressing that people have choices and are responsible for their behaviors and emphasizing the importance of an authentic therapeutic relationship.

Glasser believed that people not only need to develop a relationship with someone who cares about them but that they also need to care about others. He also suggested that people need to contribute something meaningful to society, concepts first introduced by Adler and other existentialists. Glasser believed that all behavior is an individual's best attempt to meet those needs. When people have not learned how to meet those needs responsibly, they meet them through irresponsible and sometimes deviant behaviors. In **reality therapy,** he explained that a strong client-therapist relationship based on honesty, trust, humor, and boundaries allows clients to move toward appropriate, responsible behaviors and feel more in control of their world (Glasser, 1975).

IMPLICATIONS OF EXISTENTIAL-HUMANISTIC THEORIES FOR HUMAN SERVICES DELIVERY

Existential and humanistic-based therapies can be either long or short term, depending on a client's needs. Clients who have the time and money to examine their identities and how they fit into the world may benefit from long-term existential therapy. Most clients, however, can benefit from a genuine, nonjudgmental relationship that focuses on helping clients find answers to a specific problem through clarification and empathic understanding. Reality therapy concepts are very effective for people who want help correcting their irresponsible behaviors, especially if those behaviors have landed them in jail.

One of the biggest impacts these approaches have had on the human services is the use of group counseling as a prevalent form of intervention. Group counseling is a cost effective and valuable way for clients to learn about their relational skills. Most residential treatment facilities, hospitals, and outpatient clinics conduct group therapy sessions on a regular basis. Prior to Yalom and Rogers, group therapy only referred to a bunch of clients sitting in the same room with one therapist who basically conducted individual therapy with each member while the others watched.

Behavioral Theories

Behavioral theories usually include several models for understanding both animal and human behavior. Two particularly relevant models for those in the human services are B.F. Skinner's **operant conditioning** model and Ivan Pavlov's **classical conditioning** model. Both models provide concepts that explain behavior and allow for treatment of deviant behaviors.

OPERANT CONDITIONING

B.F. Skinner's name is virtually synonymous with operant conditioning. He conducted many experiments with rats and pigeons in an effort to understand how to encourage and discourage behavior. In *Walden Two* (1948), Skinner introduced many of the concepts that he later expanded on in *Science and Human Behavior* (1953). Skinner's laboratory work with animals has been applied to people who have a variety of problems.

The basic premise of Skinner's theory is that all behavior is learned through reinforcement and any behavior can be extinguished by removing the reinforcement. A **positive reinforcement,** usually a reward or some positive stimulus, encourages a behavior to continue. Sometimes the reinforcement is the removal of a negative stimulus after a desired behavior is performed, this is called **negative reinforcement.** Along with increasing desired behaviors, this model also suggests that an individual will cease exhibiting undesirable behaviors if positive reinforcements cease to follow the behavior. Also, behavior will extinguish if the person suffers a **response cost,** the removal of a positive stimulus, after an undesirable behavior. Sometimes this theory is referred to as behavior modification.

CLASSICAL CONDITIONING

This model introduced the idea that certain states of arousal, such as anxiety, and cravings for sex, nicotine, drugs, and food, may result from learning through association. Ivan Pavlov (1927), a Russian physicist, famous for his experiments with dogs, demonstrated that when the dogs were presented with food **(unconditioned stimulus)** they would salivate **(unconditioned response).** In this part of the experiment, no learning had taken place, just a reflex response, in this case, salivation. Pavlov then gave the dogs food while ringing a bell **(neutral stimulus)** and found that they also salivated. Then Pavlov tried ringing the bell without presenting the food, and the dogs salivated, even though there was no food. This reaction he called a **conditioned response** (salivation) to a **conditioned stimulus** (the bell). His theory suggests that people learn certain arousal states because an unconditioned stimulus has been paired with a neutral stimulus. For example, a person may become afraid of the dark after having a traumatic experience as a child when the electricity went out. Another example might be a person who desires cigarettes because as a teen other kids told him he looked cool when he smoked.

Joseph Wolpe (1990) used Pavlov's theoretical model as the basis for his treatment of phobias. Wolpe's treatment, called systematic desensitization, pairs anxiety-evoking stimuli with relaxation to create what he called **reciprocal inhibition.** In commonsense terms, his treatment works on the theory that a person cannot be relaxed and anxious at the same time. If a person with a particular fear is exposed to the feared object or event while being deeply relaxed, that person will no longer feel as much anxiety when confronted with the feared situation. Consider how many people take warm baths to relieve stress. It is hard to be stressed out while in a nice, warm bath.

IMPLICATIONS OF BEHAVIORAL THEORY FOR HUMAN SERVICES DELIVERY

The behavioral models can be effective with many clients with whom human services workers might work. They work especially well with students in classrooms, inmates in correctional facilities, and patients in hospitals because workers have almost complete control over positive reinforcements and response costs in these settings. The focus for these clients is to eliminate undesirable behaviors and increase more socially appropriate behaviors.

Pavlov's model is useful for clients with phobias and certain addictions and is sometimes used with pedophiles. When people are given unpleasant stimuli while engaging in socially unacceptable behavior, they eventually begin associating the unwanted behavior with the unpleasant experience. Using this model to treat, for example, a child molester may involve that person receiving an electrical shock when he becomes aroused by looking at pictures of children. Likewise, alcoholics may be given the medication Anabuse, which causes vomiting when mixed with alcohol. If an alcoholic begins associating drinking with becoming violently ill, then the desire to drink will vanish. As far as phobias, a person may be put in a deeply relaxed and comfortable state and then is presented with the fear-producing object. The person becomes less fearful by associating what was feared with a pleasant experience.

Cognitive Theory

This approach to understanding people suggests that behavior and feelings come from the ways in which people think about their life situations. If their perceptions are distorted or unrealistic, people will generally suffer from emotional and behavioral problems. In this view, people experience feelings of shame, guilt, anger, depression, and anxiety because of their perceptions about things that happen.

Approaching people from a cognitive model first began with Alfred Adler who suggested that people first think, then they act, then they feel. Adler focused on helping people change their distorted and mistaken beliefs. He said that the way people remember their childhoods is more important in determining adult problems than what actually did happen (Adler, 1959).

Cognitive theory became very popular in the 1970s and 1980s and is still widely used by therapists. In *Reason and Emotion in Psychotherapy* (1962), Albert Ellis presented his main idea: that all people are capable of both rational and irrational thinking. Ellis believed that emotional disturbance was rooted in blame and irrational, unrealistic thoughts and beliefs. In his book he suggested methods that could change people's irrational beliefs and therefore automatically eliminate many emotional problems. Chapter 10 examines in detail the use of Ellis's model to manage stress.

Donald Meichenbaum, among others, followed Ellis in developing stress inoculation training and cognitive behavior modification (Meichenbaum, 1985; 1986). Aaron Beck is another cognitive therapist who developed a model for understanding and treating depression. According to Beck, people often use specific cognitive distortions that lead to emotional disturbances (Beck, Rush, Shaw, & Emory, 1979).

EXAMPLES OF TYPICAL DISTORTIONS

1. Arbitrary inferences involve jumping to conclusions that aren't supported by evidence or facts.
2. Selective abstraction is used to form a conclusion based on an isolated detail of an event that doesn't take into consideration the total context.
3. Overgeneralization bases extreme beliefs on a single incident. Such a distortion can lead to racism and other prejudices.
4. Magnification is perceiving a situation as being worse than it really is.
5. Personalization is believing that someone else's unrelated behaviors have something to do with you.
6. Polarization views something as being at one extreme or another—all or nothing (Beck, et al., 1979).

USING COGNITIVE THERAPY IN HUMAN SERVICES SETTINGS

Cognitive therapy can be used with clients who are old enough and have the cognitive faculties to talk about their thoughts. Typically, young children and people with brain disorders have a difficult time using this model. This model also is used in crisis intervention, a topic discussed in Chapter 8. Cognitive therapy can be used in short-term interventions, making it practical and cost effective. The goal is to help clients change their perceptions into ones that are more realistic and rational. This approach can be used by most human services workers in any situation where someone is thinking unrealistically. As with many therapies, cognitive therapy is most effective when clients are sincerely trying to change their thoughts to more rational ones. Of course, the more experience you have in helping people think more rationally, the more effective you will be with your clients.

Family Therapy Theories

These theories attempt to explain people's problems by examining them in the context of their family unit. Instead of looking only at the person who is behaving dysfunctionaly, attention is focused on the dysfunction within the entire family. In the 1950s and 1960s, Murray Bowen (1992) and R.D. Laing and Aaron Esterson (1977) studied **family therapy theories** extensively. They were all interested initially in families in which a member of the family had been labeled as schizophrenic. Their research involved observing communication patterns between patients and their parents and between parents both in the presence of the patient and alone. Prior to these studies, overbearing and over-protective mothers were thought to cause schizophrenia. The possibility that a chemical imbalance might cause the disease hadn't been fully explored. The research conducted by Bowen, Laing, and Esterson concluded that the patterns of communication observed in families of schizophrenics were also seen in families with no history of schizophrenia, making their findings useful for all families in treatment.

Families with a member identified as schizophrenic were further studied by Bateson, Jackson, Haley, and Weakland (1956) and Wynne, Tyckoff, Day, and Hirsch (1958), all of whom concluded that a family works together to a unique balance, and that the behaviors of any one family member make sense in the context of that family's rules and roles.

These studies also suggest that a family is a **self-regulating** mechanism in which rules are established to preserve the continuing essence of a particular family. Many times, family members with symptoms or other deviant behaviors are responding to obsolete rules or a lack of clear and appropriate rules. For example, a teenage girl may attempt suicide because her family rules prohibit her from having any social life. She may see suicide as her only way out. Another example might be a wife who develops agoraphobia (fear of leaving the house) in response to her husband who prevents her from having access to household expenses, from participating in raising their children, and from having a say in their social life. She may believe that agoraphobia is the only way to take back some control of her life. In both of these examples, the family's rules are faulty. If the rules were to change, the symptomatic family member might not need to go to such extremes.

USING FAMILY THERAPY IN THE HUMAN SERVICES

Family therapy is particularly well-suited for many human services, allowing workers to take into consideration various cultural differences in family units and work sensitively to overcome cultural traditions that may be creating problems for certain family members.

Family therapy approaches are helpful in educational facilities, social service and mental health settings, and within correctional agencies because most clients were raised in a family setting, continue to be involved in one, or were denied appropriate family care and are dealing with issues of neglect and abandonment. Family therapy approaches encourage brief intervention aimed at taking all family members into consideration. Those who want to explore the various family therapies in detail should examine the works of Murray Bowen (1992), Virginia Satir (1983), Salvador Minuchin (1974), Jay Haley (1976), Carl Whitaker (1976), and Cloe Madanes (1981).

Chapter Summary

In addition to knowing how to intervene with clients in need, human services workers should have an understanding of why their clients have problems. We have just learned various theories that attempt to explain why people suffer (see Table 5.1) The intervention strategies utilized by human services workers are also largely based on these causality models.

Table 5.1 Psychological Models of Causality

Therapy Model	Approach to Problem	Implications for Intervention
psychoanalytic theory (Freud)	anxiety results from conflict between the id and the superego and between pleasure and death instincts, and from fixation during psychosexual stages of development	useful as a theoretical foundation in understanding serious disorders and clients who are very low functioning or who have had long-standing problems
object-relations	deficit in relationship skills from an inability to move through normal stages of development	due to the length of time it takes, clients must have financial resources, time, desire, insight, and be able to cope with painful psychological material
neo-Freudians (Adler)	mental health and social problems come from being discouraged; people are motivated by social urges so involvement with others in friendship, intimacy, and contributing to society is necessary to overcome feelings of inferiority; how a person perceives life experiences determines adult personality	can be used with many types of clients, can be short term or long term, there is latitude in implementing this model whose focus is on conscious goals and providing encouragement, making it useful in a variety of human services settings
existential-humanistic	anxiety and defense mechanisms result from awareness of core human conditions, such as aloneness, meaninglessness, freedom, and death; people must fulfill their potential or live restricted, inauthentic lives	may be either a long-term or a short-term approach; its philosophical approach allows techniques to be flexible; may also help clients who have trouble finding meaning in life and who fail to accept responsibility for their behaviors

(continued)

Table 5.1 *(continued)*

Therapy Model	Approach to Problem	Implications for Intervention
person-centered	lacking self-acceptance, living closed and restricted lives, and looking to others for direction comes from blocks in the natural growth process and the absence of an empathic, accepting, and genuine relationship	basic attending skills, such as active listening, reflection, and paraphrasing, are essential for communicating with clients; applicable to all relationships, including parent-child, teacher-student, counselor-client, warden-convict, etc.
gestalt	problems result from immaturity; people must move from a state of environmental support to authentic self-support or they tend toward phony and phobic lives; getting stuck in problem behaviors comes from unfinished business; and an inability to be totally self-accepting leads to fragmentation	this direct approach may be useful with clients who need a strong push toward facing their anxieties; clients should be fairly high functioning and motivated to grow; a short-term approach can produce rapid results due to techniques that encourage clients to feel all their emotions in the here and now
reality	problems created by the inability to feel cared about and worthwhile; irresponsible behavior is an attempt to have those needs met	useful for motivated clients to understand how past influences affect current behavior; a short-term model can be effective for clients who are irresponsible and have socially unac-ceptable behaviors, such as criminals, juvenile delinquents, substance abusers, and those are physically and sexually abusive; because the focus is on chang-ing behavior, now!
behavioral	belief that all behaviors are learned through reinforcement (operant conditioning) or association (classical conditioning) and can be modified by changing reinforcements and associations	for clients whose environment can be controlled and who have specific behaviors that need to change, such as children, inmates, patients in a hospital, and clients in residential facilities; also used for clients suffering from illegal behaviors (pedophiles, drug addicts, etc.)

(continued)

Table 5.1 *(continued)*

Therapy Model	Approach to Problem	Implications for Intervention
cognitive	problems and deviances come from illogical and irrational thinking	can be implemented with clients with minimal intelligence and verbal skills; can be short term and cost effective; can help with stress management, crises, depression, and dysfunctional behaviors
family	problems and other dysfunctional behaviors stem from families whose rules and roles do not allow for normal development, faulty communication exists, and members' behaviors that contradict family stability are counteracted	can be used especially with clients from cultures that have traditional rules and roles; helps understand why a family discourages change and how deviant behaviors are inadvertently reinforced

Effective human services workers should know about all of these theories and methods of intervention. They utilize this knowledge with clients and employ whichever model and intervention strategy that makes the most sense with any given client. This eclectic and integrative practice often leads to effective practice. Theories of causality may be primarily biological, psychological, or social, and maybe spiritual in nature. Generalist human services practice accepts that all theories may be useful with some clients.

Suggested Applied Activities

1. Interview someone about a problem they now have or have had. Ask that person what he or she thinks caused the problem. Try to categorize the cause into one or more of the theories discussed in this chapter.

   _____

   _____

   _____

   _____

   _____

2. List the various theoretical approaches. Next to each approach, describe a problem someone might have that would best be treated using that approach. You may even use yourself as an example. I have listed below a sample of my own past and present problems as they relate to the various approaches. You may have similar issues or entirely different ones. Try to think about real issues that affect you or someone else when completing your own list. Psychoanalytic approach: "I tend to be too self-critical because my superego dominates my subconscious. So maybe I could use some insight into how I developed such a punitive attitude and allow myself to play more and permit my Id to express itself."

   Adlerian approach: "I use this model to focus on my strengths rather than my weaknesses."

   Existential approach: "This model might help me develop a stronger sense of meaning in life and encourage me to be more open to new experiences."

   Behavioral approaches: "Since I would like to lose a few pounds, I might set up a positive reinforcement schedule in which I earn a star for every day I stay on my diet. When I earn seven stars, I get to trade them in for a pedicure."

   Cognitive approach: "Sometimes I get angry at my son when he talks back and argues with me. I need to change the way I think about his arguing. Instead of telling myself that he is being disrespectful, it might be better to tell myself that he is expressing his needs and trying to assert his individuality, which is normal for a 13-year-old boy." Family approach: "Instead of thinking that my son is wrong or that I am a bad parent, I could view any of our problems as manifestations of our relationship together. I could try to look more objectively at our way of interacting and what I can do to stop participating in our 'games.'"

   _____

   _____

_____

_____

_____

_____

_____

_____

_____

Chapter Review Questions

1. What is meant by the bio-psychosocial model?

_____

_____

2. Describe the id, ego, and superego.

_____

_____

3. What are the typical tasks and relationship processes that take place during the oral, anal, and phallic phases of development?

_____

_____

4. How do Mahler's phases of development differ from Freud's?

_____

_____

5. What are three key themes emphasized in an existential approach?

_____

_____

6. With which population would Glasser's reality therapy be most useful? Why?

_____

_____

7. What is the central focus of operant conditioning?

_____

_____

8. How does the classical conditioning model explain behaviors?

_____

_____

9. Family approaches focus on dysfunctional _____ and _____.

Glossary of Terms

Anal stage is Freud's second psychosexual stage, during which a toddler learns autonomy and self-control.

Behavioral theories explain human behavior as resulting from reinforcements and associations in the environment. All behavior is learned and can be extinguished.

Biological model (or medical model) suggests that certain symptoms and other deviant behaviors are caused by biological, chemical, genetic, and neurological factors and should thus be treated with medication and other biological therapies.

Bio-psychosocial model is a causality model that uses biological, psychological, and social factors to attempt to explain various social and personal problems. Biological factors include genetics, biochemical makeup, and physiological and neurological factors. Psychological factors usually refer to how child rearing, parental nurturance or neglect, self-esteem, and cognitive function influence people in adulthood. Social factors refer to social expectations and standards that are typical in either mainstream culture or in a subculture.

Brain trauma can be caused by accident or by illness, such as a tumor or stroke, and often results in impaired cognitive and emotional functioning.

Classical conditioning uses a neutral stimulus to elicit a response when that neutral stimulus is paired with a stimulus that naturally leads to a response in an organism.

Cognitive theory points to irrational thinking as the cause of emotional disorders.

Compensation is an ego defense mechanism used to replace or make up for inabilities or disabilities with abilities.

Conditioned response is a state of arousal or a behavior that occurs in reaction to a conditioned stimulus.

Conditioned stimulus is anything that is paired with an unconditioned stimulus to elicit a response.

Denial an ego defense mechanism used to cope with an unbearable reality that denies the actual existence of a problem.

Deviant behaviors are actions and behavior patterns considered inappropriate and atypical by the majority of people in a community.

Displacement an ego defense mechanism used to channel strong emotions away from a threatening object that is eliciting those feelings and toward an unrelated, safe object.

Ego is, according to Freud, the part of the personality that operates under the reality principle. It allows people to function realistically.

Ego defense mechanisms are behaviors that allow people to function by pushing anxiety related to conflict into the unconscious mind.

Existential-humanistic theories focus on the core conditions that are essential to what it means to be human, such as freedom, anxiety, death, and meaning.

Family therapy theories suggest that behaviors of family members serve a function to maintain stability in a family.

Fixated at a stage of development occurs when a person receives too much or too little gratification and therefore remains stuck at that stage.

Fragmentation occurs when a person does not own parts of the self and avoids and hides from those alienated parts.

Genetic disorders are diseases that a baby is born with and result from duplication of chromosomes, deficient chromosomes, and mutations.

Genital stage is the psychosexual stage during which adolescents learn to accept mature adult sexuality and develop a path toward socially acceptable modes of work and play.

Gestalt therapy is a form of existential therapy developed by Perls that emphasizes self-awareness and integration of the self.

Givens are the core human conditions with which all people must struggle and that often lead to anxiety. Yalom focused on four givens: death, freedom, isolation, and meaninglessness.

Group therapy involves more than two clients and one or two facilitators who mediate among group members as they share personal information related to their lives and their feelings toward other group members. At times, facilitators self-disclose and offer feedback as well.

Id is the part of the personality, according to Freud, that contains basic instincts, impulses, fantasies, wishes, and feelings.

Individual psychology was how Adler referred to his neo-Freudian model of psychotherapy. Its focus is on how each individual perceives his or her own experiences and creates a unique style of life rather than focusing on being determined by instincts and specific phases of development.

Insight is the goal of psychoanalysis in which a person gains understanding and self-knowledge of unconscious feelings that have created psychological symptoms and dysfunctions.

Intellectualization is an ego defense mechanism used to remove yourself emotionally from the reality of a difficult situation.

Latent stage is Freud's fourth psychosexual stage in which elementary-school-aged children are free from mental conflict and can engage in learning basic social skills and school work.

Libido is the pleasure instinct, according to Freud, and is also called eros.

Medical model (see biological model)

Minimization, an ego defense mechanism used to view a problem that is in reality severe as being insignificant.

Negative reinforcement uses a negative stimulus to eliminate or decrease a behavior.

Neo-Freudians are a group of theorists and clinicians who focus on social and cultural factors to determine personality development.

Neurotransmitters, it is believed, are chemicals found in the brain that are released between messenger cells and receptor cells and that determine various feelings, thoughts, and behaviors.

Neutral stimulus is something that does not create a response.

Normal (infantile) autism, according to Mahler's object-relations developmental theory, is the phase in which infants live in their own world of impulses, drives, and instincts and exist only to survive.

Object (in object-relations theory) usually refers to the mother, father or primary caretaker who is the significant being in a child's life.

Object-relations theory focuses on how children develop personality traits and patterns in relation to how their mother (object) relates to them during their first three years of life.

Operant conditioning uses positive or negative reinforcement to increase or extinguish a particular behavior.

Oral stage, according to Freud, is the first psychosexual stage during which infants learn how to meet their needs for nurturance and trust.

Personality disorders typically create dysfunction in a person's life especially in regard to relationships. People who suffer from these disorders are considered deficient in many social skills and have unhealthy self-concepts.

Person-centered therapy, founded by Carl Rogers, relates human growth to certain characteristics, such as empathy, genuineness, and acceptance.

Phallic stage is Freud's third psychosexual stage during which preschoolers learn gender identity.

Phenomenological approach attempts to understand people from their own personal frame of reference rather than a preconceived theory.

Positive reinforcement is usually a pleasurable stimulus/reward that is given in response to a desired behavior.

Projection an ego defense mechanism used to attribute qualities and actions to others that are considered personally unacceptable.

Psychoanalytic theories attempt to explain human behavior by focusing on early childhood experiences, conflict between parts of the personality, and instincts.

Psychological theories attempt to explain a person's current behaviors and emotional states by looking at that individual's childhood interactions with family and friends, traumatic life events, and personal choices that the person makes.

Psychosexual stages, according to Freud, are specific stages that people experience as they grow from infancy to adulthood. During these stages psychological and sexual energies must be mastered. Failure to do so may lead to personality disorders later in life.

Rationalization is an ego defense mechanism used to excuse or justify certain behaviors or situations.

Reaction formation is an ego defense mechanism used to reject an unacceptable desire or impulse; the person using this defense is vehemently repulsed by that impulse or desire.

Reality therapy, created by William Glasser from his work with juvenile offenders, focuses on taking responsibility for and facing the reality of your own behaviors.

Reciprocal inhibition is based on Wolpe's idea that evoking a relaxation response while exposing a person to a feared object will eliminate the anxiety related to the object. If a client could be trained to relax and then be exposed to fear evoking stimuli while relaxed, the relaxation would inhibit the anxiety.

Regression an ego defense mechanism used to revert to an earlier and safer level of functioning.

Repression is used to push painful memories or anxieties out of conscious awareness and into the unconscious mind.

Respite care provides relief to family members who are the primary caretakers of an ill or injured relative, such as someone who has Alzheimer's disease. Human services workers often offer such relief by finding a daycare program or a qualified aide to temporarily take over the family's caretaking responsibilities.

Response cost removes a pleasurable stimulus/reward in response to an undesirable behavior. Something that is **self-regulating** maintains its own state of homeostasis and stability.

Separation/individuation is the final phase in Mahler's model during which children begin experiencing themselves as separate individuals and developing a stable, integrated sense of self.

Social problems are behaviors that often lead to dysfunctional relationships and behavior at work and at school and may also lead to illegal activities.

Sublimation an ego defense mechanism used to channel psychological energy and drives into socially acceptable outlets.

Superego, or the conscience, according to Freud, is the part of the personality that responds to the world according to a set of internalized morals, societal demands, and commands.

Symbiosis, the second phase in Mahler's theory, during which an infant develops a strong sense of relatedness to the mother/primary caretaker who meets all of the infant's needs.

Thanatos is the aggressive drive that Freud believed is often in conflict with the pleasure drive.

Toxic substances refer to any drug, poison, household spray, radiation, or alcohol that can temporarily or permanently damage brain cells.

Unconditioned response is an emotion or behavior that is a natural reaction to a stimulus.

Unconditioned stimulus can be anything that leads to a reflex or natural response.

Unconscious is the part of the mind that contains most of our mental life and is not readily available to the conscious mind. It is speculated that this mental material may flow out of the unconscious mind through the process of psychoanalysis.

Unfinished business includes any past difficulty with interactions, relationships and experiences that has not been resolved. Unfinished business often hinders people from living whole and complete lives.

Case Presentation and Exit Quiz

General Description and Demographics

Tom is a 25-year-old college student who lives off-campus with two roommates. He works part-time as a waiter at a local restaurant. His parents live close by and pay for his college tuition and books. At times, he needs to borrow additional money from them. Tom is popular, good looking, and likes to drink. Most of his time away from school and work is spent at bars drinking. He began drinking and using drugs when he was 15 years old.

Tom has a girlfriend, Kate, whom he sees at least four times a week. Tom has been unfaithful to Kate on several occasions. Even though she's aware of this, Kate continues the relationship anyway. Tom has had two previous serious relationships, both of which ended because of his drinking and unfaithfulness.

When Tom was 12 years old, he was sexually abused by an uncle during visits to his uncle's farm. Tom never told his parents or anyone else about the abuse. Tom thought he was gay for a few years after the abuse ended, but doesn't think so now. He has engaged in same-sex activity on several occasions when he was drunk. Both Tom's father and grandfather have had drinking problems.

Tom has been in college for more than seven years and doesn't know what he wants to do when he graduates. He has changed majors four times since beginning school. He feels depressed when he drinks and feels worthless when he's sober. Most people who know him describe Tom as a nice guy but don't respect him when he's drunk.

Problems That Need Assistance

For the past six months, Tom has been blacking out when he drinks. His friends often have to drag him home. He wakes up with bruises over much of his body, but he has no recollection of what happened the night before and feels terrible the next day. He often wants to drink in the morning to relieve his terrible hangovers. He knows he is an alcoholic, but tells himself that is just who he is and who he will always be.

His girlfriend has finally gotten fed up with him and has told Tom that if he gets drunk again, she is going to break up with him. Tom has told Kate that he loves her and doesn't want their relationship to end. So once again she forgives him even though he went home with a woman he met at the bar just last weekend. He was too drunk to have sex, but they did sleep in the same bed. Because Kate feels sorry for Tom, she finds it hard to leave him.

Another problem is Tom's schooling. He doesn't know what to do with the rest of his life. He tells himself he is too stupid to get a good job, and that he'll probably have to work as a waiter for the rest of his life. He sometimes thinks about killing himself, and in fact he tried to hang himself on two separate occasions when he was drunk. Tom's parents say they love him and try to be supportive. They know he drinks too much and were relieved when he moved out so they wouldn't have to see what he was doing with his life. They loan him money without question.

Lately, Tom has been feeling ashamed about having been abused. He is able to forget about it when he drinks. When he is sober, he feels scared and nervous around his girlfriend.

Tom was recently arrested for drunk driving. As a result, he's been ordered by the court to go to Alcoholic's Anonymous meetings, as well as to get individual counseling and participate in drug- and alcohol-education classes. His driver's license has been suspended, and his parents paid his $1,500 fine.

To fulfill the terms of his probation, Tom begins seeing a psychologist. His parents are paying for that as well. During the first visit, the therapist identifies several goals for Tom: reduce his drinking, improve his relationship with his girl-friend, and eliminate Tom's suicidal thoughts.

The therapist also believes that Tom must deal with his past sexual abuse. The therapist thinks that this abuse is affecting his relationship with his girlfriend and may be a reason why Tom has a hard time being faithful to her. There's also a good chance that the experience has affected Tom's self-esteem.

The therapist also feels that Tom's family and girlfriend should be involved in his treatment because they seem to be enabling Tom to continue his self-destructive behavior by covering up for him, forgiving him, and paying for his mistakes. The therapist intends to work with his family and girlfriend to help them see how their behaviors affect Tom.

To help Tom eliminate his suicidal thinking, the therapist must identify Tom's internal statements that make him feel depressed and worthless. He discovers that Tom tells himself that he is stupid, selfish, horrible, and worthless. Tom feels that no one would like him if they really knew him.

Finally, the therapist realizes that Tom must discover the adult inside himself. Tom must figure out who he is and what he wants out of life and must take a serious look at himself and figure out where he wants to go so that he can develop a realistic plan for getting there.

Exit Quiz

1. Since Tom's father and grandfather are alcoholics, there may be a strong genetic predisposition for Tom's drinking. This statement indicates that the cause of Tom's drinking is due to
   a. biological factors
   b. psychological factors
   c. social/political factors
   d. none of the above

2. Tom's depression and feelings of shame and anxiety are a result of having been sexually abused as a child. This statement indicates that his feelings are caused by
   a. biological factors
   b. psychological factors
   c. social/political factors
   d. none of the above

3. If the therapist meets with Tom's family and girlfriend and suggests that they change their enabling behaviors and set stronger boundaries with Tom, what psychological theory is he using?
   a. psychoanalytic
   b. existential-humanistic

c. family systems
d. gestalt

4. The therapist plans to confront Tom on the consequences of his drinking and make him face the fact that he has a serious drinking problem and that he has continually lied to his girlfriend and cheated on her. This is an example of
   a. reality therapy
   b. psychoanalytic therapy
   c. family systems therapy
   d. behavioral therapy

5. The therapist will be helping Tom explore the sexual abuse he was exposed to as a child and how it affects him now. He will help Tom reduce his reliance on alcohol to repress his feelings. This is an example of
   a. reality therapy
   b. psychoanalytic therapy
   c. family systems therapy
   d. cognitive therapy

6. The therapist intends to focus on Tom's negative self-talk and help him eliminate destructive thoughts such as "I am stupid" and "no one could love me if they really knew me" by offering a different way to think about himself. This is an example of
   a. reality therapy
   b. psychoanalytic therapy
   c. family systems therapy
   d. cognitive therapy

7. When the therapist gets Tom to think about what he wants out of life and to find meaning in his life, what type of approach is the therapist using?
   a. psychoanalytic therapy
   b. existential-humanistic therapy
   c. cognitive therapy
   d. behavioral therapy

Exit Quiz Answers

1. a	4. a	7. b
2. b	5. b	
3. c	6. d	

CHAPTER 6

Sociological Theories of Causality

Introduction

As you may recall from Chapter 2, societies' views and explanations of deviance and methods of dealing with deviant behavior within a society have changed from era to era in response to changes in values, political views, religious thought, and scientific discovery.

This chapter focuses on how societal norms and values affect social problems as well as the various sociological factors that create them. Factors such as **politics, culture, ethnicity,** and religion are examined as well as of the ways in which society can contribute to deviant behavior of members within certain groups.

Before specific cultures and values can be explored, an understanding of the terms relevant to **sociological theory** of causality is needed.

Sociological Factors Defined

Both the biological and psychological theories examine an individuals' internal makeup and personal experiences to determine causes of deviant behaviors and other problems. Sociological theory, however, proposes that social structure, cultural norms, history, religion, and politics play a prominent role in causing deviant behaviors and social problems.

Current human services practice is still influenced by sociological factors from the past as well as modern-day thought and values. Although many human services practitioners would like to think that current human services agencies offer services free from political and **cultural bias,** this is probably not altogether true. While there has been a trend toward **social liberalization** since the 1950s (when elimination of forced segregation first occurred), many human services agencies and workers continue to operate within a set a values that do not allow for completely unbiased practice. Admittedly, most human services workers and organizations officially operate in such a way as to demonstrate equality to all their clients. It is politically incorrect to treat people differently because of their **gender, race,** ethnicity, religion, political orientation, or sexual orientation. Unfortunately, human services agencies and political organizations that establish policies and provide funding to human services institutions sometimes still operate with biases. These biases may take on either obvious or subtle forms of **discrimination**, such as disparities in services, preconceived notions—**stigma**—about certain populations, and reinforcement of learned helplessness in some populations.

While theories and interventions in practice today are generally effective for working with the majority of clients, a significant number of people who seek services simply do not get what they need. One reason for the needs of some going unmet has to do with the origins of the theories themselves, which were created by educated, middle- and upper-class European-American males whose political and cultural values may not be applicable to other cultures' values and ideologies. Although cultural awareness and sensitivity training are now required for many college and graduate degrees, education can only do so much to influence the behavior of human services professionals. Sometimes organizations themselves prevent workers from providing culturally effective services because the **organizational culture** doesn't promote cultural sensitivity. At other times, workers themselves fail to understand or simply disagree with the need to provide culturally sensitive services.

Politics Defined

When people hear the word "politics," many think of elected officials, such as the president of the United States, or of the Republican and Democratic parties. Politics, however, also refers to power and influence. Certainly elected officials have power and influence over many matters, including the amount of funding allocated for human services agencies. Creating laws that govern the practice of human services is another area over which those with political power have influence. The ways in which our elected officials establish legislation and fund human services programs has much to do with their own personal values as well as the values of those who voted for them. Politics, then, is based largely on the values of the majority of voters and those who participate in the political process. Unfortunately, many groups in society do not participate in politics and therefore have no voice in decisions that may affect them. This imbalance in the political process can influence the cultural sensitivity of those human services agencies that depend heavily on government funding for their existence.

Culture Defined

Culture can be thought of as operating both within and outside of us. At the individual level, it refers to a person's values, beliefs, explanatory systems, and behaviors that are learned in the family and within social groups (Hogan-Garcia, 1999). The United States is home to a variety of cultural groups. Some groups are based on race and ethnicity, such as African-Americans, Asian-Americans, and Latinos, whereas others are based on religion, such as Catholics, Jews, Muslims, or Protestants. Still others are identified cultural groups based on age, economic class, sexual orientation, ability, or gender.

At the macro level, culture refers to both specific and unspoken rules under which organizations and institutions, including schools, media, government, workplaces, and mental health and criminal justice systems, operate. The policies, procedures, and practices of these organizations are their culture (Hogan-Garcia, 1999). One could refer to the "culture of the criminal justice system" when attempting to understand practices in a prison.

A major challenge for human services workers is when a client's culture clashes with the culture of the human services agency. Miscommunication and unavailability of services may result in such situations. Educating human services workers about different cultures' values, needs, and priorities and how these may differ from mainstream theories and ideas, may help agencies and workers alike provide more appropriate and effective services to all who seek help.

Foundational Definitions

Certain concepts are relevant to any discussion about cultural sensitivity. The concepts discussed below are those that human services workers need to understand and avoid acting on while providing services. It may not be possible to be completely bias free, but understanding the consequences of cultural insensitivity and of your own reactions to differences in others can help you develop a more effective way of working with all types of people.

Bias **Bias** is a preconceived point of view about a person, a group of people, or an issue. Biases may stem from beliefs of your own cultural background, your family's, or even your neighborhood's. If someone evaluating a situation or a cultural group sees it as fitting a certain pattern of behavior or demonstrating certain anticipated characteristics and qualities, then that person's evaluation may be biased either toward or against the situation or group. Bias occurs when judgment about a situation or a group is based on generalities and personal opinion rather than on an objective, dispassionate point of view

Disparity **Disparity** refers to an imbalance usually when people are treated unequally. Disparities occur all too often in human services. It may be due to someone belonging to a certain race or economic class. The result of disparity is that certain groups do not receive the same appropriate and effective services as others simply because of the cultural group to which they belong.

Prejudice **Prejudice** is the emotional and attitudinal component of group antagonism. It can refer to a negative attitude about an entire category of people and often leads to rejection of people who belong to a certain group. Prejudice usually involves a one-sided opinion based on generalities, such as disliking someone merely because of that person's affiliation with a certain group (Sears, Peplau, & Taylor, 1991; Schaefer, 1988).

Discrimination **Discrimination** is the "behavioral component of group antagonism. People discriminate against the disliked group by refusing its members access to desired jobs, educational opportunities, country clubs, restaurants, places of entertainment, and so on" (Sears, et al., 1991, p. 550). Discrimination is illegal and politically incorrect, but it is experienced all too often, especially by people of highly vulnerable groups who are reluctant to assert their rights (such as illegal immigrants). Discrimination puts prejudicial beliefs into action and prevents members of a group access to certain rights that are available to others. Not all discriminatory behaviors coincide with prejudice. One can be prejudiced but not discriminate. Bigots do not believe in equal treatment for any racial or ethnic group (Schaefer, 1988).

Stereotypes **Stereotypes** are generalized beliefs about the characteristics of a group's members. A stereotype may be positive or negative and can lead to prejudice, discrimination, and bias. Some stereotypes may include some objective truth, but basing human services practice on them is considered culturally insensitive. Instead, human services workers are encouraged to understand certain group patterns and values but always keep in mind that not every member of a certain cultural group is alike in every way.

Sexism **Sexism** is negative attitudes and behaviors toward a person because of his or her gender identity. Sexism is prejudice and discrimination against someone based only on that person's gender.

Racism **Racism** is prejudice and discrimination against someone based only on that person's ethnic or racial identity.

Ageism **Ageism** is age-specific prejudice and discrimination. In our society, elderly people tend to be victims of ageism. They are often rejected socially, receive inferior treatment by medical workers, and are asked to leave their jobs or are not hired at all because of their age.

Heterosexism **Heterosexism** are negative attitudes and behaviors based solely on a person's sexual orientation. Heterosexism is the belief that heterosexuality is superior to homosexuality.

Classism **Classism** are negative attitudes and behaviors toward a person because of the economic class to which he or she belongs. Typically, classism is most likely to be experienced by the poor and often results in a disparity of services.

Ableism **Ableism** considers people with developmental, emotional, physical, or psychiatric disabilities to be inferior (of less worth) than those who are supposedly able-bodied and -minded (Go Beyond Words website, June 2006).

Ethnocentrism **Ethnocentrism** is the belief that one's own culture and way of life are superior to all others. Ethnocentrism judges all other cultures in the context of one's own cultural group and often views other cultures as being inferior (Schaefer, 1988) and that members of these other cultures would be better off living according to the standards of one's own culture.

CRITICAL THINKING / SELF-REFLECTION CORNER

- What are some of the stereotypes you hold about African Americans? Asians? Latinos? Caucasians? Arabs? Gays? The elderly?

- Where did you learn these stereotypes?

- Toward what groups do you feel negative prejudice? Why do you think you have these prejudices? Have you ever felt someone was prejudiced against you?

- Have you ever been a victim of discrimination because of your race, age, gender, or religion? How did it make you feel?

- Do you think all people living in the United States should assimilate and adopt mainstream cultures, values, and behaviors? Why?

- What do you think the United States would be like if all races and religions completely assimilated and adapted mainstream American values and behaviors?

Specific Issues Facing Various Cultural Groups

While there may be some danger in stereotyping people because they belong to a certain cultural group, a bigger danger is not recognizing various cultural groups' particular values, needs, and ways of interacting. Although there may be an infinite number of cultural groups, the discussion here will be limited to some of the groups most frequently seen by human services workers.

Before examining those cultural groups, it may be enlightening to take the personal bias inventory in Table 6.1 to discuss various responses with others. As each item is answered, it may be worthwhile to examine the origins of one's beliefs about certain groups. Don't be afraid to respond honestly. The first step in developing cultural sensitivity is to acknowledge areas of insensitivity. Someone once said that "we are all recovering racists." It is normal to have biases and negative attitudes toward certain groups that are different from ours. The author hopes that by the end of this chapter, readers will have gained some awareness into their own stereotypes, prejudices, and biases and will endeavor to provide service to clients based on objectivity and appropriate knowledge about what each client needs.

Table 6.1 Personal Bias Inventory

Circle either true (T) or false (F) in response to each item. After you complete the inventory, review your responses and discuss them with classmates or another group of students. Compare and contrast your responses and explore where and why you responded as you did.

T	F	1. Men are smarter than women in math and science.
T	F	2. Women can cook better than men can.
T	F	3. Men do not have feelings such as sadness and loneliness.
T	F	4. Women are less capable than men of controlling their emotions.
T	F	5. More women than men are neurotic.
T	F	6. Men don't need professional help as much as women do.
T	F	7. Women are worse than men at driving.
T	F	8. Women are better than men at parenting.
T	F	9. Men are better than women at managing money.
T	F	10. Women are more dependent on men than men are dependent on women.
T	F	11. Gay men are promiscuous.
T	F	12. Lesbians want to look like men.
T	F	13. Homosexuals dress better than straight men do.
T	F	14. Homosexuality is a sin against nature.
T	F	15. Being gay is a symptom of deep psychological issues.
T	F	16. Bisexuals just have identity issues.
T	F	17. Someone who has a sex-change operation is deeply disturbed emotionally.
T	F	18. Gay men are flamboyant.
T	F	19. Most lesbians were raped or molested as children.
T	F	20. Gay people try to turn straight people gay.
T	F	21. Old people are stupid and only talk about boring things.
T	F	22. Old people shouldn't be allowed to work because they are too slow.

(continued)

Table 6.1 *(continued)*

T	F	23. New college graduates are more energetic and deserve to be hired over middle-aged people.
T	F	24. Teenagers are wild and cannot be trusted.
T	F	25. Teenagers take drugs and drink alcohol and shouldn't be allowed to drive.
T	F	26. Children should be seen and not heard.
T	F	27. Poor people are lazy and enjoy handouts.
T	F	28. Wealthy people are ruthless and arrogant.
T	F	29. Blue-collar workers have average intelligence.
T	F	30. Muslims cannot be trusted because any one of them could be a terrorist.
T	F	31. Muslims are stupid because they dress in old-fashioned clothing.
T	F	32. Buddhists will never go to heaven because they don't believe in God.
T	F	33. Atheists are immoral people.
T	F	34. Christians are the only people who will go to heaven.
T	F	35. Catholics are ignorant because they don't use birth control.
T	F	36. Protestants try to convert everyone to their religion.
T	F	37. Jewish people are greedy and stingy.
T	F	38. God will not let Jews into heaven because they don't worship Jesus.
T	F	39. Latinos are all uneducated and ignorant.
T	F	40. Most Mexicans who live in the United States are here illegally.
T	F	41. African Americans are better athletes than those of other races.
T	F	42. African Americans aren't smart enough to get into college unless they have an athletic scholarship.
T	F	43. Asians are smarter than other races.
T	F	44. Arabs are sneaky and shouldn't be allowed to live in the United States.
T	F	45. Latino men are male chauvinist pigs.
T	F	46. Asians are obedient.

(continued)

Table 6.1 *(continued)*

T	F	47. Arab women have low self-esteem.
T	F	48. Mentally retarded people are of no use to society.
T	F	49. Caucasians think they are better than all other races.
T	F	50. All Native Americans are alcoholics.

How did you do? Be honest, and discuss some of your responses with others.

Gender Issues

While the word *sex* generally refers to whether a person is biologically female or male, *gender* refers to "the psychological, social, and cultural features and characteristics that have become strongly associated with the biological categories of female and male" (Gilbert & Scher, 1999, p. 3). Many people think of men and women as opposites in their capabilities, roles, and personality types. Such thinking often leads to sexism and discrimination because some people insist on believing that all women are alike and that all men are alike. Certainly modern-day society has begun to realize that gender does not determine a person's role in life. In jobs that demand physical strength, a person's ability, not gender, should be the qualifying factor. Other modern-day realizations have changed gender roles as well. A woman can have a baby without having a man in her life. Additionally, a woman can go out to earn a living for her family, and a man can stay at home and take care of the children and the house.

Despite these many variances in gender roles, many people still hold on to obsolete gender stereotypes. Discrimination exists in human services and other businesses against both consumers and providers of service. Most of the literature on the subject has focused on sexist practices that put women at a disadvantage; however, men may also be victims of sexism.

Throughout history, women have been subjected to sexist behavior. For example, in ancient Greece (circa 300 B.C.), a woman, Agnodice, masqueraded as a man to attend medical classes, but when her gender was revealed she was arrested for practicing medicine. The magistrates studied this case and passed a law that permitted women to practice medicine but only on their own sex. Unfortunately, in the 1300s women were prohibited from practicing medicine throughout Europe (Marieskind, 1980). From the fourteenth through sixteenth centuries, many women were labeled as witches and heretics if they discussed books, theology, or politics. Throughout the seventeenth and eighteenth centuries, women were treated more as pets or as objects to be put on a pedestal, rather than human beings who had the same access to the brain power that men had. American women proved themselves worthy of respect as they battled the wild countries during the migration to settle the West. They soon began to speak out about their rights. By 1920, women had earned the right to vote, which was a huge milestone in the women's movement. By the 1970s, women worked to claim their power and equal rights by organizing to form the women's liberation movement. Unfortunately, the Equal Rights Amendment, the culmination of the work of the women's movement, never passed into law. Opponents claimed that women already had equal rights under the law. Since then, other laws have been passed that require businesses to pay women and men equal salaries for equal work, provide fair grievance processes for women who have been subject to sexual harassment on the job, and engage in hiring and firing practices that do not discriminate because of gender.

Even though it appears that society has leveled the playing field for women, sexism still operates at many levels. Rape, sexual abuse, and domestic violence against women are still prevalent, suggesting that society has not yet allowed women the same rights as men have. Because women are so frequently victimized, human services workers may work more often with women than with men. Also, more women than men are more likely to live in poverty and be their children's primary caretaker, both of which make it more likely for women to use the services of human services professionals.

Such generalizations, however, run the risk of assigning stereotypes to certain segments of a population. Women are not the only recipients of human services, nor are they the only one who are victimized and live in poverty. It's vital to avoid practicing reverse sexism in which men are not permitted to be vulnerable and to need help. A recent study (Vogel, Epting, & Wester, 2003) found that counselors emphasized themes of vulnerability and how assertive a client is more for women than for men. When discussing male clients, counselors used such terms as "being stuck" and not being "connected to others." These findings seem to fit traditional gender stereotypes of women as being vulnerable and seeking more reassurance. Likewise, the focus on men's connectedness is consistent with the widely held belief that men need to work on expressing their emotions whereas women do not. The idea of women as vulnerable goes along with the stereotype of women being emotional, and the idea of men being stuck fits the stereotype of men being stressed. The counselors in this study had no idea that their perceptions of gender were being studied, so these results are probably valid. While such perceptions do not appear harmful to clients, they may influence how a counselor proceeds with a client. If women are seen as more vulnerable, they may be given special assurances that a man might not receive, even if he also is quite vulnerable. Likewise, if men are seen as not connected, counselors may work harder on helping them to express emotions while not providing such encouragement to the female clients who might need help in that area.

In conclusion, while workers may not purposefully engage in gender-based discriminatory practices, they may unintentionally convey narrow ideas about the roles of women and men that may limit their work with clients (Hare-Mustin, 1983; Shields, 1995). The responsibility of every human services worker is to become aware of the importance of gender issues when assessing a client's needs. Of course, gender may not always be a vital issue, but gender-based stereotypes need to be identified and challenged should gender be a factor for a client. It is also very important to resist viewing clients who do not conform to traditional gender roles as being pathological. For example, a soft-spoken man is not necessarily weak-minded and passive. Likewise, not all women who are strong and ambitious have histories of abuse and therefore are out to destroy men. Sexism against men is sometimes overlooked because men have traditionally held power in society. However, human services workers must realize that the roles of men and women are changing. Men and women are almost equal in most areas. Of course, only women can give birth. On average, men are usually physically stronger than women. Beyond those facts, however, men and women are fairly equal. There is no reason that a woman cannot financially support her family. Men can be their children's primary caretakers and take care of a home. Women can be scientists and explore the universe. Men can cry and feel hurt. Men and women are human beings, and that transcends gender.

CRITICAL THINKING / SELF-REFLECTION CORNER

- What are some of your behaviors that are typical of your gender?

- What are some of your behaviors that are not considered typical of your gender?

- Have you ever been the victim of sexual harassment? How did that make you feel? Why do you think it happened?

Sexual Orientation Issues

Although society has begun to accept homosexuality in less negative ways than in years past, prejudice and discrimination are still experienced by homosexuals, bisexuals (those who are attracted sexually, emotionally, and romantically to both genders), and **transgenders** (those who have surgeries and live as a gender other than the one they were born with). Individuals who identify with one of these sexual orientations are often included in the gay, lesbian, bisexual, transgender (GLBT) community. Fear of discrimination and, at times, violence has forced many GLBT people to hide their true sexual orientation. Leading such a life is referred to as **being in the closet** and often causes feelings of depression, shame, guilt, and fear. They must always be vigilant and anxious about having their true sexual preference discovered.

Various social biases create a climate that inhibits homosexuals from living openly. Heterosexism, the belief that the only proper sexuality is between females and males, is probably the strongest bias that influences societal rejection of homosexual behaviors. This belief most likely stems from the Judeo-Christian religious foundation, on which U.S. culture is based. These particular religions propose that the Bible and other religious texts teach that homosexuality is wrong in the eyes of God. For many years, homosexuality was thought of as a sin. Later, as science began influencing cultural thought, homosexuality was considered a psychological abnormality. Homosexuality, however, has not been considered a psychological disorder since the American Psychiatric Association removed it as a diagnosis from the third edition of its *Diagnostic and Statistical Manual* (American Psychiatric Association, 1980). Nevertheless, many people still consider homosexuality to be morally wrong. Some people's fear of gays and lesbians can manifest itself as **homophobia,** an irrational fear about being around, touching, and liking homosexuals.

In fact, homosexuality has existed at least since the days of ancient Greece, where it was actually revered, and exists today in all cultures. Society, however, has only recently begun to accept gays and lesbians, as evidenced by the success of such television shows as *Will and Grace, Queer Eye for the Straight Guy,* and *Queer as Folk.* Contributing to this growing acceptance are celebrities, including Ellen Degeneres, Rosie O'Donnell, Pete Townsend of The Who, and Elton John, who are becoming increasingly open about their sexuality. When it comes to personal life, however, straight people typically socialize more often with other straight people, and gays tend to socialize more with other gays. This has to do with the differences in cultural norms between gay people and straight people. For example, gay men might be more comfortable than straight men with expressing emotions openly. Lesbians may be more comfortable than straight women in expressing physical intimacy with other women .

One of the most difficult steps homosexuals must take is **coming out**—making their sexual preference known to friends and family. This decision is difficult because it may change the way friends and family regard the person. A gay man or lesbian who comes out, risks being rejected even by close loved ones. Although such behavior is illegal, certain employers may even discriminate against an openly gay or lesbian employee (such as Tom Hank's character in the film, *Philadelphia*). Human services agencies, many of which specialize in issues faced by the GLBT community, can provide counseling to help with the emotional and psychological issues, whereas legal advocates investigate discriminatory practices at the workplace. Support groups can also provide a safe place for dealing with rejection and other issues related to coming out.

True Stories from Human Service Workers

Cultural Sensitivity at a Center for Gay, Lesbian, Bisexual, and Transgendered People

Since the 1970s, a growing number of agencies and centers have been established for gay, lesbian, bisexual, and transgendered populations who are looking for support, education, and advocacy services. The Center of Orange County in southern California is one such agency.

According to David Hart, the center's program manager, "At this agency, clients are counseled using a cultural identity model in which their sexuality is explored within society and within their own ethnic culture as well. Counselors also use traditional psychological theories with the clients that aim to empower them and reduce risks associated with the spread of HIV."

David Hart's comments suggest that human services workers must not only be aware of special issues faced by members of the GLBT community, but they also need to recognize the overall impact an individual's ethnic identity has on a person's choices and self-esteem. Some ethnic and religious cultures may possibly regard homosexuality more negatively than others do. Human services workers must keep this in mind when working with this population.

Human services workers who believe strongly that homosexuality is a sin and that those who are not heterosexual should attempt to change their sexuality should probably refer clients struggling with those issues to someone else. As mentioned in the previous chapter, imposing one's beliefs on a client is inappropriate. Unfortunately, social biases against non-heterosexuals may influence whether sufficient funding is available to programs that deal with HIV/AIDS-related problems. Those with political power have as yet failed to channel sufficient funds to programs that could potentially eradicate HIV/AIDS (which still primarily affects gay men in the United States). Perhaps this is because most Americans have conservative views about gays and do not want to see their tax dollars go to fight a disease that results from immoral behavior. The issue of HIV/AIDS is by far the greatest challenge facing the gay community due to the fact that it often leads to serious illness and death.

CRITICAL THINKING / SELF-REFLECTION CORNER

Who do you think should be first to receive treatment for diseases related to HIV/AIDS, given that funding for treatment is limited? Rank your response from the following list of client populations.

- an infant whose mother is HIV-positive

- a heroin addict who shared a dirty needle

- a gay man who had unprotected sex

- a 62-year-old woman who received a blood transfusion

Why did you rank your responses the way you did? Your ranking may illustrate the political nature of HIV/AIDS and of being gay.

Human services workers must continually examine their own attitudes about the GLBT population. It is essential to find a balance between acknowledging that people's sexual orientation can affect their needs and treating all people without disparity.

The term transgender refers to a person, usually a man, who, since childhood, has experienced himself emotionally, psychologically, and socially as a woman, despite being born biologically a male. As an adult, he may choose to change his physiology by taking female hormones to enlarge his breasts and/or undergo major reconstructive surgery to create a complete female body. He then usually refers to himself as a woman, even on legal documents. The transgender process may take many years, and many surgeons who perform sex-change procedures require their patients to receive psychological assessments and even ongoing therapy prior to this dramatic life change. Some transgendered people don't undergo the full sex-change surgery (because it is very expensive). Instead, they take hormones and live as women in appearance. Because this procedure is not common, most people in U.S. society have had little contact with transgenders. Stereotypes about transgenders often confuse them with drag queens or just consider them to be freaks. When human services workers deal with this population, they will find them to be fairly normal except that they are much more comfortable living as women than they were living as men. Some transgenders are and always have been attracted to men, whereas others may be attracted to women.

Issues of Race and Ethnicity

Just as sensitivity to gender and sexual orientation is an important part of human services practice, so too is sensitivity to ethnic and racial cultural issues. Some human needs are universal, crossing all races and ethnicities; however, when assessing a client, it is always wise to take into consideration the racial, ethnic, and cultural factors that might be influencing or affecting clients' needs. Keep in mind that most of the theories and intervention strategies, policies, and program structures have been developed using the cultural value system of mainstream America. Some ethnicities and cultures might have different values, and these differences may create conflicts between an organization's culture and a client's culture, thereby unintentionally affecting the efficacy of treatment.

The term "racial group" is often used to classify people according to their outward appearance. These physical qualities might include hair type, skin color, eye shape and color, quantity of body hair, and body type (Schaefer, 1988). Traditional racial categories put people into one of three races: Caucasoid, Mongoloid, and Negroid depending on a person's skin color, hair type, facial characteristics, and body type. It may be difficult to pinpoint the race to which someone exactly belongs because of interracial marriage and breeding.

How does **race** differ from ethnicity? Ethnicity usually refers to a group of people who share similar language, traditions about parenting and marriage, types of food and the ways in which food is prepared, values about family and home, and so forth. There are more ethnic groups than races because each race is made up of many different ethnic groups. For example, Caucasians comprise English, Irish, Dutch, German, and French people, to name only a few. Likewise, Mexicans, Puerto Ricans, Cubans, and Chileans are some of the ethnicities of the Latino race. While understanding every nuance of every ethnic group and race is impossible, human services workers should at least keep in mind common cultural themes and how mainstream U.S. culture might inhibit the free expression of different cultural views. It is important to accept and acknowledge other points of views and perhaps to use those cultural values when working with clients.

EUROPEAN AMERICAN CULTURE

American culture was founded primarily on the values and views of the Englishmen who wrote the U.S. Constitution, the Declaration of Independence, and other federal documents of the time. Men from Germany, the Netherlands, France, and other northern European countries also influenced early American culture. Because the majority of these men were Protestant, Protestantism also had a significant impact on American culture. Although many European Americans hold similar values, especially when compared to non-European ethnic groups, there was a time in American history when certain European groups were discriminated against despite their racial similarities. Some of the negative attitudes and behaviors stemmed from religious differences. For example, when the Irish immigrated to America in the late 1800s, many conflicts arose between the predominantly Catholic Irish and those accustomed to the existing Protestant-based culture. Other immigrant groups also suffered discrimination on arriving in the United States, especially when one ethnic group, such as Italians, tried to move into a neighborhood that was predominantly Polish. Eventually, immigrants from all the various countries that came to the United States in the early nineteenth century "melted" together into what has become known as a **melting pot** where most Americans have assimilated according to the norms established by the Founding Fathers.

The American way of life, according to the Declaration of Independence, is based, among other things, on an individual's right to "the pursuit of happiness." Americans are encouraged to act independently, have freedom of religion and speech, and access all the rights due to every citizen who is considered equal. The American Pledge of Allegiance teaches us that we all live in "one nation, under God, indivisible, with liberty and justice for all." These words describe the essence of American culture and help explain why American culture is often competitive because everyone is encouraged to meet his or her own needs.

The late twentieth and twenty-first centuries have brought a different type of immigrant from those who came in the late 1800s and early 1900s. Many new immigrants to the United States choose to maintain a strong traditional cultural and ethnic identity with little interest in complete acculturation. Human services workers must remain aware that many cultures differ from American views. Some cultures are more passive and cooperative. In most Asian cultures, for example, the good of the group comes before the happiness of individuals..

Of course, the reader must remember that not every person of a certain ethnic group will display the same qualities and behaviors. Many people are **acculturated**—that is, they have assimilated many of the values of and hold beliefs similar to those of mainstream culture in the United States. What is important is to find out what the client's values are and not assume that everyone agrees with mainstream values.

LATINOS, HISPANICS, AND CHICANOS

Although Latino ethnic groups, such as Mexicans, Cubans, and Puerto Ricans, may have much in common merely because all have been influenced by the Spanish language, Latino groups have different political views and migration status in the United States. They might all agree that they are Latinos, but a Cuban might become offended if referred to as a Mexican and vice-versa. Each ethnic group has a certain pride in its unique history and how it has influenced its specific cultural identity. Some people whose dominant language is Spanish refer to themselves as Latinos, or use the term Hispanic. Some prefer to use the specific country of origin with which to identify themselves, such as referring to themselves as Peruvian or Cuban. In any case, they do have certain values in common simply because of the influence of the Spanish conquerors who invaded various countries in Central and South America during the sixteenth and seventeenth centuries.

Puerto Ricans hold dual citizenship as Americans and Puerto Ricans and therefore have a different position in the United States than immigrant Latinos do. They can come and go as they please. Their communities are usually found in large urban centers, like New York City, where there are effective, natural support systems. Melvin Delgado (1998), studied these support systems and found that Puerto Ricans receive the most effective human services from local Puerto Rican vendors, people who work in beauty shops, restaurant owners, church leaders, and florist-shop owners and employees. The mainstream American notion of the necessity for government-run social services may not fit the particular needs of this population. They have developed a special resiliency to social problems because of the strong social connections in their communities.

Cubans have a different history and relationship with the United States. The first wave of Cubans who came to the United States were often well-educated and wealthy. They often tried to "de-Cubanize" themselves in an effort to blend in completely with American culture. The next wave of Cubans came after Castro and communism took control of Cuba. These Cubans often felt special because they came from a country that was largely controlled by the Soviet Union, a major world power from the 1960s through the 1980s. This differs from many other Latinos who come to America from third-world nations where they were raised in poverty.

Mexicans, who make up the largest group of Latinos in the United States (Schaefer, 1988; U.S. Bureau of the Census, 2001), have traditionally crossed the border in search of employment. Because they have had little education and they are accustomed to living in poverty, Mexicans sometimes are placed near the bottom of Latino hierarchy. Also, many Mexicans come to the United States illegally and are therefore subjected to poor treatment and discrimination. Fear of being deported keeps them from asserting their rights. Some Mexican Americans refer to themselves as **Chicanos,** which carries with it a sense of cultural pride and has strong political implications. The term became popular in the 1960s when social protest led to such phrases as **Viva La Raza** and created a more positive self-image among U.S. Latinos (Schaefer, 1988).

Despite the differences among subgroups, Latinos do have much in common. Most are Catholics, though many are becoming Protestant. Many still speak Spanish in the home and speak very little English. The divorce rate among Latinos is lower than in mainstream U.S. society, and their birthrate is higher than it is nationwide. Family *(familism)* is the most important institution for Latinos. Because they value family harmony at all costs, family conflicts may be displayed in ways unfamiliar to mainstream culture. Another unique aspect of Latino culture is *marianisma,* which is the value placed on women who are self-sacrificing and placing the needs of everyone else's above their own. *Familism* and *marianisma* may present themselves to human services workers in a phenomenon called *ataque de nervios,* which is a clinical syndrome seen primarily in women and only in the Latino community. The syndrome manifests itself as a combination of symptoms of depression, panic disorder, and generalized anxiety disorder (Kanel, 2005; Koss-Chioino, 1999; Liebowitz et al., 1994; Oquendo, 1995; Schechter, et al., 2000). This syndrome has been diagnosed in members of all different groups of Latinos, such as Puerto Ricans, Dominicans (Rubio et al., 1955), Cubans, South Americans, (Liebowitz et al., 1994), and Mexicans (Kanel, 2005). Kanel's study indicates that the perceived cause of *ataque de nervios* is family conflict. It can be hypothesized that instead of confronting family conflicts directly as mainstream American culture encourages, Latinos manifest this syndrome as a way to cope with conflicts without having to confront family members directly, thereby safeguarding family harmony. The female maintains her self-sacrificing status by suffering *ataque de nervios* so that the rest of the family won't be affected by family conflicts.

Of course, human services workers should consider other Latino cultural values and behaviors that might differ from mainstream culture clients when developing interventions for Latinos. The best advice is to listen carefully to each client and family, ask questions about how culture may be influencing a client's needs, and explore options that don't impose conflicting values onto the client. In some situations, it may be necessary to educate clients about cultural conflicts between family members and between societal institutions. Besides Latinos, this might also be necessary for Asians, Arabs, and families of other cultures in which mainstream values are colliding with traditional ones. Other conflicts may occur when one culture may see no problem with a certain behavior that may be considered morally unacceptable or even illegal by mainstream American cultural values. For example, in some cultures, it is permissible to hit children with sticks and other objects, even if they leave marks. While this behavior may be permissible in one culture, it is illegal in American culture, and people who practice such forms of discipline must be told that their behavior must change if they want to continue to live in the United States. Human services workers must explain both the practical side (avoiding jail or losing custody of a child) of assimilating this American behavior, as well as the reason for the American laws about child abuse (psychological and emotional consequences of abuse).

For example, child protective services removed the 11-year-old daughter from the home of a Nicaraguan woman after a teacher noticed the child had multiple bruises on her back and legs. The little girl's mother was accused of severe physical abuse. When doctors examined the child, they also found remnants of duct tape on her lips and wrists, suggesting the child's mouth had been taped shut and her wrists bound. When the mother was confronted with the evidence, she openly admitted that she had taped her daughter's mouth and bound her to a chair to control her. She also admitted to having hit the child along her backside with a wooden spoon. The mother stated that the child had been disobedient and was openly defiant. The mother also said that when she was growing up, all children were hit with wooden spoons and were often bound to keep them quiet.

Culturally sensitive intervention with this mother included educating her about U.S. child-abuse laws that prohibit such discipline. Her case plan included parenting education, family therapy, and individual therapy during which she talked about her own childhood and her migration experience. A culturally sensitive worker would also explore the environment in which she grew up and would not judge her actions without considering the norms established by the community in which she was socialized. On the other hand, a culturally insensitive worker would merely label her as an abusive parent and take punitive action against her.

ASIAN AMERICANS

Previously mentioned suggestions about working with clients of differing cultural backgrounds apply to a variety of groups, including Asian Americans, African Americans, Native Americans, and Arab Americans. While it's important not to stereotype, it is helpful to look at recent studies of cultural variations when first working with someone from a cultural different from one's own. Kim, Liang, and Li (2003) studied nonverbal behaviors of Asian American female counselors and of European American female counselors while working with Asian American clients. Their findings were "consistent with the literature on Asian American communication styles, which indicates that Asian Americans tend to be less expressive and more reticent and restrained in their nonverbal behaviors" (Uba, 1994). The Asian American counselors smiled less than the European American counselors, which supports the observation that Asian Americans tend to value emotional self-control and to avoid openly displaying their feelings, even if those feelings are pleasant ones (Kim, Atkinson, & Umemoto, 2001). Traditional Asian cultures value control over emotional expressiveness even among family members and consider such control a sign of strength (Hsu, Tseng, Ashton, McDermott, & Char, 1985). This behavior is vastly different from mainstream American culture that expects people to openly and directly express affection and other strong emotions to family and friends alike. These and other studies of Asian culture should help human services workers keep in mind the effect free emotional expression can have on their Asian clients and be conscious of not pushing them into doing so. Instead, workers should allow their clients to communicate in ways that are comfortable to them so that they can work through their problems and get their needs met, even if it means taking a more indirect approach than usual.

A situation in which a counselor fails to consider her clients' cultural norms is described in the following scenario: A 42-year-old Chinese American man sought counseling because he was having problems with his marriage. He told the counselor that if his wife would do what he told her to do, their lives would be fine. The counselor, unaware of the man's cultural norms, acted insensitively by asking the wife to come to the next session. At that session, the counselor told the husband to express his feelings and needs directly to his wife and then asked the wife to express how his words made her feel. Although this style of marital counseling can be useful with mainstream Americans, it was ineffective with this couple. They never returned. The author has intimate knowledge of this unfortunate scenario because it was she who made the blunder!

ARAB AMERICANS

Arab Americans are a growing ethnic group in the United States. Although they may speak different languages, they have common cultural traditions of the Middle East. Most people think that all Arabs are Muslims. In fact, Arab Americans are 42 percent Catholic, 23 percent Orthodox Christian, 23 percent Muslim, and 12 percent Protestant (Zogby, 2001). While many Arabs strictly practice their religious beliefs, not all of them do, so service providers must be careful not to make assumptions. However, a recent study of Arab Americans (Nassar-McMillan & Hakim-Larson, 2003) found some evidence that counseling and other social services for many Arab Americans can be more effective with the support of the community's religious leaders because of Arab Americans' deep religious beliefs. In addition to the support of religious leaders, the study also revealed that the support and endorsement of other community leaders makes it easier for members of the community to use mental health services. Middle Eastern culture is a collectivist one in which community acceptance is important to individuals of the culture. This also differs from mainstream American culture, which values individuality. If community leaders can proactively educate Arab Americans about how mental health services can be used to feel empowered and have better control of life circumstances, then maybe more Arab Americans may use these much-needed services. Unfortunately, human services workers who are not part of the Arab community are often mistrusted (Nassar-McMillan, 1999), which may also be true for counseling and other human services. For the Arab community, physicians, priests, fortune tellers, or other healers traditionally address issues of mental health and the family (Loza, 2001; Al-Krenawi & Graham, 2000). When working with Arab Americans, human services providers should develop a strong rapport based on personal interaction rather than on interpretation or exploration of client issues (Al-Abdul-Jabbar & Al-Issa, 2000). Overall, a multisystem approach that involves religious leaders, medical professionals, family members, and social services is the most effective way to work with this population. Traditional models must be modified to allow for flexibility around timeframe, place of service, and methods of confrontation. Arabs, like so many of us, tolerate neither open criticism, nor challenges to the patriarchal position of male family members (Nydell, 1987; Abudabbeh & Aseel, 1999).

AFRICAN AMERICANS

African Americans have a history in the United States unlike that of any other ethnic group. Most African Americans were brought here against their wills as slaves. They speak English fluently, however, their physical appearance makes them more readily identifiable than any other minority group. They have been in this country longer than any other minority group except for the Native Americans. These historical facts have influenced attitudes and behaviors that are typically observed in African American families. But because they do speak English and many of their families have been in the United States since its founding, they tend to be more acculturated to mainstream values than other minority and ethnic groups.

Probably the most important issue to keep in mind when working with African Americans is racism. Because of their history of slavery and obvious physical differences, many Americans continue to hold negative attitudes toward African Americans. On the other hand, the multitude of abuses and ill-treatment inflicted on African Americans by Caucasians have created distrustful attitudes and stereotypical beliefs toward "white" people in America. African Americans often feel singled out by police, judges, and others in authority. Unfortunately, their perceptions are often true because institutionalized racism may still exist.

Human services workers should consider these facts when beginning a professional relationship with African American clients. If a client is extremely resistant and distrustful, it may be prudent to involve a trusted minister or someone from the African American community to work with the client. Religious institutions have been a sanctuary for this ethnic group since the days of slavery and continue to be a natural support system for African Americans. Music and athletics have also been trusted and valued institutions for this cultural group, and involving coaches and other role models may be an effective way to work with a client. However, not all African Americans need such traditional support systems. Many middle-class and professional African Americans easily accept mainstream interventions, most likely because they have found ways to circumvent racism and discrimination. The important thing is to approach each client as an individual and to be culturally sensitive to a client's needs. The reality of racism must always be acknowledged but never assumed.

NATIVE AMERICANS

Although land owned by the Navajo nation extends into Arizona, New Mexico, and Utah and is home to about 175,228 Navajo, which is the largest U.S. on-reservation population, an estimated 4,366,000 of all Native Americans live outside of Indian-owned lands (U.S. Census Bureau, 2004). Approximately 978,000 Native Americans are school-aged children (U.S. Census, 2004). Sadly, only 29.2 percent graduate from high school (U.S. Census Bureau, 2004), compared to 65 percent nationwide.

Lack of sufficient education may contribute to their high rate of unemployment and poor standard of living (O'Brien, 1992). In addition, they have less access to resources such as medical and dental care, medications, and rehabilitation services, which may result in the high rates of chronic disease and disability found in Native American populations (Seekins, 1997). Four out of every 1,000 Native American babies are born with fetal alcohol syndrome (FAS), compared to less than one out of 1,000 in the Anglo population. They also suffer higher rates of hearing loss and visual impairment, 85 percent of which are preventable (Native American Research and Training Center, 1995).

Native Americans' ideas about child rearing, change and intervention, medicine, and healing are different from those found in mainstream American culture (Allison & Vining, 1999). Of course, as with any ethnic group, not all Native Americans think alike. Some incorporate mainstream American practices into their own belief systems, whereas others—often those within the same family—prefer using traditional practices (Dufort & Reed, 1995).

Most Native Americans live in extended families that include, besides their immediate family members, grandparents, aunts (often referred to as mother), uncles (often referred to as father), and cousins (often referred to as brothers and sisters), as well as adopted relatives. As these families relocate away from reservations and to urban settings, they face a constant struggle between sustaining their traditional culture that is built on spirituality, socialization, and language and adopting more mainstream values that emphasize competition and independence. Tribal communities are small and close knit, encouraging dependence within members. These traditions also conflict with mainstream values that encourage children to become independent of their families (Allison & Vining, 1999).

Because many tribes have autonomy within their reservations to intervene using their own traditions, many people whose needs may best be met outside their tribal community do not receive assistance. While autonomy has its benefits, it also has a downside. Communities that live outside government's constraints have difficulty when availing themselves of government-funded resources. When Native Americans do seek services outside of their communities, problems occur because most human services workers cannot speak their language, trained interpreters are rare, and most service providers do not understand Native American culture (Mattes & Omark, 1984).

Human services workers who encounter this population must be sure to communicate their ignorance and ask the client if Native American tradition is a part of the problem and how it might be a part of the solution.

Religious Issues

The traditional bio-psychosocial perspective has recently expanded to include a spiritual component. Many human services workers have found spirituality helpful to clients' overall well-being. In the past, workers may have been reluctant to discuss religion and spiritual beliefs with clients for fear of imposing their beliefs on their clients. Others, however, believe that "addressing spirituality within the therapy is not optional. Human beings are spiritual by nature. If spirituality has no place in therapy then we leave out this part of our humanity and are therefore incapable of best serving the full needs of our clients" (Zylstra, 2006, p. 4). Edward Canda (website, Feb. 2006), created an entire course of social work study that he calls "Spiritual Aspects of Social Work Practice." Canda states on his course outline "that social work practice adopts a holistic person-in-environment perspective that requires taking into account the biological, psychological, socio-logical, and spiritual aspects of human needs, strengths, and experience" (2005). His rationale for creating the course was that "minority spiritual perspectives have been especially neglected given the Eurocentric assumptions common in social work" (Canda, 2005).

This section on religious beliefs provides some basic information and can be used to help clients explore their own spirituality and religious beliefs. Perhaps the bio-psychosocial model might be renamed the bio-psychosocial-spiritual model.

Mainstream U.S. culture has been based largely on Christianity, in particular Protestantism, although religious freedom has been and is still encouraged. While a politician's religious background may seem irrelevant, all of the U.S. presidents have been Protestant, with the exception of John F. Kennedy who was Catholic. So while religious freedom is a basic American value, social and political views may largely favor Protestant values.

PROTESTANTISM

The word "Protestant" originated from the word "protest," referring to those who protested the power and hierarchy of the Catholic Church during the fourteenth and fifteenth centuries. Protestants typically adhere to the teachings of the Bible, in particular the teachings of Jesus, which encourage forgiveness and concern about one's neighbors. Of course, not all Protestants behave the same or hold the same beliefs. Human services workers should explore their clients' religious beliefs and spirituality and how these factors may or may not affect a person's needs and problems.

CATHOLICISM

Catholics differ from Protestants in that they look toward the Pope to lead their values and behaviors. While they accept the Bible and the teachings of Jesus, they also worship saints and the Virgin Mary. Priests hold powerful positions and are given more respect and authority than Protestants give their clergy. The Catholic Church prohibits certain behaviors, such as using birth control, and mandates certain rules, such as going to confession, that are generally not followed by Protestant churches. Some people may find such traditions offensive. Human services workers should, however, be aware of the effect such practices have on a client's needs and problems.

JUDAISM

Those who call themselves Jewish may be referring to their religious beliefs or their cultural heritage. The Jews have been oppressed for thousands of years, and this oppression plays a large part in their culture. Hostility toward Jewish people, often called **anti-Semitism,** can be traced back to early Christianity when Jews were blamed for the death of Christ (Schaefer, 1988). Jews do not believe Jesus to be the Messiah and, as a result, are often rejected by mainstream American culture.

When a person labels himself as Jewish, he is not always referring to being affiliated with the religion of Judiasm because being Jewish is more than a religious belief, it is a culture and a way of life. Just as early history shaped Jewish thought and tradition, the horrors of the Jewish Holocaust implemented by Nazi Germany and carried out all over Europe during World War II affected Jewish perspective today. Jews tend to be politically active and fight for rights of the downtrodden. Jewish people have always valued education and are often considered to be skilled businesspeople. Jews attend synagogue usually during the high holy days as well as to participate in various religious ceremonies, such as to celebrate the coming of age of a 13-year-old child, called a *bar mitzvah* for a boy or a *bat mitzvah* for a girl.

Orthodox Jews strictly follow the old traditions, dietary laws, and commandments as they were written in the Old Testament, the Torah, and the Talmud. Some Jews, however, prefer to practice Reformed Judaism, which is less rigid and considered by many Orthodox Jews as being only a little better than being nonobservant (Schaefer, 1988). In general, being Jewish transcends nationality, religion, and culture to include a shared identity and history of oppression and resilience.

MUSLIMISM/ISLAM

Muslims believe in many of the same prophets of the Old and New Testaments. Mohammed (born about 500 A.D.), however, is the most sacred and the focus of the Islamic faith. Not all Muslims are Arab, and not all Arabs are Muslim. Muslims do not support terrorism. Terrorism is a result of political extremists who sometimes use the Muslim faith to fuel terrorist activities. While it may be true that Muslims believe in a different type of heaven and entrance to heaven than Christians, they do not support violence and revenge. They do have strict rules, sometimes requiring women to cover themselves in public, but Muslim women regard this as a sign of respect toward men and for themselves. It is important not to stereotype Arabs and Muslims as violent terrorists. Most devout religious people do not engage in violence. Instead, they seek peace as did their prophets. Keep in mind that war and violence is usually a political issue, not a religious one.

BUDDHISM AND HINDUISM

These religions are practiced in many Asian countries, particularly in India, China, and Japan. They focus on meditation, compassion, and kindness as a way to achieve Nirvana. Both religions believe in reincarnation (people return to Earth as another life form after death). Worship is usually done in private at a temple rather than in a church with a congregation and a sermon. Buddhists follow the philosophical teachings of Buddha, who lived his life doing good works for others. Hindus believe in three forms of God: Brahma is the Creator, Vishnu is the Sustainer, and Shiva is the Destroyer. In addition to these main deities, they also believe in nine other forms of God who possess various characteristics (Hindu Universe website, Jan. 2006).While there are many differences between Buddhism and Hinduism, both seem to encourage compassion toward others, communion with God or the universe, and spirituality in daily life.

ATHEISM

This ideology is rarely included with other religions. "Theism is defined as the belief in a god or gods, while atheism literally means without theism or without the belief in a god or gods. One who does not believe in the existence of a god or supernatural being is properly designated as an atheist. Another way to think of an atheist is someone who does not believe in the existence of a god, rather than someone who believes that a god does not exist. It is more of an absence of belief" (Smith, 1989, p. 7). A common stereotype about atheists is that they are immoral or that they worship Satan. Atheists are as unlikely to believe in Satan as they are to believe in a god. Atheists are just as likely as any religious person to lead ethical, moral, and compassionate lives. The important thing for human services workers to keep in mind when providing services to atheists or, for that matter, to anyone who has a particular set of beliefs is to avoid letting one's own religious biases interfere with providing services.

Age, Class, and Disability

Three other types of bias that often occur in human services institutions and in society in general involve age, socioeconomic class, and disability. Most of the psychological theories that have been used over the past 100 years to provide mental health services, social services, criminal justice services, and education focus on young, middle-class, able-bodied, and educated people.

AGE

Although more recently, theories on the study of aging, or **gerontology,** have begun to emerge, bias against the elderly still exists. Many people hold negative attitudes toward elderly people, perhaps because of their own fears about aging. American society, unlike many other cultures, does not respect its elderly population. The young do not seek out elderly people to benefit from their wisdom and years of experience. American society accepts the practice of having elderly relatives who can no longer care for themselves live in retirement and nursing homes rather than having them live with their extended family. Much of this has to do with the high value American culture places on being independent. Also, American society values youth, as can be evidenced by the increased use of plastic surgery by people who are trying to stay looking young. Sadly, doctors and other service providers treat many elderly people like children. It's as if some people will not give the elderly credit for understanding anything. Also, elderly people who are physically vulnerable and prone to illness may hesitate to assert their rights for fear of being abandoned or mistreated. One place where elderly do have clout is at the voting booth come election time, and politicians, aware of their voting power, do court their vote.

True, older people may have slower reaction times, might be slower in learning new ideas, but they do offer an historical perspective on life that's unavailable to younger people. A little patience is required when working with elderly clients, and unfortunately, many workers, faced with institutional deadlines and other demands made by our fast-paced society, simply cannot provide the types of services or offer the kind of attention that an elderly person may need.

CLASS

People of lower socioeconomic classes may also be discriminated against and find disparity in the services they receive. American culture values education and wealth, so it's not surprising that those who are uneducated and poor are treated as if they are immoral or just lazy. The unfortunate reality is that wealthy people receive all kinds of better services than poor people do. People without much money must make do with what is given to them, "beggars can't be choosers." This creates disparity in service, but seems to be intrinsic to the American capitalistic economic and societal structure. "Money talks" really does seem to be a reality. It is unfortunate that the poor usually don't participate in elections and therefore don't assert their political power as much as they could. This may be due in part to their lack of education about political power and to learned helplessness.

DISABILITIES

Throughout history, people with disabilities have been victims of stigma, prejudice, mistreatment, discrimination, social isolation, inferior status, and inferior services. Just 50 years ago, mentally retarded people were called idiots, feeble-minded, imbeciles, and morons. At times, disabled people may be viewed by others unrealistically; others either overestimate the degree of disability, or they underestimate the special needs of the individual (Doyle, 2007). Finally, the Americans with Disabilities Act of 1990 was enacted into law to challenge discrimination against persons with disabilities. This provided the legal muscle the disabled need when they face discrimination.

Some common reactions, even from human services workers, to persons who are disabled are fear, repulsion, anxiety about loss and dependence, embarrassment, and avoidance of social contact. Working with the disabled might be considered by some as being less prestigious. It is vital to keep in mind that this population needs meaningful attention and services rather than being stigmatized or patronized.

Poverty, the needs of the elderly, and the issues facing those with disabilities will be more thoroughly examined in subsequent chapters.

Concluding Remarks about Causality

Much of the time, politics and the values of those in power determine who receives services. In the case of deviance, these values are based on what society attributes the cause of the behaviors and whether it is perceived as being under a person's control. Throughout history, the manner in which society has attributed causes of problems has been cyclical; at times deviant behaviors have been attributed to either biological, psychological, or sociological factors. Society's views about whether deviant behavior is under a person's control has also fluctuated.

If popular opinion believes a problem is not under a person's control, people tend to be more sympathetic and motivated to provide charity and help for that person. When a problem is considered controllable, people often respond in anger, and react punitively or with rejection. Despite scientific studies about biological, psychological, and social factors, many people still approach social problems from this causality model. Social pressure and values often dictate funding for interventions, which, unfortunately may inhibit necessary programs for certain populations (heroin addicts, for example).

Table 6.2 provides an opportunity to explore one's own values and how they influence how one perceives the causes and the most appropriate treatment for them. Before reading about various client populations in Chapter 7, take a few minutes to respond to the inventory in Table 6.2. Answer each item by circling the chosen response. Start with column entitled "emotional reaction" and continue to the end of the row. Order what you believe to be the primary, secondary, and tertiary causes of each client' problems. Then decide whether or not the client described in the left-hand column has control over a particular problem. If you struggle or become confused, don't worry too much. Social scientists have been studying these problems for centuries and still don't know for sure what causes them or exactly how to prevent them or help those burdened by them. This exercise might be good preparation for the often ambiguous causality theories used by modern-day human services workers.

After reading about each of these client populations in Chapter 7, try retaking this inventory to see whether any responses have changed.

Table 6.2 Personal Causality Theories and Reaction Inventory

Client Population	Emotional Reaction	Bio-Psychosocial Causality Ranking	Attribution of Causality
poor, homeless, welfare recipients	pity/sympathy anger/punitive	biological 1 2 3 psychological 1 2 3 social/political 1 2 3	out of the person's control under the person's control
abused children	pity/sympathy anger/punitive	biological 1 2 3 psychological 1 2 3 social/political 1 2 3	out of the person's control under the person's control
child molesters	pity/sympathy anger/punitive	biological 1 2 3 psychological 1 2 3 social/political 1 2 3	out of the person's control under the person's control
parents who physically abuse their children	pity/sympathy anger/punitive	biological 1 2 3 psychological 1 2 3 social/political 1 2 3	out of the person's control under the person's control
spousal abusers	pity/sympathy anger/punitive	biological 1 2 3 psychological 1 2 3 social/political 1 2 3	out of the person's control under the person's control
battered women	pity/sympathy anger/punitive	biological 1 2 3 psychological 1 2 3 social/political 1 2 3	out of the person's control under the person's control
abused elderly	pity/sympathy anger/punitive	biological 1 2 3 psychological 1 2 3 social/political 1 2 3	out of the person's control under the person's control
physically disabled	pity/sympathy anger/punitive	biological 1 2 3 psychological 1 2 3 social/political 1 2 3	out of the person's control under the person's control
mentally retarded	pity/sympathy anger/punitive	biological 1 2 3 psychological 1 2 3 social/political 1 2 3	out of the person's control under the person's control
schizophrenics	pity/sympathy anger/punitive	biological 1 2 3 psychological 1 2 3 social/political 1 2 3	out of the person's control under the person's control
emotional disorders/ personality disorders	pity/sympathy anger/punitive	biological 1 2 3 psychological 1 2 3 social/political 1 2 3	out of the person's control under the person's control

(continued)

Table 6.2 *(continued)*

Client Population	Emotional Reaction	Bio-Psychosocial Causality Ranking	Attribution of Causality
anorexics/bulimics	pity/sympathy anger/punitive	biological 1 2 3 psychological 1 2 3 social/political 1 2 3	out of the person's control under the person's control
cocaine addicts	pity/sympathy anger/punitive	biological 1 2 3 psychological 1 2 3 social/political 1 2 3	out of the person's control under the person's control
rape victims	pity/sympathy anger/punitive	biological 1 2 3 psychological 1 2 3 social/political 1 2 3	out of the person's control under the person's control
rapists	pity/sympathy anger/punitive	biological 1 2 3 psychological 1 2 3 social/political 1 2 3	out of the person's control under the person's control
criminals	pity/sympathy anger/punitive	biological 1 2 3 psychological 1 2 3 social/political 1 2 3	out of the person's control under the person's control
AIDS patients	pity/sympathy anger/punitive	biological 1 2 3 psychological 1 2 3 social/political 1 2 3	out of the person's control under the person's control
pregnant teens	pity/sympathy anger/punitive	biological 1 2 3 psychological 1 2 3 social/political 1 2 3	out of the person's control under the person's control
gang members	pity/sympathy anger/punitive	biological 1 2 3 psychological 1 2 3 social/political 1 2 3	out of the person's control under the person's control
Alzheimer's patients	pity/sympathy anger/punitive	biological 1 2 3 psychological 1 2 3 social/political 1 2 3	out of the person's control under the person's control
alcoholics	pity/sympathy anger/punitive	biological 1 2 3 psychological 1 2 3 social/political 1 2 3	out of the person's contro under the person's control
heroin addicts	pity/sympathy anger/punitive	biological 1 2 3 psychological 1 2 3 social/political 1 2 3	out of the person's control under the person's control

Chapter Summary

While there is a growing trend among human services providers to increase cultural sensitivity, there is still room for growth in this area. Most of us would agree that all races, ethnic groups, religions, genders, sexual orientations, ages, and social classes should be treated equally. American culture is founded on the notion of liberty and justice for all. If each of us consciously works to reduce the biases and prejudices in our own lives, maybe discrimination and bigotry can be eliminated permanently.

Suggested Applied Activities

1. Interview a few people whose race, ethnicity, religion, sexual orientation, gender, age, or class are different from yours. Find out if and how their subculture differs from mainstream culture. Ask about their experiences with racism, sexism, heterosexism, classism, or religious discrimination.

   _____

   _____

   _____

   _____

   _____

   _____

2. Divide a circle into sections and label each with the name of an ethnic group living in the United States. Describe some of the positive elements that each group contributes or has contributed to mainstream culture. Divide and label sections of another circle listing the negative aspects of each group.

   _____

   _____

   _____

   _____

   _____

   _____

   _____

3. Make a list of the pros and cons of mainstream American culture as you perceive it. How would you change American culture if you could?

_____

_____

_____

_____

_____

_____

_____

Chapter Review Questions

1. What does disparity mean? What are some of its causes?

_____

_____

2. What is heterosexism?

_____

_____

3. What two factors are important to keep in mind when working with the following groups:

Latinos

_____

_____

African Americans

_____

_____

Asian Americans

_____

_____

Arab Americans

_____

_____

4. Mainstream American culture was primarily founded on the values of
   _____, _____, and _____.

5. What is the most important aspect of culturally sensitive human services
   practice?

_____

_____

Glossary of Terms

Ableism refers to a dislike of all people who are disabled.

Acculturate is someone who adopts mainstream values and behaviors as one's own.

Ageism refers to a dislike of people because of their age.

Anti-Semitism is a dislike of all Jewish people.

Ataque de nervios is a syndrome diagnosed in Latinos who have symptoms of anxiety, depression, and panic.

Being in the closet refers to homosexuals who hide their sexual orientation from society.

Chicano refers to a Latino, usually a Mexican American, and implies pride in that person's ethnic identity.

Classism is negative attitudes and behaviors based on a person's socioeconomic class.

Coming out (of the closet) refers to a person who reveals for the first time his or her homosexuality to family, friends, and coworkers and lives an openly homosexual life.

Cultural bias makes judgments that are based solely on a person's background and ethnicity.

Culture refers to attitudes, behaviors, traditions, family structure, and values of a group of people.

Discrimination occurs when a group of people (of the same race, ethnicity, religion, gender, age, social class) are denied the same rights and privileges that are available to others. Discrimination can be either overt when it occurs openly, or covert, when the discrimination is not readily apparent.

Disparity refers to a condition of being unequal, as in the amount or quality of services received.

Ethnicity refers to the culture traditions, language, history, and country of origin that a group of people share.

Ethnocentrism is the assumption that one's own culture is superior to all others.

Familism among Latinos refers to valuing the family above all else.

Gender refers to the psychological, social, and cultural features and characteristics associated with being biologically female or male.

Gerontology is the study of aging and the services that elderly people need.

Heterosexism is an active dislike of people based on their sexual orientation.

Homophobia is the fear of homosexuality and homosexuals.

Marianisma is the value placed on Latina women who are self-sacrificing and put the needs of others before their own.

Melting pot is a term used in the late 1800s and early 1900s to describe the mix of cultures that came together to form an integrated U.S. society.

Organizational culture refers to the accepted policies, rules, and behavior under which an organization operates.

Politics refers to the seat of power and influence. Politics exist in all organizational groups.

Prejudice is a negative attitude toward an entire category of people or a particular belief about a person based on the group to which he belongs.

Race usually refers to a group of people who are similar in physical appearance that differ from other groups of people.

Racism is an active dislike of people based on their ethnicity or race.

Sexism is an active dislike of a person based only on that person's gender.

Social liberalization accepts all perspectives, cultures, and behaviors without discrimination or bias.

Sociological theory focuses on a society's political, cultural, and religious factors to understand human behavior.

Stereotypes are preconceived, generalized characteristics (true, false, positive, or negative) of a particular group.

Stigma is a negative label given to a person because of an affiliation with a particular group, religion, culture, or lifestyle, or because of a physical or a mental disability.

Transgender refers to a person who may undergo surgery, take hormones, and alter dress and appearance so that he or she can live in the gender that is different from the one that person was born with.

Viva La Raza is a Spanish phrase that means "Long Live the Latino Race," which became popular among activists during the 1960s and 1970s.

Case Presentation and Exit Quiz

General Description

Jack is a case worker at the AIDS Services Foundation. He has worked there for almost two years. Jack has a bachelor's degree in human services and is currently working on a master's degree in social work. Jack had done his undergraduate internship at the center before he was a case worker.

Today Jack has five new cases. He will interview these clients, assess their problems and needs, and develop a treatment plan. As the cases are described, try to focus on the social/cultural and political aspects involved in each one.

Client 1: George

Jack's first client is a 48-year-old Caucasian man named George who has just been told by his physician that he is HIV-positive. Jack asks George how he thinks he got infected. The client tells Jack that he probably got it from an encounter he had at a bath house he visited while vacationing in San Francisco last year. George tells Jack that he has been living an openly gay life for the past 20 years, and until about a year ago, he had been in a long-term relationship that lasted 15 years.

Jack asks George what is most difficult about learning that he's HIV-positive. George says that now he feels like he's just any other gay man, promiscuous and irresponsible. Jack explains to him that many people contract HIV, not just gay men. George feels ashamed about telling his parents, who are very religious Catholics and can barely tolerate his being gay. But now he fears they most certainly will reject him. Jack encourages George to rethink this position and suggests that since his parents are such strong Catholics, they may have learned about sin and forgiveness. Also, they are his parents and love him.

George is also worried about the stigma attached to having HIV/AIDS and being gay. Jack empathizes and tells his client that while many people still hold negative views toward gays, society has changed its ideas about HIV/AIDS since it was first diagnosed in the United States. Knowledge of the disease is now part of the mainstream population and is not looked at the way it was 20 years ago. Jack recommends that George join a support group for HIV-positive people. Jack also encourages him to have an honest talk with his parents, who may even pray for him rather than reject him. Jack will see George next week to follow up with these plans.

Client 2: Elena

Elena is a 23-year-old woman who tearfully tells Jack that she doesn't think she can cope with being HIV-positive. She is from the Middle East and a practicing Muslim.

Elena is sure that if her family finds out they will hate her, and she sees no choice but to kill herself. She tells Jack that she thinks she contracted the virus from her boyfriend, but is too afraid to ask him about it. Elena was a virgin prior to having sex with him, but only he knows that they had sex. She believes she will disgrace her family if they find out she had sex before marriage. Elena does not feel they can get married now.

Jack lets her know that her situation is very complicated, but he will help her get through it. He says that her choices will not be easy considering her background. One of Jack's first concerns is to get her boyfriend tested, but he doesn't want to push Elena to talk to him by herself. Jack is concerned about her physical and emotional safety and realizes he must help this client find out what she wants from this relationship. Jack decides to focus on Elena's physical health first.

He talks to her about medications and healthy lifestyle practices. He asks if she has a personal doctor she trusts to talk to about this. He suggests that until she's decided what to do, she should avoid sexual contact with her boyfriend by telling him that she would feel better waiting until they are married.

Client 3: The Wilsons

The Wilsons are an African American couple who have both tested positive for HIV. They have been living together for 14 years. Both are longtime heroin addicts and most likely contracted HIV through needle sharing. They are very hesitant to talk to Jack, who is Caucasian. They tell him that he doesn't understand "what's up." Jack listens and says very little at first. He asks them if they would prefer to see a different counselor. They tell him that he's just trying to get rid of them like everyone does.

Jack listens again and asks if there is anything they would like from him today. They ask him why he wants to help them. He says simply "because I can and I want to." They begin to open up about how they have tried to kick the drug habit but always end up going back to it. Jack talks about various residential facilities for HIV-positive IV-drug users. He asks if they would be interested. They tell him they'll think about it. Jack recommends that they talk with any family, friends, clergy, or anyone else about this as a possible lifestyle change. He sets up an appointment for next week.

Client 4: Thomas

Thomas is a 36-year-old Latino male who has tested positive for HIV. He refuses to tell his wife of eight years that he is HIV-positive. He says that she doesn't need to know anything because she's just a dumb woman. He is in charge, and if he is infected, then it's ok if she is too. Besides, he tells Jack, during sex he's been withdrawing before he ejaculates in her. Thomas believes that since his wife has no symptoms, she probably won't get sick. All he wants from Jack is the medication.

Jack keeps his opinions to himself but feels very upset after hearing all of this. He asks Thomas if they have children. The client says they have three children, ages two, five, and six. Jack asks more about the children, and Thomas expresses great pride when talking about them. Jack asks Thomas if his wife is a good mother. He says yes she is. Jack educates him about how HIV can be contracted even if a man withdraws during sex. Jack also says that if Thomas's wife is positive, both of them can live long lives as long as they take medication and live a healthy lifestyle. Jack points out how important that would be for his children.

Client 5: Fred

Fred is a 70-year-old man who has tested HIV-positive and desires counseling and medication from the center. When Jack asks how he might have contracted the virus, Fred replies, "I must have gotten it from that pretty little hooker I called several months ago." Jack asks how the man is feeling and what his main concerns are. Fred says that he is worried about getting sick and dying. Jack tells him that many people worry about dying when they first find out they are HIV-positive, but it really isn't a death sentence anymore because of advances in medications. He refers Fred to a support group and discusses medication issues with him.

Exit Quiz

1. One of George's primary issues has to do with
   a. coming out as gay
   b. being embarrassed about going to a bath house
   c. the Catholic church
   d. societal heterosexism

2. Jack shows sensitivity to the religious beliefs of George's parents when he
   a. tells the client that his parents love him
   b. suggests that his parents might know something about sin and forgiveness
   c. says that society has changed its ideas about being gay
   d. says that the client should try to talk with his parents

3. Jack shows cultural sensitivity to Elena when he
   a. holds off having the client confront her boyfriend
   b. cares about her medical issues
   c. asks how she contracted the virus
   d. tells her that her family will not hate her

4. The Wilsons might be hesitant to open up to Jack because of their experience with
   a. ageism
   b. familism
   c. racism
   d. heterosexism

5. When dealing with Thomas, what concept does Jack use to try to persuade his client to tell his wife so that she might get tested?
   a. classism
   b. familism
   c. racism
   d. ataque de nervios

6. When Jack meets Fred, he treats him like any other client who is HIV-positive, thereby avoiding the risk of
   a. classism
   b. ageism
   c. racism
   d. ethnocentrism

Exit Quiz Answers

1. d	3. a	5. b
2. b	4. c	6. b

CHAPTER 7

Populations That Utilize Human Services

Introduction

People who seek assistance from many and various human services agencies have many and various needs, problems, strengths, values, backgrounds, and culturally acceptable behaviors. Sometimes, there is a clash between what the client needs and what can be offered at human services agencies. Typically, though, human services agencies have developed programs that can meet the vast array of their clients' needs. Much research has been done that can help human services workers understand the needs of people who typically use human services as well as effective interventions for those populations. This chapter discusses a variety of client populations in an attempt to assist the reader in developing a beginning understanding of these populations.

People Living in Poverty

Historical Background

Meeting the needs of people based on economic status has long been the focus of government as has been presented in Chapter 2 (Elizabethan Poor Laws). Being poor, or living in **poverty** has been viewed in a variety of ways throughout history. At one time it was thought to be due to immorality. Some people think that poor people are lazy. Others have proposed it is part of a government plan to control the economy. All of these explanations may have some truth to them. It probably depends on the particular situation of each person who is poor.

Definition of Poor/Poverty

Over the years the economic standard of living as well as government guidelines that determine level of income have changed the definition of poverty. In general, people are considered poor if they can't earn enough money to support themselves and their families. Support includes having a clean, safe place to live, enough food to feed each family member at least twice a day, and clothes that are appropriate for the climate. Support also includes being able to pay for health and dental care and for children's school supplies. Most welfare programs either assist poor people to earn enough money to support themselves, or provide money, services and products to permit a minimal standard of living.

The U.S. government defines and sets poverty thresholds according to income and family size. These definitions are updated annually by the Census Bureau and are used nationwide as a statistical yardstick and to determine government funding for people who fall within the parameters of the thresholds. The first thresholds were based on the U.S. Department of Agriculture's statistics on food budgets for families under economic stress in 1963 to 1964 and from data on how much families spend on food. If total family income was less than the threshold appropriate for that family's size, then that family was considered to be living in poverty (U.S. Census Bureau website, March 2005).

Prevalence

Poverty rates have decreased since the 1950s from 22.4 percent of the entire U.S. population to 11.7 percent in 2001. Poverty rates differ by subgroup and are higher than the national average among African Americans and Hispanics and

Table 7.1 2004 U.S. Health and Human Services Poverty Guidelines for the 48 Contiguous States and the District of Columbia

Size of Family Unit	Income Allowed
1	$9,310
2	$12,490
3	15,670
4	18,850
5	$22,030
6	$25,210
7	$28,390
8	$31,570
For each additional person, add	$3,180

(Source: *Federal Register,* vol. 69, no. 30, February 13, 2004, pp. 7,336–7,338.)

lower for Caucasians and Asian Americans. The poverty rates for African Americans and Hispanics in 2001 was 22.7 and 21.4 percent, respectively, while for Caucasians and Asian Americans it was 9.9 and 10.2 percent, respectively. Poverty rates are highest for families headed by single women and for children, with about 11.7 million children living in poverty in 2001 (*Federal Register,* 2003).

Not all people living in poverty are unemployed, in fact more than 40 percent work full time. Approximately 48 percent became poor because their work hours were reduced, and 18 percent became poor because of losing the family bread-winner through divorce. Of all those who manage to work their way out of poverty, 50 percent fall back into poverty within five years (Oswald, 2005).

Causality Models

Psychological and sociopolitical factors are usually considered to cause poverty. It would be the rare social scientist who believed that genetics or biochemical imbalances caused poverty. Some people consider poverty to be under a person's control, and others believe that certain people who live in poverty (such as children) have no control over their economic situation. Those who believe that people have control over their situation often feel angry and don't want assistance available for them. Some people think that poor people are merely lazy and are looking for an easy handout. However, it is doubtful that many people would begrudge a small child financial and medical assistance because people usually believe that children cannot control their standard of living.

Most people believe that able-bodied adults should work and support themselves without governmental assistance, unlike children or people with disabilities who are physically unable to work and support themselves. Government welfare assistance has been based on this philosophy since Queen Elizabeth created her programs in England during the late 1500s and early 1600s.

Psychological factors, not genetics and biology, are considered causes of poverty. This is where biology might interface with poverty. Some people are thought to be unable to work and sustain their own basic needs due to depression or other emotional disorders. It is possible that some of these disorders are due to biochemical imbalances and genetic predisposition. Specific mental disorders and their causes will be discussed later in this chapter. So, in an indirect way, biological factors may have a part in poverty.

Learned helplessness is a popular psychological concept used to explain the cause of poverty. Learned helplessness is often caused by depression, low self-esteem, lack of coping skills, ineffective role-modeling from parents, and inability to mature and develop emotionally. From a psychoanalytic standpoint, people living in poverty have failed to accept their position as adults in society and are fix-ated at a primitive, infantile way of functioning. Perhaps their dependency needs were never fully met in childhood and are seeking this fulfillment later on in life.

Some believe that some poor people may have chosen poverty as a lifestyle because they are lazy. But what psychological factors lead to such laziness? To consciously decide to live in poverty does not seem enjoyable, so what would make a person lazy enough to desire it? Humanistic theorists might suggest that these people are searching for need fulfillment and have simply not found a safe environment to explore their potential and have just given up trying to succeed.

A behavioral perspective might suggest that people stay poor because they are encouraged to stay dependent on others. If someone can receive money and food stamps without working, as long as that person has children, that may be enough incentive for single mothers to remain unemployed. The behavioral model might also suggest that poor people continue to live in poverty because that is what they learned growing up. Acceptance of poverty was role-modeled by parents, and children raised in these homes learn to adapt to having very little. Their coping skills might range from stealing, to borrowing, to begging. Some social scientists refer to the transmission of poverty from one generation to the next as a **cycle of poverty**. These children grow up thinking that this is the only way in which they will ever live and cannot see any other existence possible. They are raised to adapt to the norms and values often seen in poor families, such as "lack of expectations," "make-do with what you have," and "life is a struggle so take what you can." Being raised in poverty might also make the children feel deprived and therefore grow up feeling entitled to assistance, especially if they grew up in a home in which the mother received welfare to raise her children. The idea of being financially independent might not even occur to these children.

Poverty is also thought to have several sociological, cultural, and political factors. Racism, sexism, and ageism play a big part in keeping certain groups poor. Many people are unable to find work because of these factors, or if they do work, the pay is not enough to meet their needs. In general, unemployment does lead to poverty for many people, but it is especially tough for those who are also discriminated against because of race, ethnicity, age, or gender. As stated previously, only 9.9 percent of Caucasians in the United States are poor, compared to 22.7 percent of African Americans and 21.4 percent of Hispanics. It is not a stretch to suggest that race is a factor in poverty.

Many times, people's lack of education prevents them from finding jobs that pay enough to support them. Certain cultures may value work more than education and so people from these cultures are encouraged to quit school and start working as soon as possible. Often, this creates a vicious cycle of poverty.

For example, a married couple from Mexico have immigrated to California in an attempt to find work and escape the devastating poverty in their country. They both start working at a farm, picking fruits and vegetables, each earning $40 a day for 10 hours of work. To them, this seems like a lot of money compared to what they'd earn in Mexico. The couple moves in with cousins and share food and rent. Soon, they start a family and expenses increase. The wife must quit working to take care of their children. The husband secures employment at a factory and makes minimum wage. They move into their own apartment but can barely make ends meet. The wife has three more children, and they are living just below the poverty threshold, but because they were raised in stark poverty, they adapt. The children start school and by the time the eldest is old enough to go to high school, his parents ask him to quit school so he can get a job to help support the family. After all, that is what both his mother and father did in Mexico when they were his age. He quits school, gets a low-paying job, and begins helping out. As this boy grows up, he must now rely on job skills to secure future employment. Because he never finished high school, his chances of finding work that pays enough to raise his standard of living are low. This family's cycle of poverty may continue for several generations until someone breaks out of the mold to complete high school and maybe even continue on to college, giving that person the chance to earn a decent salary and move up the socioeconomic ladder.

Some suggest that there is a political motive, that keeping people poor allows the rich to stay rich. By creating tax laws that benefit the wealthy and keeping unemployment high, individuals living in poverty may consider themselves lucky to be working at all, even if it's only for minimum wage. As a result, "many poor people accept lower-paying work than their abilities enable them to perform because work at their level of skill and training is unavailable." People who accept such jobs are considered to be **underemployed** (R. C. Wallace & W. D. Wallace, 1985, p. 295).

Needs and Issues

Different types of people live in poverty and therefore have needs and issues that vary. Whether poverty results from suddenly being unemployed, being raised in a culture of poverty, or being disabled, assistance of some type is usually needed, but not always sought.

The so-called **deserving poor,** children, elderly, and disabled, usually receive government funding directly. This assistance usually does not cover all of a person's expenses, so additional assistance with health care, child-care, housing, transportation, and food is available. Because of physical disabilities and age, these deserving poor cannot work and so are given priority for receiving assistance. Children also receive free meals at schools to ensure they're getting proper nutrition.

When a person living in poverty is an able-bodied adult, financial assistance is not easily obtained. These people are deemed able to work and to take care of themselves, and so only short-term programs, such as homeless shelters and the Salvation Army, are available that focus on helping people find work and improve their job skills. Sometimes these people are eligible for food stamps, but often they look to churches and other charitable organizations to survive. Shelters and other agencies that help the destitute often can provide clothing to those who need it. These individuals often need a boost in self-esteem and supportive counseling while they transition from being homeless to being self-supporting. They may still live in poverty, but at least their dependence on outside assistance has lessened.

Educational programs are also available for single mothers, especially teenage mothers. The intent of these programs is to end the cycle of poverty by encouraging the mothers to be able to secure decent-paying jobs. Often these women and girls need guidance and encouragement regarding their ability to succeed in the work world. They may need education about how to end the cycle of poverty and how to be a role model for their own children.

Many people living in poverty are also addicted to drugs and alcohol, and need to be motivated to get into detox and drug-treatment programs. Similarly, people who are depressed or have other emotional disorders need access to counseling services and possibly medication simply to have the motivation and energy to take care of his or her own needs.

Problems of Children, Disabled Persons, and the Elderly

Historical Background

People in these groups were the first to receive government financial and social welfare assistance. What do these groups have in common that make them deserving of aid? Members of each group have physical limitations that prevent them from working, from defending themselves, and from living independently, all of which puts them at risk for being poor, abused, and taken advantage of. Society considers their vulnerability to be out of their control and therefore takes responsibility for providing for their needs and protecting them from harm.

Definition: Children, the Disabled, and the Elderly

From a legal standpoint, children are minors until their eighteenth birthday. Once children turn 18, they are considered adults and no longer have the protection and assistance they had as children. People are considered elderly at age 65. People described as disabled may have many types of physical and mental challenges, some of which were present at birth. Disabilities that usually receive assistance and protection are typically biologically based, such as mental retardation, blindness, cerebral palsy, and other physical handicaps, but also may include mental illness.

True Stories from Human Service Workers

The Needs of Those Living in Homeless Shelters

Because of the many needs of individuals and families living in poverty, agencies that serve this population typically offer a multitude of services. As with any human services agency and any population, needs are assessed and then clients are referred to one or more services aimed at meeting those needs.

For example, Cindy Snelling, assistant director of a homeless shelter in southern California, says that "the specific needs of this population is stability, safety, increased self-concept, a job, housing, food, and clothing."

The shelter offers safe and clean housing and food for at least 45 days. This time period creates some stability while its residents look for work. People staying at the shelter are also encouraged to participate in support and educational groups that often improve participants' self-esteem.

Prevalence

At the time the Americans with Disabilities Act was enacted into law (1990), about 43 million Americans had at least one physical or mental disability. This is about 5% of the total population of that time which was 248,709,873 (U.S. Census Bureau, 1990). As of 1995, 52.5 percent of people 65 years and older reported having at least one disability, and 33 percent reported having at least one severe disability (Doyle, p. 129, found in Kanel, 2007). Since the elderly population is growing, it is likely that human service workers will be assisting not only more elderly people, but more elderly people with disabilities. Advances in medical care have prolonged the lives of many who, in past years, would have died at a much younger age.

Not only does advanced medical care increase the lifespan of the disabled elderly, it increases all of our lives. The 2000 U.S. Census reports that in the United States, about 35 million people are age 65 and older, of whom 4.2 million are 85 and older. By 2050, an estimated 90 million people will be over the age of 65 (federal interagency forum on aging related statistics website).

During 2002, an estimated 1.8 million reports of child abuse or neglect were received by state and local child-protective agencies. Of those 1.8 million reported incidents, 896,000 were confirmed cases of abuse or neglect, nearly double the number of confirmed cases reported in1986 (Sedlack & Broadhurst, 1996).

Causality Models

It is quite evident that the primary cause of a person being a child, elderly, or disabled is biological. Because of this biological reality, these populations cannot control their circumstances, and therefore society regards them with charity and sympathy. There may be exceptions, such as a gang-related shooting in which a gang member becomes permanently disabled, but for the most part, these three groups tend to be seen as vulnerable and worthy of human services assistance.

Scientific research has proven the genetic origins of certain disabilities, such as blindness, mental retardation, epilepsy, cerebral palsy, Alzheimer's disease, and muscular dystrophy. Likewise, people who are in wheelchairs because they have lost the functioning of their legs and arms have biologically based disabilities. It may be true that lack of stimulation during childhood exacerbates mental retardation or that lack of mental stimulation throughout one's life can bring on Alzheimer's disease sooner, but the bottom line is that they are biologically caused. Despite society's willingness to provide services for people with disabilities, societal rejection of the disabled contributes to problems of the disabled, often causing feelings of shame and loneliness among this group.

While it is obvious that being young or elderly is a biological fact, the issues facing them might be viewed by some as psychological or sociocultural in nature. The fact that both of these groups are so often victimized might be viewed as a sociocultural phenomenon. American culture in particular holds negative attitudes toward the elderly. As has been discussed previously, this is ageism and often leads to poor medical care, manipulation of the elderly person's finances, and outright physical and sexual abuse of the elderly. Some believe that the elderly stop being worthwhile to society and therefore can be treated as less than a real person. Psychologically, the elderly may experience low self-esteem because they are no longer working or are suffering from poor physical health. This combination of low self-esteem and society's negative regard of the elderly create situations that are ripe for abusing elderly people.

Similar theories regarding the causes of victimization of children can be observed. Socioculturally speaking, many people in our society believe that children are to be seen and not heard. Some parents view children as not worthy of adult respect, and believe that the parents have the right to punish or sexually violate them in any way the parents see fit. It wasn't until 1974 that the federal government stepped in and created laws against child abuse. Traditional cultural and societal values held that families had the right to privacy, and that children were property of their parents.

Psychological causes of victimization relate to a person's coping skills, such as self-esteem and inner strength, that people develop in childhood from their parents. If children are raised to feel badly about themselves and are not equipped with the coping skills to manage life's stresses, they become vulnerable to being victimized. Sadly, even children who have developed healthy self-esteem may be victimized simply because the adult abusing them is bigger, smarter, and able to manipulate them psychologically.

Most people also believe that parents determine whether their children will have criminal behaviors. Laws are very lenient for children because their problems are viewed as resulting from a faulty psychological upbringing rather than from a deliberate decision to be deviant. Juvenile delinquency is also blamed on social factors, such as poverty and racism. At a certain age (usually 16), however, the criminal justice system begins treating children like adults because 16-year-olds should be able to make decisions on their own. Fortunately, that age is still 18 when it comes to providing protection from parental abuse because it is believed that child are not psychologically capable of coping with abuse until they reach legal adulthood.

Needs and Issues

These three populations are so often linked because of the similarities of their needs. All seem to be emotionally impressionable and therefore easily manipulated. Their physical limitations make them vulnerable to abuse. Because they often lack coping skills and are financially dependent on others, they are also at risk for being neglected. They simply cannot take care of their basic needs without assistance from others.

Children need guidance from stable and emotionally healthy adults to grow up physically and psychologically healthy themselves. They need both physical and intellectual nurturance. When this is not provided by their own parents, human services workers must intervene to ensure each child has the opportunity to grow and develop into a functioning adult. The earlier intervention takes place, the better it is for a child. Human services workers attempt to meet the need children have for a trusted adult who will protect them and help build their self-esteem. While it is true that society does address the need to protect children (e.g., child-abuse reporting laws), breaking up a family, even in a child's best interest, is usually discouraged. This may deny children access to the safe environment necessary for developing into happy and healthy adults. Providing the types of services children, especially those born into extremely disadvantageous circumstances, is costly. Sadly some children's race or socioeconomic status may prevent them from receiving the same services that are available to other children. We must never close our eyes to the effect that societal racism and classism have on all children.

In addition to emotional and psychological guidance, children also have basic needs, such as food, clothing, shelter, and medical attention. They are incapable of meeting these needs on their own and so must rely on others to meet them. When their own family cannot or will not provide for them, human services programs must intervene and meet those basic needs. Some children require extensive assistance, while others may only need help with medical care or food. Social service agencies have been created to protect children from abuse and to provide assistance for these basic needs.

The elderly also have difficulty meeting their basic needs, especially if they are suffering from illness or physical disabilities. Many elderly, often referred to as the **frail elderly,** require daily assistance to eat, get to the bathroom, get dressed, go to the doctor, or walk. Some elderly do not have enough money to support their needs entirely by themselves, and so they depend on others to supplement their income. Because they can no longer work and bring in new income, they must rely on retirement income, savings, or family financial assistance. Elderly also suffer from more medical illnesses than other segments of the population. They often need assistance simply to get to a doctor or pharmacy because many don't drive.

As of the writing of its pamphlet in 2004, according to the Alzheimer's Association an estimated 4.5 million Americans were suffering from Alzheimer's disease. This association states that the number is growing because the longer people are living, the greater the risk factor is for developing Alzheimer's. One in 10 people over the age of 65 and nearly half of those over the age of 85 are affected. A person with Alzheimer's disease can expect to live an average of 8 years and as many as 20 years from the onset of symptoms (Alzheimer's Association, 2004). Elderly people suffering from this debilitating disease usually require a daycare facility or 24-hour family care. This creates much stress on the caregivers, and, in the beginning phases of the illness, on the elderly person as well. The financial burden of caretaking can be as stressful as the emotional burden. Caretakers need to set realistic goals and expectations. They need to make time for activities that bring them joy and satisfaction and to get adequate exercise, nutrition, and rest. They may need to join a support group where they can be honest (Orange Caregiver Resource Center, No date).

Not all elderly are frail, but many of them still have special needs. Because of negative social attitudes about aging, the elderly are often left out and lonely. This makes them vulnerable to depression and suicide. They need social interaction and intellectual stimulation to feel alive and able to contribute to the world.

The elderly also need protection from physical, sexual, and financial abuse (sometimes called fiduciary abuse). Their physical weakness and susceptibility to manipulation of their financial holdings may increase the likelihood of their being the target of their own adult children or mail-order schemers. Unfortunately, sometimes residential facilities may take physical or sexual advantage of an elderly person. Government-run **adult protective services** agencies attempt to stop these abuses and prosecute the abusers.

Adult protective services also protect disabled adults when abuse is an issue. Issues of violence and abuse are the highest health priority for women with disabilities (Berkeley Planning Associates, 1997). These women are more likely to experience abuse by more **perpetrators** over longer periods of time than able-bodied women (Young, Nosek, Howland, Chanpong, & Rintala, 1997). They are less likely than those without disabilities to reap the benefits of the criminal justice system due to lack of mobility, communication barriers, and the social and physical isolation that exists for many disabled people. Unfortunately, disabled women who have been assaulted are often too ashamed to report the incident because the perpetrator may be a family member or a caregiver, and they may fear that there will be no one to care for them if they report the abuse (U.S. Department of Justice, 2001).

Many individuals who have been disabled since birth also receive services from **regional centers,** which are federally funded agencies that specialize in developmental disabilities and follow clients from birth to death. The type of needs a disabled person has depends on the type of disability. Some are capable of working and making enough money to support themselves but still need such services as protection from abuse. Some need advocacy services to ensure they aren't discriminated against. Others, however, do require services to take care of all basic living needs, such as food, shelter, clothing, medical care, and daily living care. Some people with disabilities prefer not to be referred to as disabled, but rather "differently abled," such as hearing impaired individuals. They usually can work and don't require financial assistance. However, they may be eligible for other forms of assistance due to their disability.

Some persons with disabilities need counseling to deal with depression and anxiety associated with their disability. The families of this population may need counseling to help them deal with feelings of sadness about their family member's disability. Self esteem may be an issue for the person who is disabled, and so counseling often focuses on the person's strengths and what they can contribute to society. There may be feelings of anger that the disabled person or the family needs to express and learn to manage. They may feel the disability is unfair and suffer from feelings of resentment. Unfortunately, if a person who is disabled carries a chip on his or her shoulder, he or she inadvertently pushes people away, increasing the feelings of isolation that often accompany being disabled. Facing the reality of having a disability is also an issue to be dealt with in counseling. Once the person or family comes out of denial, they then must deal with anger, depression, until they finally come to accept the disability and integrate it into their lifestyle.

In sum, all three groups need protection, assistance with basic needs, improved self-esteem, nurturance and emotional support, and encouragement to focus on their strengths and how they can be used to lead a productive life.

CRITICAL THINKING / SELF-REFLECTION CORNER

- What do you think would happen if the government did not provide financial assistance or medical care to people who could not afford to pay for their basic needs on their own?

- Do you think society would be better off without government-sponsored social welfare assistance?

- Do you think everyone is capable of working and taking care of themselves? If not, what types of people, in your opinion, cannot take care of themselves? Should they be entitled to government assistance?

- How do you feel about your tax dollars going to help protect abused and neglected children, the elderly, and people with disabilities?

- How do you feel about the government's using your tax dollars to provide food, housing, and income for unemployed, single mothers and their children?

- Do you think the government should provide medical care, housing, and food to unemployed men? Why?

Victims of Abuse

History and Background

People have been victimized throughout time. Perhaps it relates to survival of the fittest. The strong survive, and the weak submit, are abused, and even killed. Men do more victimizing than women do. Women are victimized more than men are. Protection for victims is a fairly new phenomenon. It wasn't until the 1980s that the United States enacted laws that made spousal abuse a crime. Mandatory child-abuse reporting laws weren't enacted at the federal level until 1974 when the Child Abuse Prevention and Treatment Act was passed (Nelson, 1984). Penalties for rape have become increasingly more severe, but many incidents are either never reported or never go to trial because of societal attitudes and biases that let rapists escape prosecution.

Identifying Abuse Victims

As mentioned earlier, the vulnerability of children, elderly people, and disabled people makes them all targets of abuse. Additionally, women are subject to being victimized both physically and sexually. This section addresses children who are abused and women who are victims of domestic violence and sexual assault. Although these groups all have much in common as victims of abuse, differences among the three groups exist and so each group will be presented separately in this section.

CHILD ABUSE

There are three types of child abuse. Physical abuse occurs when children are hit, burned, grabbed, choked, or punished in some other way that leaves a visible mark, such as bruises, scars, welts, or broken bones. These injuries must be sustained by other than accidental means. Sexual abuse occurs when an adult, or a minor who is capable of adult sexual gratification, engages in sexual behaviors aimed at gratifying either the child or the adult sexually. This may include sexual intercourse, masturbation, finger penetration, insertion of objects, or exhibition of genitals. General neglect is the other type of child abuse. This occurs when parents fail to provide for a child's basic needs, such as food, shelter, clothing, medical care, and supervision. Emotional abuse also occurs when adults repeatedly criticize a child and purposefully tear down the child's self-esteem.

DOMESTIC-PARTNER ABUSE

This section focuses on females who are abused by male partners. While men do live in abusive relationships with women, most would agree that women are at far greater risk of severe if not fatal injury from partner abuse than men are. This is due in part to a man's physical size and strength, which make him less physically intimidated by a woman. However, men may be subject to emotional abuse by women at the same rate as women are by men. So while this section focuses on women being abused by men, keep in mind that domestic abuse can occur in situations where two men are living together, two women are living together, and to men who are living with an abusive woman. When abuse occurs in these other relationships, the emotional needs are similar to those discussed in this section in which women are being abused by men.

People who are abused by domestic partners live in ongoing relationships in which they are beaten, choked, threatened, stalked, controlled, or raped. This is referred to as domestic violence, and may include women who are not married, but merely dating or living with someone.

SEXUAL ABUSE AND ASSAULT

Most sexual-assault victims are females, though men can also be victims of sexual assault, especially in prison. This section deals only with adult victims of sexual assault. Sexual assault occurs when one person forces any sexual behavior on another. This can include many types of forced physical contact, including rape (forced vaginal or anal penetration), forced oral copulation, and other sexual acts that one person is forcing on another.

Prevalence

According to worldwide estimates, at least one in three women has been beaten, coerced into sex, or otherwise abused during her lifetime (Heise, Ellsberg, & Gottemoeller, 1999). According to a study conducted by Silverman, Raj, Mucci, and Hathaway in 2000, approximately one in five female high-school students report being physically and/or sexually abused (2001). Many agencies and researchers have gathered statistics regarding the prevalence of rape in the 1990s. It has been discovered that during that time period, three out of four women who reported being raped and/or physically assaulted at least once after age 17, said the assailant was either a current or former husband, domestic partner, or date (U.S. Department of Justice, 1998). Based on research obtained in the 1980s and early 1990s, it has been discovered that an estimated 683,000 women are forcibly raped each year in the United States, meaning that every minute, 1.3 women are being raped (Kilpatrick, Edmunds, & Seymour, 1992). Child abuse reports, as stated in the previous section, reached almost 1,800,000 in 2002 and almost 900,000 cases were substantiated.

Causality Models

DOMESTIC ABUSE

In the past, people often blamed the victim for the assault, speculating that the woman "asked for it." If she was being battered by her husband, she must have done something to provoke him. Many women who sought help from clergy or their own mothers, were advised to "just be more loving to him," or "just try to keep the children quiet and have dinner ready," or "pray and hope things get better." Unfortunately, these suggestions do not solve the problems of spousal abuse. While modern-day thought puts more of the responsibility on the abuser, some people still blame the victim.

The causes for a woman being battered are not generally thought to be biological. However, many battered women are depressed, and so they are often the focus of mental health treatment. Since depression is often thought to be biochemically based, there may be some indirect link between biology and being battered. It is more likely, however, that psychological factors, such as low self-esteem, dependency, and fear, play a bigger part in being battered and continuing to live with a physically abusive spouse. Walker (1984) proposed that women stay in battering relationships because they suffer from **battered-women's syndrome,** which results from repeated episodes of abuse. The woman comes to believe that the situation is hopeless and that she can't do anything to fix it. She is afraid to leave because her husband may kill her or the children, for fear that she cannot survive on her own or that family and friends will reject her if she leaves. She may also believe that she loves her husband and that the children need their father. Many of these beliefs are irrational and can be altered through cognitive therapy. These feelings of helplessness, hopelessness, and worthlessness, cause women to live in a chronic state of emptiness and shock, and focus only on survival rather than escape. This lifestyle is similar to that of a prisoner of war. Both tend to blame themselves and seek their captor's approval without thought of escape.

Societal and political causality models also explain domestic violence. Many feminists believe that women are battered because society permits it. According to this causality model, punishment for domestic violence is not severe enough to deter it. The media portrays women as victims and men as aggressors. Women are taught since childhood that they aren't complete unless they have a man in their life. This often means that a bad relationship is considered to be better than no relationship at all.

SEXUAL ASSAULT

Feminist theory also suggests that the media, pornography, and overall socialization all contribute to the high rate of sexual assault on women. While some may still blame the victim for being raped, claiming that she is promiscuous, or a scorned lover, or that she was provocative, most social scientists do not hold these views. Instead, the rape victim is viewed as not having anything to do with being raped. She is simply a victim of a rapist who has needs to control and humiliate. Her only role is being female, weak physically, and perhaps too trusting. Some propose that a woman who is raped may not have the psychological resources to protect herself. She may be in shock once attacked and not be able to yell or fight. This may be a survival mechanism that could save her life.

Since date rape is the most common type, a woman may simply not know she is being raped. Some women believe that if they agree to talk with a man, kiss a man, get close physically with a man, or even engage in heavy petting, they are required to "go all the way." They do not know that they have the right to say "no" at any time. Lack of knowledge, then, is another factor that may play a part in sexual assault.

CHILD ABUSE

Unlike women who are battered and victims of sexual assault, children who are abused are not usually viewed as being the cause of their own abuse. Rather physical weakness and psychological insecurities and ignorance make them vulnerable to abuse by men and women who have abusive personality structures. Children in particular are often dependent on the abuser for their very survival and so they usually do not tell anyone they are being abused. While this doesn't cause the abuse, it does contribute to its continuation. Although most people, except for the abuser, do not blame the child for being abused, some people believe that children who are abused are bad and deserve to be punished physically, but social scientists vehemently disagree with this belief and instead believe that no abuse is acceptable or warranted because of something a child does or does not do.

Sadly, sexual abuse of children may be influenced by the media. Beauty contests, magazine ads, and movies often depict young girls and boys in adult roles and dress. Children are exposed to sexual activities at a younger age than in the past and may appear more sexually sophisticated than they really are. This may make sexual predators feel less guilty about engaging in sex with a child. Both boys and girls are vulnerable to being sexually exploited because of lack of psychological resources. They often do not understand the emotional implications of engaging in sexual acts. They may enjoy the attention at first, but then as they mature experience misgivings for having participated.

As far as neglectful treatment of children, it is doubtful that anyone would blame the child. Neglect is sometimes due to poverty, but is more commonly a result of the parent's psychological make-up.

Needs and Issues

Victims all need to feel empowered. They need to understand that they have survived the abuse and that they are not damaged. Victims may often suffer from **damaged goods syndrome,** in which they carry chronic feelings of being dirty, bad, and worthless. Being victimized leaves the person feeling powerless. Victims need to experience situations in which they are in control and able to make choices.

They also need to acknowledge the existence of the abuse. Denial is a typical reaction to being abused. Victims may not want to admit they were abused because they may feel ashamed or as if it were their fault. They need to understand that the perpetrator has the problem and they were victimized through no fault of their own.

Often, victims need to be educated about domestic violence, child abuse, or sexual assault. They need to be told that these are crimes. They also need to have a safe place where they can express their feelings and thoughts. Group therapy is extremely useful because many victims need to see that others have gone through the same experiences.

In general, victims need safety, trust, and someone to understand what happened without judging them. They need to see that they can have a happy life despite being abused. This often means helping them rebuild self-esteem and self-confidence. They also need help in reconnecting with people. After being victimized, some people close off to those they love or put walls around themselves to prevent others from getting too close. They truly need help in reaching out to others and feeling comfortable being close to others.

True Stories from Human Service Workers

Working with Battered Women at a Shelter

Battered-women's shelters exist throughout the nation. These agencies provide a multitude of services for women and children who leave their homes because the mother has been a victim of physical, sexual, or emotional abuse by boyfriends and husbands. The women and children often stay at the shelters for about 45 days, long enough to develop psychological and emotional coping skills and social resources to be able to live independently.

Example: Rosalba Acosta, the director of residential services at a battered-women's shelter in southern California says that, "The clients at the shelter have several needs. They have basic needs, such as shelter, clothing, and food. They have community resource needs, such as county assistance for financial aid and food stamps. They need counseling for post-traumatic stress disorder, suicide prevention, and referrals to mental health workers for serious mental health problems. They may also need help in transitioning to independent housing."

Clearly, these women exemplify the multi-needs client, and the agency appropriately offers a generalist and multidisciplinary team approach.

Criminal and Violent Behavior

Historical Background

Human services workers often work with people who break the law. Some of these clients behave violently and have harmed others, while others seem to be less violent and aggressive. People who commit crimes are often referred to as perpetrators. This term is most often used when discussing those who commit violence against others, such as child abusers. People who fall into this group have also been called criminals, deviants, and sometimes sociopaths. Society has always had to deal with this type of person. As we learned in Chapter 2, corrective action with this group has ranged from humanistic compassion to execution. Our current society still reacts similarly to this population.

Definition of Crime/Violence Perpetrators

Anyone who breaks the law has committed a crime. Crimes range in severity from misdemeanors to felonies. Misdemeanors are not punished as severely as felonies are. Felonious acts are often violent in nature, such as armed robbery, kidnapping, murder, and drug distribution. A misdemeanor might include such first-time offenses as minor drug possession, drunk driving, or passing bad checks. Our system tends to be easier on first-time offenders than on those who have a history of criminal behavior. California's three-strikes rule, established in the 1990s, mandates that if someone is charged with three felonies, that person will be prosecuted to the full extent of the law, which could mean receiving a life sentence.

Defining what constitutes a crime may be difficult because that which constitutes a crime differs from state to state. Some crimes, such as spousal abuse have only been crimes since the 1980s. Other crimes, such as murder, have been against the law since the beginning of civilization.

Causality Models

Why do people commit crimes? This question has been studied for the past 100 years by social scientists. Some believe that aggressive behaviors are caused by abnormal biochemistry that causes **bipolar disorder** or **attention-deficit hyperactivity disorder** (ADHD). Some scientists believe that people with these disorders are not in control of their behaviors. They would need medication to create balance in their biochemistry.

While it may be true that some perpetrators do indeed suffer from biochemical imbalances, others are probably more influenced by psychological and social factors. Psychoanalytic theory suggests that chronic criminality is due to **antisocial personality disorder.** People with this disorder have not developed proper superego capacity and do not feel remorse or guilt for aggressions against others, much like a 2 year old does not feel guilt if he or she hits someone. These people go through life as if the rules don't apply to them. They behave in ways to meet their needs without regard for others' needs.

Another personality disorder thought to be associated with certain crimes is referred to as narcissistic. Psychoanalytic theory suggests that this type of person is fixated at an early stage of psychological development (around age 3). His or her behavior is an attempt to satisfy primitive needs for recognition, power, control, and validation. **Pedophiles,** spousal abusers, and child abusers are often thought to be suffering from **narcissistic personality disorders.**

Some perpetrators were abused as children and often attempt to gain some type of restitution by violating another when they become adults. This payback theory is part of the psychoanalytic theory that proposes that people displace anger and aggression onto safer targets because they feel powerless to express their anger on the person who abused them. While being abused may be one cause of becoming a perpetrator, it is not the only cause. Humanistic theory might suggest that these perpetrators were not given enough love or nurturance and are deficit in self-esteem development. They were not raised by parents who were capable of providing a safe or realistic environment.

Social and cultural theories also attempt to explain why people perpetrate crimes. Poverty is thought to lead to crime. When people see others living within a standard of living above theirs, they often engage in behaviors, such as theft, robbery, burglary, and drug sales to get what others have. Living in violent neighborhoods may also lead to criminal behaviors. It may be the norm in certain communities to engage in violent acts against others, such as gang violence and partner abuse. If one is raised in an area where guns are prevalent, that person may think it is normal to possess and use guns. Likewise, if someone is raised in an area where people openly sell and use drugs, this behavior seems normal. Some communities have a culture of learned helplessness where people grow up believing that they cannot get out and advance their way of life. They may not even know that there is a different way of life. Using drugs, engaging in criminal activity, and acting out aggression may be seen as exciting. The idea of spending time incarcerated may not even bother this type of person.

Needs and Issues

Because perpetrators range from first-time offenders to chronic offenders, their needs and issues will vary from perpetrator to perpetrator. If someone does suffer from an antisocial personality disorder, that person has been committing crimes since childhood. People with antisocial personality disorders are difficult to treat with counseling and need to face the reality of what they are doing and face the consequences. If motivated to change, they can receive help and try to learn that positive results can happen if they can change their behavior. Reality therapy is a type of counseling in which the counselor attempts to create a safe, involved relationship in which the client can feel cared about by a responsible person. The focus is on helping this person meet his or her needs for feeling worthwhile, successful, and loved. It is very difficult to completely cure this type of disorder, but criminal behaviors can be controlled with proper intervention.

Other perpetrators need help gaining access to resources, such as education, employment, and other social welfare assistance. They may need intense guidance on how to become a successful contributor to society as well as intense monitoring on maintaining a structured lifestyle that does not include involvement with other perpetrators of crime.

Perpetrators of family violence and rape often need intense counseling. They must learn how to empathize with others and learn how to control their own needs. They often have many irrational thoughts and distorted beliefs about their behaviors that have permitted them to engage in violence against those whom they love. These need to be addressed in group, individual, and family counseling. Some of these perpetrators need to spend time incarcerated to keep society safe while they work on these issues. They may also need punishment, such as jail, to help them truly understand that there will be consequences for their criminal behaviors. To be truly helped, perpetrators must deal with their childhood traumas and learn how to successfully meet their needs as adults.

Substance Abusers

Historical Background

The use of mind-altering substances has been part of human behavior ever since man first discovered that certain plants induce euphoric states. It is widely known that opium was smoked thousands of years ago by ancient civilizations, such as the Chinese and Egyptians. Wine consumption was discussed in the Bible and was an integral part of ancient Roman ceremonies. Alcohol has been the number one used substance in the United States since its creation. At one point, there was an attempt to make alcohol use and distribution illegal. This didn't work however, and so alcohol remains the number one drug used because it is the only legal mind altering substance accessible without a physician's prescription. Other drugs, such as cocaine, opium-based drugs, and marijuana, can be traced back to the 1890s in the United States. At first, they were used medicinally. People then started using these drugs for pleasure and to enhance work performance. These drugs became illegal during the early 1900s under the Harrison Drug Act. Synthetic versions of these drugs have been created during the past 100 years and are also illegal. Despite the strict laws prohibiting drug use, many people still abuse drugs. Some are illegal drugs; others are legally prescribed by physicians. We are in general, a society of alcohol and drug users. Many social events revolve around drinking and using drugs.

Definition of Substance Abusers

The *Diagnostic and Statistical Manual IV (DSM-IV)*, (APA, 1994) puts people with **substance abuse** in one of two categories: **substance dependence** or **substance abuse.** Dependence means that without the drug, users suffer physical withdrawal. This person needs increasingly larger amounts of the substance to feel its effects. The dependent drug user suffers from one or more medical consequences as a result of using the drug. Abuse means that the drug is taken most of the time and creates impaired social, work, academic, or daily functioning. Abusers include both those who drink alcohol and those who take mind-altering drugs. Although nicotine and caffeine are addicting, they will not be addressed in this text.

Alcohol, amphetamines, cannabis, cocaine, hallucinogens, inhalants, opiates, and sedatives are all discussed in this section as they are the most commonly abused substances. Some are more addicting than others. Table 7.2 provides a brief look at the effects of different drugs.

Prevalence

In 2003, an estimated 21.6 million people (9.1 percent of the total U.S. population) 12 years of age and older were classified as having substance dependence or

Table 7.2 Substance Abuse

Drug	How Taken	Addiction Potential	Pleasurable Effects	Negative Effects
Alcohol	ingested	very addicting, may cause convulsions, shakes, hallucinations during withdrawal	euphoria, disinhibitions, pleasant taste	slow reaction time, too much causes nausea, blackouts, slurring, falling down, liver damage
Marijuana (Cannabis)	smoked, ingested	psychologically, not physically, addicting,	euphoria, silliness, laughter, sleepy, hungry (munchies)	a motivational syndrome, paranoia, depersonalization, kills brain cells, leaves tar in lungs
Cocaine, crack, crystal methamphetamine	snorted, smoked, IV injection	physically addicting, during withdrawal feels sketchy, paranoid, depressed, agitated	high energy, increased confidence, weight loss, diminished need for sleep	can't concentrate, poor social interaction, poor sexual performance, heart attack, stroke
Heroin	snorted, IV injection	very physically addicting, during withdrawal, feels sick, vomits, shakes	euphoria, release from all stress and pain	nodding out, needle marks, hepatitis, risk of HIV
Sedatives	ingested	very physically addicting, during withdrawal feels sick, convulsions, hallucinations, seizures	euphoria, sleepy, lack of anxiety, relaxed	feels out of it, can't function without the pills, liver damage, emotionally vacant
LSD	ingested	not addicting	euphoria, feelings of unreality, distortions of reality, increased visual and sensual pleasure	bad trip, paranoia, psychotic feelings of depersonalization, panic, anxiety
Ecstasy	ingested	not addicting	euphoria, heightened sensual pleasures, mind feels open and creative	heart palpitations, unconsciousness especially when used with other drugs, poor impulse control

(continued)

Table 7.2   *(continued)*

Drug	How Taken	Addiction Potential	Pleasurable Effects	Negative Effects
Inhalants	sniffed	addicting	euphoria, a rush of excitement	drowsiness, poor muscle control, suffocation, nausea, vomiting, damage to brain and central nervous system

abuse. Of those, 3.1 million used both alcohol and illicit drugs, whereas 3.8 million were dependent on or abused illicit drugs only, and 14.8 million were dependent on or abused only alcohol. Of the illicit drug users surveyed, 4.2 million, or 61.4 percent, used marijuana, .2 million used heroin, 1.5 million used cocaine, and 1.4 million used pain pills accessed illegally (National Survey on Drug Use and Health, 2003).

Causality Models

While there is probably not a genetic code inside people that makes them drink or use drugs, it is probable that certain people do have genetic codes that increase the chance that once a substance is used, they will become addicted to the substance. This appears to be especially true for alcohol.

There are also biochemical alterations in the brain as a result of ingesting certain drugs. Stimulants tend to increase the release of dopamine, which keeps people alert. Sedatives and opiates tend to release the chemicals, serotonin and endorphins, which create a sense of well-being and mediate pain. People become lazy and rely on drugs to make them feel good instead of engaging in other activities, such as exercise, work, and recreational activities.

Psychological theories suggest that substance abusers have various psychic imbalances resulting from deprivation as children and unresolved emotional pain. Substance abuse is seen as an attempt to blot out the awareness of anxiety and shame experiences. Family theories propose that substance abuse regulates family functioning. Having an addict in a family often leads to the creation of roles, such as enabler, hero, scapegoat, and victim, for various members in the family. There does seem to be some truth to this theory because when the abuser stops using, the family often goes into crisis mode until family members learn new ways of relating to one another. People who have difficulty with intimate relationships may use substances to cover up the anxiety they experience being close to others. When the abuser becomes sober, family members must now relate to each other in emotionally intimate ways, which can be felt as emotionally threatening.

Society might also play a role in substance abuse. Movies, television shows, magazines, and social events often encourage alcohol usage. Of course mainstream media does not support illegal drug abuse, but certain communities encourage people to try drugs. This is particularly true with teenagers. Peer pressure has long been thought to be a factor in substance abuse.

Needs and Issues

The main thing substance abusers need is to stop using! They must learn how to live a sober life. This requires learning how to cope with feelings that may have been denied for many years. They need to identify distorted thinking patterns and face life more realistically. Denial of having a problem is the number one obstacle in dealing with both the user and his or her family. They all must accept that there is a problem and work through feelings of shame and guilt.

Substance abusers must also develop a new lifestyle with new social connections. Often, their only social ties are with other abusers. They need to learn how to feel pleasure through socially acceptable activities. This process may take years to complete. Some believe it is an ongoing process that is never complete. The philosophy of Alcoholic Anonymous suggests that all addicts are merely recovering and are never cured.

People with Mental Disorders

Historical Background

As previously discussed in Chapter 2, mental illness has been viewed from a variety of perspectives throughout time. Whether mental illness was thought to indicate demonic possession, imbalances of bodily humours, or immorality, mental illness has existed from the beginning of humankind. Scientists today believe they are finally getting a handle on what causes mental disorders and how to regulate symptoms. However, the causes of mental disorders are still in dispute, which leads to disagreements about the best methods of treatment. Additionally, much of mental health treatment is based on managed care and state-funded programs. Unfortunately, these funding sources control who receives treatment and what kind of treatment is administered. There are laws that ensure certain rights for mental health patients as well as professional ethical codes. These ethical standards and laws were implemented because of the history of maltreatment of those afflicted with mental disorders. Ethical codes will be discussed in Chapter 11.

Definition of People with Mental Disorders

The term "mental disorder" refers to a variety of syndromes and diagnoses. It has been defined as "a clinically significant behavioral or psychological syndrome or pattern that occurs in an individual and that is associated with present distress or disability, or with a significantly increased risk of suffering death, pain, disability, or an important loss of freedom. In addition, this syndrome or pattern must not be merely an expectable and culturally sanctioned response to a particular event, for example, the death of a loved one. It must currently be considered a manifestation of a behavioral, psychological, or biological dysfunction in the individual" (APA, 1994, p. xxi). Table 7.3 lists some of the more common mental disorders and the general category under which each falls in the *DSM-IV.*

Prevalence

According to Comer (1995), 13 percent of people in the United States suffer from **anxiety disorders,** 65 percent with serious depression, 5 percent with personality disorders, 1 percent suffer from schizophrenia, 1 percent with Alzheimer's disease, and 10 percent suffer from drugs and alcohol difficulties.

Causality Models

Some disorders result from biological factors more than other factors, such as **schizophrenia,** delirium, dementia, and delusional disorders, bipolar disorder, major depressive disorder, **panic disorder, obsessive-compulsive disorder,** ADHD, and **pervasive developmental disorder.** There is believed to be a strong genetic component to each of these disorders. Scientists believe that neurotransmitters, such as dopamine and serotonin, are not released in sufficient amounts in people who suffer from these disorders. While it may be true that all disorders have a genetic component to them, some are considered to be more the result of psychological and social factors.

Personality disorders are considered to result from early childhood deprivations and deficits in relationship skills. These people didn't receive adequate nurturance, boundaries, or guidance from their parents and therefore do not have the skills necessary to function in society as adults who work and sustain themselves, or who can sustain healthy and satisfying relationships.

Many of the other disorders are also considered the result of inadequate parental love. Anxiety disorders can also be traced to early experiences of serious trauma, such as child abuse, a natural disaster, or war. Some anxiety and depression results from being rejected by peers during childhood. **Phobias** often come after experiencing a scary event (such as being bitten by a dog). **Eating disorders**

Table 7.3 Categories of Mental Disorders

Disorders Usually First Diagnosed in Infancy, Childhood, or Adolescence	Delirium, Dementia, and Amnestic and Other Cognitive Disorders	Schizophrenia and Other Psychotic Disorders	Mood Disorders	Anxiety Disorders	Dissociative Disorders	Gender-Identity Disorders	Eating Disorders	Adjustment Disorders	Personality Disorders
mental retardation	delirium	schizophrenia	depressive disorders	panic disorder	dissociative amnesia	sexual dysfunctions	anorexia nervosa	with depressed mood	paranoid
learning disorders	dementia	schizoaffective disorder	bipolar disorders	agoraphobia	dissociative fugue	paraphilias	bulimia nervosa	with anxiety	schizoid
motor skills disorders	amnestic disorders	schizophreniform disorder		specific phobia	dissociative identity disorder	gender identity disorders		with mixed anxiety and depressed mood	schizotypal
communication disorders		delusional disorder		social phobia	depersonalization disorder			with disturbance of conduct	antisocial
pervasive developmental disorders		brief psychotic disorder		obsessive-compulsive disorder				with mixed disturbance of emotions and conduct	borderline
attention-deficit disorder and disruptive-behavior disorders		shared psychotic disorder		post-traumatic stress disorder					histrionic
feeding and eating disorders		psychotic disorder due to medical condition		generalized anxiety disorder					narcissistic
tic disorders									avoidant
elimination disorders									dependent
									obsessive-compulsive

(Source: American Psychiatric Association (1994). *DSM-IV.* Washington, D.C. Disorders related to substance abuse are omitted from this table.)

are believed to be an attempt to be perfect to compensate for feelings of inadequacy or to feel in control. Perhaps a person with an eating disorder was raised in an extremely controlling family, and controlling the amount of food that's eaten is the only way to feel powerful.

Some counselors believe that dysfunctional family systems reinforce mental disorders to keep the family regulated. Certain disorders might help the family focus on the client instead of the problems between the husband and wife (e.g., a child "acts out," and the parents focus on the child rather than on their marital conflict).

Adjustment disorders usually occur when people do not have the coping skills necessary to deal with an unexpected situation. Although they may try to cope for awhile, without help, they will be overwhelmed by feelings of depression and anxiety, and their functioning will become impaired.

Society and culture may have some influence on mental disorder. For example the media's depiction of pencil-thin models may contribute to eating disorders in adolescent girls. Certain cultures permit behaviors that may seem like a mental disorder to mainstream culture (*ataque de nervios* found in Latinos) as was discussed in Chapter 6.

Needs and Issues

Most people with mental disorders need a safe place to talk about their problems. They need to know that help is available and that they are not alone. Privacy is vital, as is trust. Some may need medication and counseling, whereas others may need to be hospitalized.

The purpose of counseling is to create a relationship in which clients can be open, honest, and genuine when discussing their life experiences. Sometimes, clients need to discuss childhood traumas. Other clients need to discuss a current situation that they cannot cope with, and learn adaptive coping skills. Some people need to learn how to relax and learn stress management skills that include cognitive restructuring as well as behavioral changes. When the problems are due to dysfunctional family rules, clients may need family counseling to help change crazy rules and roles into more adaptive rules and roles.

CRITICAL THINKING / SELF-REFLECTION CORNER

- Do you think people who abuse children, commit rape, and abuse their partners should be treated similarly to people who have mental disorders? If not, should they be treated like criminals and be sent to prison?

- Should substance abusers be considered as having a mental disorder?

- Do you think people who abuse illegal drugs should go to prison or go to counseling?

- Should other criminals, such as burglars, forgers, and kidnappers, go to counseling or prison?

- How are these crimes different from child abuse, rape, and domestic violence?

- Do you feel that substance abusers and perpetrators of abuse and crimes should receive pity and charity, or rejection and punishment?

- Is it possible to rape someone, abuse a child, or batter a spouse without having a mental disorder? How so?

AIDS and HIV Patients

Historical Background

Acquired immunodeficiency deficiency syndrome (AIDS) was first diagnosed in the United States in the early 1980s. And almost since that time, human services workers have been involved because of the psychological and social impact this disease has on its victims. Stigmas have been attached to those diagnosed with human immunodeficiency virus (HIV) and with AIDS because of the way in which HIV/AIDS is usually transmitted. People who have HIV/AIDS may often be ostracized by society, discriminated against at work, and made to feel guilt and shame about having the disease, all of which could prevent people from being diagnosed and treated. To make it easier for those with or who suspect they are ill, special services that specialize in dealing with issues related to HIV/AIDS have become available in most communities. Although HIV/AIDS is not regarded as negatively as it was 20 years ago, the stigma still does exist. The notion that only gay men, drug addicts, prostitutes, and sexually promiscuous people contract HIV is still common among the misinformed who have not bothered to educate themselves about the disease.

Definitions of HIV and AIDS

HIV has been identified as causing AIDS. Someone who is infected with HIV is said to be seropositive or HIV-positive, whereas AIDS is the full-blown, active illness.

"AIDS means that the virus has invaded the body and disrupted the immune system so that it can't protect the body from various deadly infections, like cancer or pneumonia. It is a life-threatening disease that sooner or later kills most everyone who has it" (Kanel, 2007, p. 153). An opportunistic infection has invaded the body or T-cell count is very low, usually under 200.

Prevalence

In 2000, the number of U.S. residents living with HIV was estimated between 850,000 and 950,000, including approximately 180,000 to 280,000 who did not know they were infected (Fleming, Byers, Sweeney, et al., 2000). In 2003 alone, the estimated number of people diagnosed with AIDS in the United States was 43,171, of which, 31,614 were adult or adolescent males, 11,498 were adult or adolescent females, and 59 were children under the age of 13. During that same year, AIDS-related deaths totaled 18,017. From 2000 through 2003, an estimated 929,985 people in the United States have been diagnosed with AIDS, and approximately 524,060 people died from the disease during that same time period. (CDC website, 4/29/05).

Causality Models

There are five ways that HIV can be transmitted from one person to another: during sexual contact involving the exchange bodily fluids; by using dirty IV (intravenous) or tattoo needles that had been used by someone who has HIV/AIDS; from an infected mother to her baby during pregnancy, labor, delivery, or by breastfeeding; from a transfusion of infected blood or blood products; and through the bloodstream if contact with the feces or vomit of an infected person.

What causes someone to engage in behaviors that may lead to HIV/AIDS? Some people are considered innocent victims of HIV because their illness was not the result of promiscuous behavior. Infants who become infected from their mothers and those who have become ill from a blood transfusion are considered innocent, and social attitudes toward them are different from the way HIV-positive IV-drug users are regarded. The behavior considered the riskiest for contracting HIV is still unprotected sexual contact between two men. The second-riskiest behavior is sharing IV-needles. Drug addicts' need for a "fix" is often stronger than the possibility of being infected by a deadly virus. The third-riskiest behavior is unprotected sexual contact between a man and a woman (U.S. Centers for Disease Control, 2005).

Sexual urges, especially when mixed with alcohol or drugs, can also drive people to engage in risky behaviors, such as having unprotected sex with strangers or passing acquaintances. Discussions about sexually transmitted diseases are avoided because such talk may be considered rude in some subcultures. Also, using condoms during sex, which can protect people from infection, is prohibited by some religions. Although for the most part, society has opened up the dialogue about sex and HIV, however, many parents still do not talk to their children about sex, and children remain ignorant about the consequences of unprotected sex.

Until society condones open and frank discussions about sex and disease and makes sexual protection available to teenagers, sexually transmitted diseases will continue to spread. Society also needs to educate people about drug addiction and how it is one of the ways that HIV/AIDS can be spread to the heterosexual population. Although in 1999 gay men made up the largest segment of the U.S. population (42 percent) who were infected with HIV/AIDS, it's important to keep in mind that 33 percent of those with the disease were infected during heterosexual intercourse, and 25 percent became ill as a result of their IV-drug use (Centers for Disease Control and Prevention, 2002). Society must let people know that all people are susceptible to contracting HIV/AIDS.

Needs and Issues

People infected with HIV but who do not yet have full-blown AIDS need to first deal with being diagnosed with a potentially life-threatening disease. They often feel they've been given a death sentence. They need to be fully educated about how to live with HIV rather than die of AIDS. Knowing about available medications and how proper nutrition and exercise can improve their chances of survival can be helpful. They also need to deal with disclosing their diagnosis to any other intimate partners they may have had. This may mean disclosing dishonest behaviors, such as marital infidelities or drug use. Sometimes this may result in relationship break up and so the person needs a lot of support emotionally and sometimes financially. They also need to deal with their fears about lifestyle changes, such as becoming sober and celibate or using condoms during sex. For some newly infected HIV patients, suicide seems like the only way out, and these feelings must be monitored by counselors and case workers.

Once someone has AIDS, they have different needs and issues. They now must deal with the possibilities of death and dying. They may need help making out a will and coping with a life of ongoing illness. This will require medical care that may cause a person to be depressed. Being dependent doesn't come easily for some people, and they must learn to adapt to financial dependency and physical dependency. They may have to stop working and have someone take care of them daily. Again, suicide might be an issue and must be monitored (Kanel, 2003, p. 170).

In general, HIV/AIDS patients need emotional support, social involvement, and normal treatment. They need physical contact with others and to be as productive as possible for as long as possible, which for some may be 20 years or more.

At-Risk Behaviors in Adolescents

Historical Background

As society became less agriculturally based, teenagers became an increasing problem for families. Because they weren't busy working the farms from sun up to sunset, the newly freed adolescents had time on their hands. Teenagers aren't quite adults but do have the physical and mental abilities to engage in many adult behaviors unlike younger children. Adolescents have sexual urges similar to adults as well as the need to feel in control of themselves. Unfortunately, in their <u>search for independence</u>, their <u>emotional immaturity</u> can get them into trouble.

Defining the Problems

Of course teenagers deal with all sorts of problems, too many to list here. The issues and needs that underlie gangs, teen pregnancy, teen runaways, and teen self-mutilation and suicide apply to many other problems that teenagers face. These particular problems are examined here because they are considered to pose the greatest risk to adolescents' well-being. They are at risk of incarceration, dying prematurely, and of developing a dysfunctional lifestyle. If they can be dealt with before they reach adulthood, it is hoped that these dire consequences can be prevented.

GANGS

Many Latino, Asian, and African American adolescents join gangs of their peers for a sense of belonging and of family, especially if their lives at home are troubled. Gangs engage in various, often illegal, activities. Gang members must swear a loyalty oath that supersedes loyalty to their family. Gangs are known for engaging in violent behaviors and turf wars between other gangs. Gang members often wear a certain color or style of clothing that indicates affiliation with their gang. Of course, any race or cultural group can form a gang, such as white supremacists whose gangs are referred to as skinheads.

PREGNANCY

Teen pregnancy usually refers to pregnant females under the age of 20, whether or not they are married. When teenage girls have babies, they often are at risk of dropping out of high school, depending on welfare throughout their lives, abusing drugs and alcohol, being victims of domestic violence, abusing their children, and being unemployed (Simpson, Pruitt, Blackwell, & Sweringen, 1997).

RUNNING AWAY FROM HOME

Teenagers are considered runaways when they leave their legal residence without parental consent. Teens often run away because of a heated argument or to escape abuse. Sometimes, runaways do so to use drugs freely, commit crimes, or to experience what they imagine are the glories of freedom.

SELF-MUTILATION AND SUICIDE

Adolescence can be a very difficult time for many young people. Pressures from peers, parents, and school may seem overwhelming. In an attempt to cope with this barrage of demands, some teens cut their bodies with razors, knives, or needles to gain a sense of release from these pressures. This habit often becomes addictive and can create a cycle of self-loathing. For other teenagers these pressures are intolerable, and they see suicide as their only alternative .

Prevalence

In 2002, 433,000 teenage girls had babies (U.S. Census Bureau, 2004–2005). That figure doesn't even include those pregnancies that ended in abortion or miscarriage.

Surveys show that gangs exist in most cities and towns in the United States. In 175 cities with populations between 50,000 and 250,000, 84 percent had gang-related problems. Between 1970 and 1995 reports of gang-related problems in U.S. cities increased by 640 percent (Kenner, 1996).

In 1999, an estimated 1.7 million children and teens had either run away or were thrown out of their homes. Of those, 37 percent were missing from their caretakers' homes, and missing-persons reports were filed on 21 percent in an attempt to find them and bring them home. Adolescents between the ages of 15 and 17 made up about two-thirds of those children (*National Incidence Studies of Missing, Abducted, Runaway or Thrown-Away Children,* 2002).

After car accidents, suicide is the second-highest cause of death in adolescents between 15 and 19 years old (Wyman, 1982). Although this statistic may seem dated, Rogers, et al. (2001) state that despite suicide prevention efforts over the past 40 years, suicide rates have remained relatively stable.

Self-mutilative behaviors are seen in about 4 percent of the general adult population and in 40–61 percent of adolescents in psychiatric inpatient settings (Darche, 1990; Diclemente, Ponton, & Hartley, 1991) and in 14–39 percent of adolescents in the community (Lloyd, 1998; Ross & Heath, 2002).

Causality Models

For the most part, these adolescent problems are not considered to have a biological basis; however, that may not be true for self-mutilation and suicide. Teens with these behaviors may suffer from depression caused by a biochemical imbalance and are therefore biologically predisposed to engaging in such impulsive, self-destructive behaviors.

But for the most part, researchers and practitioners agree that psychological and social factors contribute to problematic behavior in adolescents. Adolescents are struggling for independence yet still need guidance and emotional support as they venture forward toward **autonomy.**

Having a baby may be the only way a teenager believes she can receive the nurturance that her parents were unable to provide. Becoming pregnant may also be a defiant act by some teen girls and their only way to **differentiate** from over-controlling parents. Additionally, a teen girl may believe that having a baby will make her feel better about herself or make her relationship with the baby's father more secure. Teenage girls might also become pregnant because they see no other future for themselves other than having babies and being taken care of by others. Perhaps she is unsuccessful in school and becoming a mother may seem to be a way out of hard work and study.

Simpson, et al. (1997) have identified several factors that put adolescent girls at high risk for becoming pregnant. These include living in poverty, being a member of a minority, and being the daughter of a teenage parent. Teen pregnancy can sometimes be thought of as part of the cycle of poverty.

Gang membership is also thought of as being caused by lack of needs being met in the teen's family. Drass (1993) found that kids who come from dysfunctional homes where they have been neglected or abandoned are most likely to join a gang. Gang members also tend to have grown up with little verbal communication, lack of structure, and no sense of belonging. In addition, most gang members come from one-parent families in which children and the parent have very little interaction. Drass also found that poor self-esteem, no sense of personal safety, and little if any adult guidance, combined with boredom and social alienation also increased the chances of gang involvement Other contributing factors included a lack of job opportunities and living in poverty. In many cases, the teen might be raised in an area where his or her parents are part of a gang as well as the majority of people in the neighborhood. Joining a gang may be expected and even necessary for actual survival if one is to live in that neighborhood.

Running away from home is also a way to achieve autonomy and independence. Some feel abandoned by their parents and seek the acceptance of anyone, so they run away to find a sense of belonging elsewhere. Others are seeking independence, but ironically they usually end up being controlled by pimps and other abusive people. The streets are neither safe nor glamorous, but are sometimes seen this way by confused and stressed-out teens.

As with all of the above problems, teens that self-mutilate or attempt suicide are usually attempting to deal with the tremendous stress of growing up. They either do not feel proper nurturance from their parents and peers or feel too much pressure from both groups. Adolescents are known for being impulsive, so it is no wonder that they attempt suicide often. They are second only to elderly, single men in suicide attempts.

Needs and Issues

All pregnant women need prenatal care and education, but this is especially true for teenagers that are pregnant. They are often misinformed or ignorant about how to care for themselves or their children and need guidance and medical care. They also need to learn to communicate their needs and to figure out ways to continue their education and find employment especially considering their upcoming lifestyle change. Overall, they need to become more independent but also need to learn how to access resources. Some teens may wish to terminate their pregnancy or give up their babies for adoption. These girls need support, guidance, and information so they can make the best choice for themselves and the baby. Of course, preventing future pregnancies is another issue for this group. They need access to birth control and counseling about abstinence.

Preventing gang membership, like pregnancy, is more effective before the fact than after a gang is joined. At-risk teens need to be identified early on, before they enter high school. Children of minorities who come from single-parent, poor homes need special guidance, encouragement, after-school programs, and role-models to help them increase their self-esteem and believe that they have a future outside of gang membership. They may need tutoring to help with school work. They usually benefit from intervention that works on strengthening parent-child communication.

In general, the parent-child relationship determines whether an adolescent can get back on the right track. Although peers have a strong influence on teens, parents must not give up. Some parents feel that once their child is a teenager, their parental duties are finished. Not so. This is the time when parents must increase communication, get to know their teens as people, show respect for them, and maintain structure, supervision, and allow for some autonomy. When parents demonstrate these behaviors with their teens, many problem behaviors can be avoided or reduced significantly.

CRITICAL THINKING / SELF-REFLECTION CORNER

- Would you be afraid to touch a client or be in the same room with a client who has been diagnosed with HIV/AIDS? Why?

- Do you hold any prejudices or stereotypes about people who are HIV-positive?

- What are your thoughts about immorality leading to the AIDS epidemic?

- Could you provide a pregnant teen with information about pre-natal care, adoption services, or abortion services in an objective manner? If not, do you think human services workers should offer unbiased advice?

- What stereotypes do you hold toward gang members? How might these affect your ability to be empathic with this population?

Chapter Summary

Many people in society might benefit from human services. Certain problems seem to be the focus of human services workers more than others. Individuals and families living in poverty often use services to help them survive. There seems to be a cycle of poverty that continues without some form of assistance by human services workers. Children, the elderly, and people with disabilities also seem to utilize human services frequently due to their vulnerable and dependent status in society. They often need financial assistance and protection from abuse. Adolescents have other special needs due to their developmental needs to individuate from their family. While adolescents may have physical strength and intellectual knowledge to survive on their own, they are often emotionally unprepared to manage the world around them, which may lead to a variety of problems necessitating the services of human services workers.

Other populations that need human services include both victims and perpetrators of abuse, individuals who abuse drugs and alcohol, individuals suffering from a variety of mental disorders, and people suffering from the social and psychological ramifications of HIV/AIDS. The prevalence rate of all of the above mentioned groups is high and the specific needs vary from group to group.

Suggested Applied Activities

1. Watch a movie or a television show that focuses on one of the populations described in this chapter. Write down the main issues and needs facing one of the characters.

---

2. Choose five people to interview briefly. Have them agree to share a minimal amount of information about themselves. During each interview, find out whether the person has had some exposure to substance abuse either personally or because of a family member or close loved one. How many have been victims of some form of abuse? How many know someone who is infected with HIV? How many have had experience with teen pregnancy, gangs, running away, or teen suicide or self-mutilation? How many have or know someone or know someone who has a mental disorder? Of course, they can share as little or as much as they feel comfortable. Don't use anyone's real names if you write down their information. Keep all conversations private. Make sure the people are emotionally healthy enough to share such information. Perhaps choose friends or family members you know well. You can even include yourself. How many of these issues have you dealt with in your life? This exercise may help you understand how common these problems are in our society, hence the need for human services workers.

Chapter Review Questions

1. What are the types of child abuse? Describe each.

   _____

   _____

2. Why are children, the elderly, and the disabled at risk of being abused in our society?

   _____

   _____

3. What does learned helplessness mean and how does it relate to being poor?

   _____

   _____

4. How might psychoanalytic theory explain why certain individuals abuse and violate others?

   _____

   _____

5. What needs do adolescents have that often result in pregnancy, gang membership, running away, and self-destructive behaviors?

   _____

   _____

6. What is Alzheimer's disease?

   _____

   _____

7. What is the difference between substance dependence and substance abuse?

   _____

   _____

8. Name five mental disorders and their symptoms.

_____

_____

9. What is the difference between having AIDS and being HIV-positive?

_____

_____

10. How does HIV spread from one person to another?

_____

_____

Glossary of Terms

Adult protective services are government-funded agencies established to protect the elderly from abuse and neglect, whether they are living in nursing homes or are being cared for by family members at home.

Antisocial personality disorder is a pattern of behavior that displays a lack of regard for people and rules. People with this personality disorder lack feelings of guilt, seem to have no conscience, and usually have a history of criminal behavior.

Anxiety disorders are a group of mental disorders in which the primary symptoms are anxiety, fear, worry, and panic.

Attention-deficit hyperactivity disorder (ADHD) is found in young children who exhibit restlessness, inability to concentrate, impulsivity, and misbehavior.

Autonomy is a sense of self-sufficiency and independence

Battered-women's syndrome is seen in women who repeatedly find themselves in abusive relationships. They often begin to lose hope about ever escaping the abuse and focus only on survival within the abusive relationship.

Bipolar disorder previously known as manic depression, is an illness in which sufferers experience extreme mood swings, from feelings of elation to those of deep depression.

Cycle of poverty occurs when living in a state of poverty becomes an accepted way of life that is passed down from parents to children.

Damaged-goods syndrome is an emotional and cognitive response to having been raped or molested as a child so that the victim feels dirty and ashamed for having been abused.

Deserving poor are those who are poor through no fault of their own, such as children, disabled people, or the elderly.

Differentiating is the process of becoming autonomous in one's thinking and feeling.

Eating disorders are a variety of food-related disorders in which sufferers become obsessively involved with body image and what they are eating and how it will affect their bodies. They usually have unrealistic body images.

Frail elderly refers to older people who are in poor health and therefore physically weak, requiring assistance in activities of daily living.

Learned helplessness is the inability to escape poverty or an abusive relationship and instead accepting and living with the situation as if it's the only alternative.

Narcissistic personality disorder is characterized by a constant need for admiration and validation from others to counteract feelings of insecurity and a weak sense of self. People with this personality disorder are usually selfish and incapable of empathy for others.

Panic disorder is an emotional disorder that involves recurring experiences of shortness of breath, sweating, chest discomfort, nausea, among other things, along with feelings of going crazy and of losing control.

Perpetrators are people who commit crimes and violate rules.

Personality disorders are a group of mental disorders that impair a person's ability to interact and experience the world rationally. They are typically caused from deprivations in early childhood.

Pervasive developmental disorder is used to describe the symptoms of autism, such as head banging, poor eye contact, and an inability to interact with others.

Phobia is an anxiety disorder that causes people to have fearful reactions to an object or a situation that are so extreme that they cause people to avoid the object or situation at all costs.

Poverty is a state of extreme economic distress that results in a substandard quality of life. Poverty, as defined by the government for the purpose of determining the amount of assistance that people need, changes depending on the economic standard of living in society.

Regional centers are government-funded agencies that assist people who are physically and mentally disabled from birth.

Schizophrenia is a psychotic disorder that causes people to have delusions and hear voices and prevents normal functioning.

Substance abuse occurs when a person uses drugs or alcohol to the extent that they cause impaired social, behavioral, occupational, or academic functioning and whose friends also overuse drugs and alcohol.

Substance dependence occurs when users suffer medical consequences of drug and alcohol abuse and are physically addicted to the substance.

Underemployed is used to describe a person whose job skills and earning potential exceed that individual's current employment situation.

Case Presentation and Exit Quiz

Introduction

While the following case may seem extreme and even outlandish to some, it is based on actual events. The names have been changed, but the details and events are real.

Case History and Demographics

Debbie is a 38-year-old Caucasian woman. She was born into a Mormon family and has practiced her faith throughout her life. She has been married for 12 years and has three boys, ages 10, 8, and 4. Before she married, Debbie worked as a hairstylist. She stopped working outside the home when her first son was born and hasn't worked since. Her husband worked and paid the bills after she quit. Her husband was married previously and his 12-year-old daughter has been living with them for the last five years. Her husband has a tense relationship with his parents and thinks they are very controlling. His parents were strict disciplinarians and were often physically abusive.

Debbie and her husband live in a lower-middle-class home, which was bought by her in-laws' and so they own it, although Debbie and her husband pay the mortgage. All their children's needs have been met, and Debbie and her husband socialize either with his parents or with other people from their church. When the couple have had financial problems, her husband's parents, as well as the church, have come to their assistance.

Last year, Debbie's husband hurt himself on the job and was no longer able to work. He received $300,000 from workmen's compensation, and additional funding for training in a new occupation at a local community college. He put all of the money in his parents' bank account. He shows no income on his income tax returns.

Recently, her husband was charged with physical abuse of his daughter. She arrived at school one day with welts on her legs and told the school counselor that her father whipped her with a belt because she talked back to him. The case was referred to child protective services, and her father was ordered to attend 16 parenting classes and seek personal counseling for six months. He complied with these orders, and both daughter and father were allowed to remain in the home as long as Debbie was there to ensure the daughter was protected.

Current Problems

Debbie and her husband have had a history of marital violence. Her husband has hit her on several occasions and more recently attempted to choke her and gave her a black eye. Two days later, when Debbie called a battered-women's shelter hotline, she was told to come to the shelter and to bring her children. Since the daughter was not legally hers, Debbie called the child's biological mother who was not interested in taking care of her daughter. So Debbie took all four children to the shelter too. While at the shelter, Debbie spoke with the bishop of her church who advised her to go home and try to be more patient with her husband. He recommended that she keep the family together and try to be a better wife and mother. When the shelter workers heard of Debbie's plans to return home, they told her that if she tried to come back to the shelter after another episode of domestic violence, they would have to call protective services and her children would be taken from her because of the emotional abuse they were suffering as a result of Debbie's inability to protect them.

Despite those warnings, Debbie returned to her husband, and for a while things were calm. Unfortunately, a few months later, her husband threw a telephone at her, which broke her wrist. Debbie became very frightened and as soon as he left the house, she took her children to the shelter. After she explained to the shelter staff what had happened, they told her they would have to inform child protective services as they had told her they would if she returned. A social worker from child protective services came to the shelter, interviewed the children and Debbie. She decided to place Debbie's three boys in foster homes and to send her stepdaughter to live with her biological mother. Debbie was allowed to stay at the shelter for 45 days.

After her stay at the shelter was up, Debbie had nowhere to go. Her husband's parents had sold her home. Her husband was living with his very affluent parents and had filed for divorce, with his parents' money. Debbie had very little support system. She was estranged from her parents who were very abusive to her as a child. They wanted nothing to do with her. She met a man at a bar one night and he offered to let her stay with him until she could get on her feet. Within one month, he began battering her, so she left him. She found a job as a hairstylist and made enough money to live in a motel. She eventually rented a room from a woman.

The Department of Social Services referred her to a counselor so the counseling was free to her. She was very depressed and often considered suicide. The church gave her some food and money from time to time, but that stopped when her car broke down and was no longer able to attend church. She didn't have enough money to fix it. The social worker from protective services developed a case plan that ordered Debbie to get counseling and set up a visitation schedule for her and her sons at their foster homes, which were 30 miles away from where Debbie was living, making it very difficult for her to visit them regularly without a car. From the social worker's point of view, Debbie wasn't following the case plan, and they began to have a hostile relationship.

The husband was able to visit his sons because his parents' car was at his disposal. He was also ordered to attend parenting classes. He hired an attorney who got the domestic violence charges reduced to disturbing the peace, so he didn't have to attend any batterer's treatment groups. Since he had been complying with the social services case plan to visit his sons, he was eventually awarded full custody of them. After all, he lived in a nice home with his parents in a nice neighborhood. Even though he didn't work, he had means to support his children.

Debbie was given visitations every other weekend. She wasn't entitled to any of the $300,000 that her husband put in his parent's bank account. She wasn't entitled to receive any welfare benefits because her children didn't live with her. Because she worked, she had to pay the husband child support!

As unbelievable as these events may seem, they did actually take place. Before moving on to the quiz, take some time to think about the situation calmly and your emotional reactions to it.

Exit Quiz

1. Debbie has a variety of needs because of
   a. poverty issues
   b. child-abuse issues
   c. depression
   d. all of the above

2. Debbie's poverty resulted from
   a. her being lazy
   b. her lack of motivation
   c. her being underemployed
   d. all of the above

3. To help Debbie avoid future violent relationships, the counselor should focus on
   a. reducing Debbie's dependency on a man
   b. empowering Debbie
   c. understanding why Debbie finds unconscious satisfaction in being abused
   d. all of the above

4. When Debbie's sons were taken from her, the social worker probably believed
   a. that her husband was a better parent than Debbie was
   b. that Debbie would beat them because she was abused
   c. that witnessing their father beat their mother was causing them emotional harm
   d. all of the above

5. For the counselor to help Debbie's depression, Debbie probably needs to
   a. talk about her problems with her own parents
   b. be evaluated by a psychiatrist for schizophrenia
   c. be confronted about her attempt to take advantage of the system
   d. none of the above

6. The shelter staff demonstrated
   a. sensitivity to Debbie's religious beliefs
   b. insensitivity to Debbie's religious beliefs
   c. unethical behaviors by reporting the case to child protective services
   d. none of the above

7. The husband's abusive behavior probably resulted from
   a. being married to an incompetent wife
   b. having bad children
   c. being raised by controlling and abusive parents
   d. inflated self-esteem

Exit Quiz Answers

1. d	4. c	7. c
2. c	5. a	
3. b	6. b	

CHAPTER 8

Micro- and Mezzo-Level Assessments and Interventions

Introduction

Many of the problems that bring clients in to see human services workers can be dealt with using three levels of intervention, two of which are examined in this chapter. **Micro**-level interventions focus on working with an individual, **mezzo**-level interventions involve working with families and small groups, and macro-level interventions involve working with organizations and communities (Alle-Corliss & Alle-Corliss, 1999). Chapter 12 examines macro-level interventions, which usually require change throughout a broad societal spectrum and within communities.

Human services workers must assess all the needs of an individual or of a group, decide which type of intervention is most appropriate, and then assist them in accessing services to meet the needs or to personally provide services to meet the needs. Knowledge of various interventions is vital when assessing a client's needs as it guides the human services worker through the **assessment** and subsequent referral process. Also, human services workers often work collaboratively with others to best meet the needs of clients, and so the assessment process includes considering which community agencies and which types of human services workers should be involved in the case. Assessment includes determining the needs of a client and the appropriate services to meet those needs.

Primary, Secondary, and Tertiary Intervention

People who seek services have various types of needs or problems. Just as clients' needs ranges from extreme to minimal, interventions range from preventative to life maintenance.

Primary Interventions

Primary prevention usually includes efforts to prevent the occurrence of a disorder or a problem. These efforts are typically used with people who appear to be either functioning normally or at-risk but have not yet demonstrated a need for human services. Broadly speaking, this type of prevention includes social policy development aimed at reducing environmental stress and enhancing life opportunities and educational programs that offer adaptive skills and alternatives to at-risk populations (Price, Cowen, Lorion, & Ramos-McKay, 1988). Some well-known examples include the **D.A.R.E.** (Drug Awareness Resistance Education) program offered to elementary-school children, **Scared Straight** (a program in which at-risk teens visit prison and speak with convicts), **Project Head Start** (a program for low-income, disadvantaged preschoolers), and parenting classes for adolescents in high school.

Secondary Interventions

Secondary interventions include efforts to assist people who have already demonstrated early signs of dysfunction or problematic behaviors. Such interventions should be immediate, and if provided early enough, the problem's **prognosis** is good. **Crisis intervention** is one of the best examples of secondary intervention. The goal is to prevent people from developing **chronic** problems and to maintain functioning in as many areas as possible. Many of the problems that are suited for this level of intervention result from situational stress. Some are emergency situations and may have a life-threatening component, such as an attempt at suicide or the onset of psychotic behavior. Others may not necessarily be considered emergencies, but should still be dealt with quickly. The crises may arise from normal transitional and developmental situations, such as the birth of a baby, marriage, or adolescent rebellion. Crises may also result from unexpected traumatic events, such as rape, divorce, unemployment, death, diagnosis of an illness, or extreme natural or human-caused disasters, as in the terrorist attacks of September 11, 2001, and Hurricane Katrina's destruction in New Orleans in 2005).

Tertiary Interventions

Tertiary interventions are typically used with people who suffer from chronic problems and have difficulties caring for themselves. Many of these people are in a state of chronic distress and need ongoing rehabilitation and possibly even long-term institutionalization. Examples of tertiary care include long-term stays at psychiatric hospitals, ongoing attendance at Alcoholics Anonymous meetings, incarceration, and indefinite periods in **residential facilities.**

Unfortunately, secondary and tertiary programs receive the largest portion of government funds (Newton, 1988). It might be more useful to fund programs that prevent problems from occurring rather than waiting for problems to materialize before fixing them.

Assessment

To best meet a client's needs, human services workers must identify what a client's specific needs are. The purpose of such an assessment, then, is to determine the most appropriate intervention plan for each client. In conducting an assessment, human services workers should include the following:

1. Identify a client's presenting problems: Why did the client seek services at this moment in his or her life?
2. Identify a client's specific needs: Clients usually have more than one need.
3. Identify whether the problems are serious, moderate, or minor: This will help workers decide what type of intervention—primary, secondary, or tertiary—is required. Severe problems can impair a client's functioning in one or more areas, such as work, academics, relationships, and activities of daily living, such as eating and sleeping.
4. Identify how frequently these particular problems occur: Problems that are chronic—long-term, ongoing—usually require tertiary intervention.
5. Identify who is most suitable to provide some or all the services needed to assist clients with the problem. At times, human services workers may need to refer a client to other workers and find multiple resources to assist a client.

Prioritizing Problems and Collaborating with Others

Another aspect of the assessment process relates to prioritizing needs, sometimes called **triage.** Because a client's needs often differ in severity and importance, human services workers must help their clients decide which needs must be dealt with first, second, third, and so on. Clients whose chronic problems receive ongoing tertiary intervention also may have emergencies and crises that require immediate intervention, beyond the established tertiary measures. For example, an individual suffering from schizophrenia who lives in a board-and-care home (tertiary intervention) may have attempted suicide. This is an emergency requiring secondary, or crisis, intervention and emergency hospitalization. Another example might be a client who has had a long period of sobriety and had been going regularly to Alcoholics Anonymous meetings but was recently arrested for drunk driving. His immediate needs include emergency medical and legal assistance, then crisis intervention (secondary intervention). His involvement in AA is still important, but is secondary to the crisis and emergency at hand. Commonsense dictates that if someone is lying in a hospital bed, vomiting up an overdose of pills after a suicide attempt, a human services worker should not be encouraging the client to discuss low self-esteem issues. Rather, the client needs first to deal with the medical emergency at hand. After the emergency aspect has passed, the client might be ready to talk about what was the reason for the overdose of pills (secondary intervention).

Because clients often present with more than one problem, they must receive services from a variety of human services workers. This requires **collaboration** among workers to best meet the overall needs of the clients. Frequent consultation, open communication, and flexibility among the various workers are vital in providing effective intervention for clients. The multidisciplinary approach is paramount in ensuring that all or most of a client's needs are met. Although human services workers are generalists, and are capable of working with many problems, there simply isn't enough time in the day to meet all of a client's needs by oneself. The generalist knows how to detect needs, how to manage immediate needs, and how to utilize the vast array of resources available in the community for ongoing assistance. Being practical and resourceful are two of the human services worker's most effective qualities.

During the assessment phase of an interview with a client, the human services worker attempts to identify the problem, and design a plan to solve it. Maintaining a state of mind that permits flexibility, that allows for a holistic approach, and that embraces the idea of working with other human services workers for the sake of the client, leads to the most effective intervention.

Micro-Level Intervention Strategies

Deciding on an intervention strategy depends on the function and role of the assessing human services worker at his or her agency. Sometimes, workers provide all the services as part of their job duties. At other times, a worker's duty is to merely identify problems and connect the client with an appropriate resource to solve it. Regardless of the specific duties of any worker, knowledge of community resources is essential in providing effective intervention. In addition to resource utilization knowledge, human services workers must have knowledge about many different types of problems, their causes, and their specific needs. Workers must also have a basic understanding of what causes a client's problems. Knowing all of these facets can help human services workers provide the most appropriate and effective intervention available. The concept of "generalist" truly comes into play when designing and implementing interventions.

Crisis Intervention

This is a short-term counseling approach. However, workers do not necessarily have to be counselors to provide crisis intervention, which can be conducted by many types of workers, including social workers, correctional officers, and school personnel, in a variety of settings. This is because crises occur regularly in the lives of most people. In providing crisis intervention, workers must assess the client's presenting needs, offer some new perspectives on the problem, and help the client decide on the interventions that will be most helpful in effectively managing the crisis. Sometimes workers refer clients to outside agencies and workers, and at other times the crisis can be managed in-house, without input from others. An important part of the assessment phase is determining how much intervention will be provided by the worker doing the assessment and how much will be provided by others.

Crisis intervention focuses on identifying the precipitating event (a situational or developmental stressor), and how clients' perceptions of this event have led to negative, painful feelings and impairment in functioning. Once the nature of the crisis has been identified, the crisis worker then offers new ways of thinking about the situation and offers new coping skills. The usual duration of crisis intervention is no more than six weeks. Many agencies and facilities follow this model and offer 45-day-treatment programs.

THE ABC MODEL OF CRISIS INTERVENTION

The **ABC Model of Crisis Intervention** (Kanel, 2007) offers a helpful guide for conducting short-term, problem-focused counseling.

A: Basic Attending Skills: These interactions include active listening, paraphrasing, reflection, and open-ended questions (discussed in Chapter 4). Such questions create a sense of safety and trust that help encourage clients to discuss their problems freely and openly. The crisis worker wants to develop a strong relationship with the client rather quickly to ensure that the client accepts the counselor's suggestions and referrals.

B: Identifying the Problem: To properly design appropriate intervention, counselors must understand what triggered the crisis, how the client perceives and feels about the situation, and the areas in which the client is having trouble functioning. Once the nature of the crisis is appropriately identified, the crisis worker must offer the client new ways of thinking about the situation. Often this requires education, cognitive restructuring, and empowerment. Once clients perceive the crisis differently, they will be better able to accept various coping solutions offered by the worker because the client will be feeling better. Crisis theory suggests that feelings of distress are closely linked to how a person perceives the situation, so if the perceptions are changed, the emotions will be changed as well.

C: Coping: Solutions may be offered during this stage and include suggestions, such as keeping a journal, exercising, going to **support groups,** connecting with other human services workers, and working on assertive communications and stress management (both of which will be described in Chapter 10).

Crisis intervention is provided for many problems because it is immediate and useful in assisting people to function in as many areas as possible in their lives. It is cost effective and encouraged by most agencies. It can be by phone, such as when a client calls a suicide hotline, or in person during a normal office visit. It can last as long as two hours, such as when someone is severely suicidal and may need to be hospitalized, or be resolved in 10 minutes as is often done in residential living facilities, such as when a resident has a conflict with another resident and a worker steps in to help resolve the conflict.

Suicide Assessment and Intervention

An assessment skill used in crisis intervention as well as when working with clients who are not in crisis is assessing for **suicide risk.** This skill is vital for any human services worker who has direct involvement with clients. The goal of **suicide assessment** is to determine whether a client is actually intending on doing himself or herself harm. Suicide prevention is the goal once the risk level is assessed. The prevention strategy differs depending on the assessed risk level.

Not every client who feels suicidal will openly disclose this to a human services worker. These thoughts and feelings must often be explored in connection to other complaints and presenting issues. Some typical statements made by clients who may be suicidal include:

"Life's just not worth living anymore."
"Why should I bother to try? Nothing ever goes my way."
"I wish I could just sleep and never wake up."
"I have to find some way to get out of my depression." (Sometimes a person's depression lifts because they have decided to kill themselves as a way out of it.)
"I'm so alone, and no one cares if I live or die."

Of course some people actually say, "I think about killing myself." In addition to assessing for suicide when a client discloses one of the previous statements, suicide assessment is a good idea whenever someone states that he or she feels very depressed. Other factors that may make someone at risk for killing or harming themselves include living alone, drinking alcohol excessively, taking drugs, attempting suicide in the past, knowing someone who has committed suicide, and suffering from chronic physical pain.

STAGES USED IN SUICIDE ASSESSMENT

Assessing for suicide risk usually is done in stages (see Table 8.1). Human services workers that suspect a client may be thinking about suicide must first ask whether this suspicion has merit. The stages progress logically from first thinking about suicide, to making a **plan,** to identifying what **means** are needed to carry out the plan, and to wondering what, if anything, can persuade a client from carrying out the plan. While many risk factors are associated with committing suicide, the following are the essential factors that human services workers must assess to determine an effective intervention strategy. Remember, the goal of a suicide assessment is to gather enough information to understand the risk level of a client at the time of the assessment. Once the risk level is assessed, the best intervention plan can be implemented.

Stage 1: Are There Thoughts of Suicide? The first stage is assessing for **suicidal ideation.** When clients present with one of the previously mentioned factors or appear to be considering suicide, workers should ask clients directly whether they have had thoughts of harming or killing themselves. Some possible questions are, "Have you had thoughts of hurting yourself?" "Have you thought about committing suicide?" or "You mentioned that you are very depressed; sometimes people who are depressed think about suicide and death. Have you?" Workers who are just starting their careers often worry that such questions will make someone want to kill themselves. However, this does not typically happen. If someone has no thoughts about suicide, asking them may help them realize that maybe his or her problem is not so bad after all. He or she will usually respond with an emphatic "no." However, clients who have had such thoughts may feel relieved to talk about them openly.

If a client denies any suicidal ideation, a worker can assess the client's needs and proceed with basic counseling, crisis intervention, or case management, depending on what intervention is appropriate. A client at a low level of risk can usually benefit from a variety of services. A brief description of common interventions follows the section on suicide assessment. If a client reveals ongoing thoughts about suicide, the worker must then proceed to the next stage of assessment.

Stage 2: Is There a Plan? This next stage of assessment determines whether a client has a plan for committing suicide. This refers to the method of suicide a client intends on using. Typical plans include overdosing on pills, hanging, shooting oneself, driving off a cliff, and cutting oneself with a razor blade. If someone has thoughts of suicide but has no plan, that person may still be assessed as low risk and should be monitored regularly to make sure that he or she still does not have a plan. If a client admits to having a specific plan, the worker must proceed to the next stage of suicide assessment.

Stage 3: Are the Means Available? The next piece of information needed is whether the client actually possesses the means to carry out the plan. Once a plan is disclosed, workers must find out if a client has a gun, pills, rope, razor blades, and the like. If a client does not have whatever is needed to carry out the suicide plan, then that person may still be considered at a low risk for suicide. When clients have **suicidal ideation** and a plan, they should be monitored closely to ensure that the means to carry out their plans have not been obtained. A verbal **no-suicide contract** is a good idea. The client is asked to make a verbal contract with the worker, promising not to commit suicide. If a client agrees, it is a good idea to shake hands and solidify the contract. This client should continue in a relationship with one or more human services workers until the ideation subsides completely. A client who has the means moves into the next level of risk, middle risk. Assessment must proceed to the next stage.

Stage 4: What Is the Level of Determination? It is vital to find out how determined a client is to carry out the plan. Many times a client who has suicidal ideation, a plan, and the means is ambivalent and hasn't carried out the plan because there might be something that offers hope of feeling better. At this stage of assessment, a worker must explore reasons why the client has not attempted suicide, despite having a plan and the means to carry it out. What a client says at this stage helps workers establish their clients' levels of **determination,** which helps establish whether a client is at middle or high risk. The more reasons a client has for living, the better, especially if a specific experience is discussed that would definitely make a difference. For example, if a client says "I won't want to kill myself if I knew I would find a job in the next six months," a worker has a chance to assist the client in finding a job. Another example might be a client who says, "I haven't killed myself because it would hurt my grandmother. She's always been so loving and kind to me." A worker might encourage this client to focus on this loving relationship and even use the grandmother as part of treatment, perhaps in a family watch.

If something can stop a client from committing suicide, the risk level remains middle risk. Interventions at this stage may include making a written no-suicide contract (see Figure 8.1) with a client, frequent sessions with the client, referral for **medication** assessment, removal of the means, and involvement of family members. If a client is adamantly determined to commit suicide, making such comments as, "I'm going to leave here and kill myself," then workers must proceed to the next stage of the assessment.

Stage 5: Voluntary or Involuntary Hospitalization? When a client is determined and has the means to commit suicide, that client is assessed a high-level suicide risk. A worker can then offer a client one of two options: **voluntary or involuntary hospitalization**.

If a client agrees to being hospitalized for further assessment and for that person's own safety, the worker proceeds in finding an appropriate placement, usually determined by medical insurance and other resources. Some high-risk clients realize that they need protection from themselves and will enter into a facility voluntarily. Other high-risk clients, however, may refuse to voluntarily enter a hospital, and they may need involuntary hospitalization to ensure their safety.

Typically, when a high-risk client refuses hospitalization, specific, usually state-determined, steps need to be taken. In some U.S. states, police are called, along with a member of a psychiatric emergency team (PET). PET workers are trained to assess whether high-risk clients need to be held in a protective facility for a brief time period until further psychiatric assessment can be made. It is important to keep in mind that only qualified people can have someone involun-

Any human services worker can make a written no-suicide contract with a client. Of course it is not legally binding, but it is psychologically binding and can be effective.

I (client's name) _____

agree that I will not cause any harm to myself or intentionally allow harm to come to me at least until I speak personally with (worker's name) _____

I agree to this contract for the next two weeks.

Date _____ client's signature _____

Date _____ worker's signature _____

Figure 8.1 Sample No-Suicide Contract

tarily hospitalized. In California, for instance, only state-certified PET workers and hospital psychiatrists have the authority to do this. All human services workers must understand how to work collaboratively when conducting suicide assessment and prevention. (Kanel, 2007; Wyman, 1982).

Table 8.1 lists the stages involved in suicide assessment and provides intervention plans for each level of risk. This table can be useful to human services workers in a variety of situations.

CRITICAL THINKING / SELF-REFLECTION CORNER

- Do you think human services workers should always prevent suicide?
- Are there any situations in which you think people should be allowed to commit suicide?
- What are your initial feelings about asking clients whether they have been thinking about killing themselves?
- Do you think that other professionals should be responsible for ensuring that people don't commit suicide? Which professionals?

Other Intervention Strategies

In addition to suicide assessment and interventions, many clients benefit from a variety of other interventions. Part of effective assessment includes determining if

Table 8.1 Suicide Assessment

Stage	Response	Risk Level	Intervention
1. Is there suicidal ideation?	no	low	crisis intervention, support
	yes		proceed to stage 2
2. Has a plan been made?	no	low	crisis intervention, support, verbal no suicide contract
	yes		proceed to stage 3
3. Are the means available?	no	low	crisis intervention, support, regular monitoring or suicidal thinking and plan, written no-suicide contract
	yes	middle	proceed to stage 4
4. Will the plan be carried out?	no	middle	family watch, written no-suicide contract, frequent contact, medication evaluation, take away the means
	yes	high	proceed to stage 5
5. Will hospitalization be voluntary? or involuntary?	yes	high	Assist in finding a placement, ask family or friends to transport client to hospital.
	yes	high	Call appropriate authorities to evaluate for involuntary hospitalization

and where a client should be referred for ongoing services. Following are some brief descriptions of interventions typically found in most communities. Once the human services worker has assessed the specific needs of a client, the severity and chronicity of the client's problems, and the economic and social resources available to the client, the worker may connect the client to one or more of these services. This is an example of "brokering," which was first discussed in Chapter 3.

OUTPATIENT TREATMENT

Outpatient treatment usually refers to private or group counseling held at an agency or a therapist's office. Sessions usually take place once a week for about one or two hours at a time. The client continues to work and live at home during this treatment.

Example 1: A 28-year-old man begins seeing a psychologist because he's been very depressed and having trouble concentrating at work after his girlfriend of two years broke up with him. His therapy focuses on his loss and how to deal with being alone. He participates in therapy for the next eight weeks and begins to socialize more, concentrate better at work, and feels less depressed. He spent most of the time expressing his feelings and talking about what went wrong in his last relationship.

Example 2: An 18-year-old woman sets up an appointment to attend educational and support groups at a nonprofit agency that helps women who are recovering from substance abuse. Groups are run by marriage and family therapy (MFT) interns who are supervised by licensed MFTs. She attends weekly, hourlong educational and support groups. Because she is unemployed, she can only pay the minimum of $8 for each group. After 16 weeks of group counseling, she gets a job and terminates her participation in the groups. Of course, she continues going to AA meetings, which she intends to do for many years to come (tertiary prevention).

PARTIAL HOSPITALIZATION, DAY TREATMENT, AND DAYCARE

Some recipients of human services need treatment more frequently than once a week. Instead, they need daily programs in which they participate in various groups and receive services, such as lunch and medical exams. These clients usually live at home under the care or supervision of family when they're not at their day-treatment facilities. Clients who participate in **partial hospitalization, daycare, or day-treatment** services have various difficulties including people with Alzheimer's disease who have become dangerous to themselves when home alone and those who are severely depressed and need supervision because they are suicidal. If the setting of service is a hospital, the intervention is referred to as **partial hospitalization** because the patient sleeps at home and doesn't attend on weekends. Day-treatment programs may occur at hospitals or other centers and clinics, but basically include a full day of group activities and lunch.

Example 1: A 58-year-old woman has been at high risk for suicide. She was recently released from a psychiatric hospital after a three-day involuntary hospitalization following a suicide attempt. Because she still has suicidal ideations, she and her psychiatrist believe she needs intensive treatment but feel comfortable with her sleeping and eating dinner at home with her husband who is willing to monitor her for suicidal behaviors. The client attends various educational and support groups at a hospital from 8 a.m. until 5 p.m. She eats lunch at the hospital but goes home before dinner. She attends these groups Monday through Saturday for the next six weeks until her suicidal ideation disappears.

Example 2: A group of people diagnosed with schizophrenia attend a variety of groups run by mental health workers at a local community mental health agency from 9 in the morning until 5 in the evening. After which, they return to their board-and-care homes to eat dinner and sleep.

Example 3: A 78-year-old man suffering from Alzheimer's disease has begun to wander when left alone at home. Both of his grown children must work all day, but can afford to have him go to a daycare program where he participates in various social and occupational groups from 7 a.m. until 6 p.m. His daughter and son take turns picking him up at the daycare center. He eats dinner and sleeps at one of his children's homes at night. The children alternate taking care of him so neither gets too burnt out from caretaking responsibilities.

INPATIENT TREATMENT

This type of treatment involves a client being admitted to a hospital or other residential facility. An aim of **inpatient treatment** is to protect clients from harming themselves and others and to ensure clients' basic needs, such as eating and medical care, are provided. They receive intensive group and individual therapy, medications, and often participate in a therapeutic milieu model in which the entire hospital program is aimed at changing behaviors. Some clients function at such low levels that they remain hospitalized permanently, though this approach is not considered fiscally sound. Others are released from inpatient care and referred to board-and-care homes, to their families, or to partial hospitalization or daycare programs after a two- to four-week stay at the hospital.

Example: A 45-year-old woman has been excessively self-mutilating and recently told her therapist that she was going to kill herself. Because she refused to be hospitalized, she was involuntarily admitted to a psychiatric hospital. She stayed in the hospital for the next six weeks, attending group and individual therapy and taking new medications. Because her suicidal ideation was not subsiding, she stayed longer than the usual length of treatment.

MEDICATIONS

Many clients behaviors and coping abilities improve by taking medication (sometimes referred to as chemotherapy). Although medication may be the best option for certain clients, most clients on medication are also encouraged to participate in other services. Medication may be prescribed by a client's primary care physician or psychiatrist.

Example 1: A 27-year-old man, diagnosed with bipolar disorder, recently suffered an intense manic episode during which he assaulted someone at a local bar. When he went to court, the judge put him on probation and ordered him to see a psychiatrist and stay on his medication. He went to a court-appointed psychiatrist and began taking Depacote (an anticonvulsant drug). After three weeks, he was stabilized and no longer had drastic mood swings.

Example 2: A woman suffering from severe panic attacks went to a therapist who thought she should see a psychiatrist, who could evaluate her need for medication to treat her panic attacks. The therapist continued with counseling, and the psychiatrist prescribed Paxil (an antidepressant) and Xanax (an anti-anxiety drug) for her panic disorder.

RESIDENTIAL TREATMENT FACILITIES, HALFWAY HOUSES, AND BOARD-AND-CARE HOMES

Certain facilities provide housing and therapeutic care for a variety of clients who have serious problems and are at risk for severe deterioration in functioning if they do not have daily monitoring and care. They may live in the halfway house for six months to two years. During their stay at residential facilities and halfway houses, clients are usually required to participate in group and individual counseling. They often receive job-skills training as well as social-skills training by human services workers who do not live at the facility, but rather work in three different shifts to provide 24-hour supervision.

Board-and-care homes are privately owned homes that usually house up to 6 residents who are provided with food and shelter. The board and care owners monitor the taking of medications and contact professionals if clients appear to be deteriorating. Some clients live in **board-and-care homes** for the rest of their lives. Others, such as abused children, might live in a foster home for one to two years while their parents complete a rehabilitation program. Although the owners of the board-and-care homes and foster homes do not provide counseling services, they often work with counselors to ensure continuity of care for clients.

Example 1: A 32-year-old man was recently released from prison after serving three years for first-offense drug trafficking. Because he had been a model prisoner, he was let out on good behavior two years before his sentence was up. The judge ordered him to live in a halfway house for those two years so he might have a stable environment to learn job skills, learn new social skills, and receive counseling for his substance abuse problems.

Example 2: A 39-year-old woman recovering from methamphetamine addiction applied to live at Phoenix House, a well-known residential facility for recovering addicts. This environment allowed her to stay sober, learn job skills, learn basic independent living skills, and participate in counseling. She stayed for one year until she got a job and had more confidence in her ability to stay sober.

Mezzo-Level Intervention Strategies

Twelve-Step Programs

These groups are run by group members, not professional human services workers. They have proven to be successful for people struggling with addiction and are a great referral resource for clients because attendance is free (though voluntary donations are asked at each meeting), and clients can attend daily meetings if they choose. In 1935, Bill Wilson founded Alcoholics Anonymous (AA), which was the first of many **twelve-step programs** that followed. The AA program of recovery suggests using 12 steps (listed below), which can be used in any way members find helpful.

1. We admitted we were powerless over alcohol—that our lives had become unmanageable.
2. Came to believe that a Power greater than themselves could restore us to sanity.
3. Made a decision to turn our will and our lives over to the care of God as we understood Him.
4. Made a searching and fearless moral inventory of ourselves.
5. Admitted to God, to ourselves, and to another human being the exact nature of our wrongs.
6. Were entirely ready to have God remove all these defects of character.
7. Humbly asked God to remove our shortcomings.
8. Made a list of those persons we had harmed and became willing to make amends to them all.
9. Made direct amends to such people wherever possible, except when to do so would injure them or others.
10. Continued to take personal inventory and when we were wrong, promptly admitted it.
11. Sought through prayer and meditation to improve our conscious contact with God, *as we understood Him,* praying only for knowledge of His will for us and the power to carry that out.
12. Having had a spiritual awakening as the result of these steps, we tried to carry this message to alcoholics, and to practice these principles in all our affairs. (*Source:* Alcoholics Anonymous website)

Since its founding, many other **12-step programs** have used AA's principles to treat other kinds of problems. These programs are for people with other types of addictive behavior, such as eating disorders (Overeaters Anonymous), sexual promiscuity (Sex Addicts Anonymous), and gambling (Gamblers Anonymous). In addition, there is Ala-non, which is for spouses and families of addicts, Co-Dependents Anonymous, Co-DA, for people who find themselves in co-dependent relationships, and Incest Survivors Anonymous, or ISA, for people who have survived incest.

Support Groups

Support groups comprise people who all share common problems and issues. Sometimes these groups are lead by counselors who facilitate group discussions. The focus is usually on current daily living problems that are usually the result of deeper problems. Some support groups are lead by volunteers, paraprofessionals, or members take turns leading the discussions, such as with Compassionate Friends, a group for parents who have lost a child to death.

Example 1: A 20-year-old woman is raped by a friend of her brother. She is scared to press charges but wants to talk about the rape with people that she doesn't know. The rape crisis hotline refers her to a local support group. A volunteer counselor runs the group for women who have been raped by an acquaintance.

Example 2: A counselor has about four women in their late 70s who are all depressed and feeling lonely since their husbands died. She decides to start a support group where they would all come to see her at the same time instead of individually so they could share their common feelings with each other. One of the positive outcomes of this support group was that some of the women decided to start a bridge club. Some began to meet at the local mall to walk in the mornings.

HMOs

Health maintenance organizations (HMOs) are a special breed of assessment and intervention model. Originally, their main focus was on keeping families healthy, and early intervention when a family member became ill, to prevent the need for long-term care. HMOs have existed since the early 1900s but have received more impetus for growth since the passage of the Health Maintenance Organization Act of 1973, which was considered a building block in a national system for maintaining health rather than a system for treating illnesses (DeLeon, Uyeda, & Welch, 1985). Recent estimates put the number of Americans enrolled in HMOs at well over 50 million. HMOs provide specific health services to enrollees for a prepaid, fixed payment. If the HMOs can find ways to keep enrollees healthy rather than providing them the various health services to which their payments entitle them, the HMOs stand to profit considerably. Keeping enrollees healthy sounds like an admirable goal, however, many therapists and physicians complain that their decisions about who needs services and for how long are being micromanaged by HMOs. The policies mandated by an HMO often reduce the autonomy by which many mental health workers typically practice. Because people pay less for HMO mental health services, private practice clinicians may feel in competition with HMOs. Some HMOs are located in a particular building as is often the case with the HMO called Kaiser Permanente. Patients, whether they're being treated for medical or psychiatric problems or receiving preventive educational services, all go to the same building for services. Other HMOs contract with individual providers who service patients at their own offices. Although clients are seen at various locations, all providers must follow the policies and practices of the HMO. This includes filling out specific forms, obtaining authorization to treat people, and providing justification for treatment.

Despite some of the complaints by providers about losing autonomy, HMO involvement has increased knowledge about how mental health practitioners other than physicians play a vital role in the overall care of many multi-need clients. HMOs tend to operate within the multidisciplinary team model because of the variety of providers contracted with an HMO. Providers have access to the names of specialists and may refer their own clients to those who have contracted with the HMO. Not only is it easier for physicians to call on mental health clinicians to aid in treating various medical conditions, but mental health clinicians also may have easier access to physicians to aid in the biological components of emotional conditions (Tulkin & Frank, 1985).

The line separating patients' physical health from their emotional health has grown thinner since medical doctors began working closely with psychotherapists within HMO systems. The role of the psychotherapist within that system may be seen as behavioral medicine specialist rather than merely a psychotherapist as mental health providers do so much more than simply provide psychotherapy. This phenomenon is a function of the growing evidence that 60 percent of visits to physicians are really to treat emotional problems (DeLeon, Uyeda, & Welch, 1985). Including mental health providers in the traditional physicians' world has reduced medical costs because mental health clinicians are trained to treat emotional problems more successfully than general physicians are (Herr & Cramer, 1987). HMOs also allow a variety of clinicians to collaborate on the needs of an entire family and not exclusively on an individual's needs.

HMO policies have encouraged mental health practitioners to create treatment models that are brief and cost effective. Clinicians who have been trained in long-term models, such as psychoanalysis, often object to limits being put on them by insurance policy makers. HMO policy has dramatically affected how mental health providers work with clients. Crisis intervention skills, family therapy models, and cognitive behavioral models have come in handy for providers contracting with HMOs because they are usually short-term models that effectively help clients within 20 weeks. Some mental health providers still object to cost-effectiveness being the ruler of mental health treatment, but it is, for now, a huge reality in the provision of mental health services.

HMOs usually have services available for many complaints. They have educational groups, support groups, individual therapy, family therapy, and medication services. Additionally, most HMO plans are contracted with psychiatric hospitals and partial hospitalization services. Most of the human services workers employed by HMOs are licensed therapists, such as licensed clinical social workers (LCSWs), licensed, marital and family therapists, psychologists, and psychiatrists. Some interns may also be employed. HMO hospitals often employ medical social workers to assist with patient discharge plans and other social issues.

CRITICAL THINKING / SELF-REFLECTION CORNER

- What are your thoughts on administrative workers giving psychiatrists and psychologists and other mental health providers permission to treat a mental health client?

- Do you believe that most mental health providers could treat clients appropriately and effectively without administrative watchdogs?

- What are your own experiences in being a patient at an HMO?

- How does service from an HMO provider differ from services received from other types of agencies?

The Intake Process

An initial assessment is often referred to as an **intake.** The initial assessment is typically recorded on an intake form provided by the agency. The information gathered on an intake form varies from agency to agency and from profession to profession. In general, an intake interview may be conducted by phone, or it may be conducted in person. An intake interview may be conducted by a worker who will continue to provide ongoing services to the client, or a designated **intake worker** may conduct nothing but intake interviews. The purpose of an intake interview is to get a brief idea of the reasons the client is seeking services. Demographic information, nature of the problem, and history of similar problems is typically assessed during an intake interview and recorded on an intake form. A few examples from different types of agencies are presented in Figures 8.2 through 8.5

Intake Assessments Example 1: Suicide Hotlines

Workers who answer hotlines calls usually make their intake assessments by phone. Hotline workers may use a specific form for gathering intake information and ask the client questions to record on the form. Of course, not every caller is willing to provide all the information asked for, but a counselor can at least try to get the information.

Intake Assessments Example 2: Child-Protective Services

Most communities have standard child-abuse reporting forms that are completed prior to calling the information in to a child-protective services worker. Social workers receiving the call complete their own version of an intake form that includes the information in the child-abuse report that the caller will eventually send to the department of social welfare. Figure 8.3 is an example of intake information gathered from the Child Abuse Registry/Child Protective Services in southern California.

Name (if possible) _____   phone number (if possible) _____

Date and time _____

Are you having suicidal thoughts? Yes _____   No _____

Do you have a plan? Yes _____   No _____

Do you have the means? Yes _____   No _____

Have you ever attempted suicide? Yes _____   No _____

Have you ever been treated for emotional problems? Yes _____   No _____
If so, who were you seeing? _____

Are you still in treatment? Yes _____   No _____

Name of therapist (if different from previously named) _____

Are you taking any medication? Yes _____   No _____   What type? _____

What is stopping you from committing the act? _____

Will you make a commitment with me not to harm yourself? Yes _____   No _____

Will you follow up with a therapist? Yes _____   No _____

Referrals given _____

Follow-up plan_____

Figure 8.2 Suicide-Prevention Hotline: Sample Intake Information

Intake Assessments Example 3: Battered Women's Shelters

An initial intake that comes in through a shelter's hotline is answered by an advocate worker who asks callers a variety of questions to ascertain whether they are eligible for acceptance into the shelter or to provide referral information when they are not. Following is an example of the questions on a typical intake form:

Party making the report: Name/title _____

Address _____

Phone _____   Date of report _____

Party receiving the report: police department, sheriff's office, county welfare, or county probation

Address of receiving party: _____

Official contacted: _____

Phone number: _____

Date and time of report: _____

Victim(s): Name, address, birth date, sex, race, present location of child, phone number

_____

_____

Siblings of victim: Name, birth date, sex, race

_____

_____

Parents of victims: Names, birthdates, sex, race, address, phone numbers

_____

_____

Date/time of incident: _____

Place of incident: _____

Type of abuse: _____

Narrative description/summary of what the abused child or person accompanying the child said happened: _____

Known history of similar incidents for this child: _____

Figure 8.3 Child Protective Services: Sample Intake Information

Name: _____

Location: _____

Number of children and ages: _____

Are you currently in danger? _____

When was the last abusive episode? _____

What happened? _____

Have you ever been to a shelter to escape abuse? _____

When and where? _____

Are you being treated by a psychiatrist or therapist? Yes _____   No _____

Name of therapist _____   For how long? _____

What medications are you taking? _____

Do you use drugs or alcohol? _____   How much? _____   For how long? _____

Are you employed? _____

Do you have access to any money? _____

Do you need to leave now? _____

Tentative Plan_____

Figure 8.4 Battered Women's Shelter: Sample Intake Information

Intake Assessments Example 4:
Outpatient Mental Health Clinic

If clients have HMO insurance, they will probably phone the HMO plan and speak with an intake worker who will gather brief information to properly refer the client to the best counselor. If clients seek mental health services from non-profit agencies, community mental health services, or from private practitioners, they will most likely be asked to complete a brief intake form before their first appointment. The type of information usually gathered on a mental health intake form is presented in Figure 8.5.

Once an intake session is conducted, workers begin the process of developing a plan for intervention.

Treatment Planning

Most human services agencies require workers to complete formal treatment plans. These plans may be written on a form provided by the agency or in some cases, workers may merely write up their version of the treatment plan. Some agencies might refer to these treatment plans as **case plans.** An effective treatment plan includes clear and specific needs and problems to be worked with, goals and objectives, interventions, and timelines for completion of the plan. Human services workers should include as many interventions as are available in the plan. In this way the clients have a better chance of achieving their goals.

Figure 8.6 provides a sample treatment plan for a mental health agency.

Figure 8.7 offers a sample case plan for a case at a child protective-services agency.

Progress Notes

In addition to treatment and case plans, human services workers must also maintain ongoing **progress notes** for every client. These notes not only help workers remember each case and each session with clients, but they also serve as a form of protection for workers. Proper documentation should include information that demonstrates ethical and competent practice. Notes should be written in an organized manner, clearly, and objectively. These notes provide continuity in the care of clients. Continuity of care is essential because many times new workers take over the case from a previous worker, or clients transfer to different areas. Having detailed information about a client's treatment with one worker is helpful for another worker who may be called upon to provide services to the client for

Name: _____

Date of Birth: _____

Social security #: _____

Address: _____   Phone: _____

Insurance: _____

Physician name and address: _____

Previous mental-health treatment? _____

By whom? _____   When? _____

Presenting problems: _____

History of similar problems: _____

Informed Consent: (this part explains to clients their rights to voluntary treatment, voluntary termination, any risks involved in treatment, fees, cancellation policy, and confidentiality rights. This section should explain that a counselor is mandated to report abusive behavior to children, elders, disabled-adults, and dangerous behavior to others. Clients should also be made aware that the counselor may breech confidentiality if a client becomes suicidal).

Figure 8.5 Out-Patient Mental-Health Clinic: Sample Intake Information

different problems as well. The progress notes also help the client and worker see when a client has completed the plan and no longer needs services. Finally, many funding agencies, such as Medicare, require certain information in a client's chart to provide proof that appropriate services are being provided for appropriate problems. Following is an example of a widely accepted form of progress notes referred to as **SOAP.**

The SOAP Method of Progress Reports

- S = subjective This refers to the subjective view of the client. The workers documents what the client says during an interview.

Name of client: __Jane Doe__

Intake Date: __03/27/2006__

Symptoms/Complaints	Goals	Interventions	Proposed timeline
Uncontrollable crying daily	Reduce crying	Refer to psychiatrist	4 weeks to once a week
Suicidal ideation	Eliminate S.I.	Crisis intervention Verbal no suicide contract	2 weeks
Feels hopeless and worthless	Increase feelings of hope and self-esteem	Cognitive therapy	4 weeks
Conflicts with husband and children	Learn more productive communication	Family therapy	4 weeks

Multiaxial Diagnosis per DSM IV–R
AXIS I: Major Depression, recurrent, moderate
AXIS II: No personality disorder noted
AXIS III: No physical illness related
AXIS IV: Occupational stress, conflicts with husband and children
AXIS V: Current GAS- 55 Highest in past year- 75

Figure 8.6 Mental Health Treatment Plan

- O = objective This refers to the worker's objective view of the client's state. The human services worker often describes emotions observed, interpersonal behaviors, hygiene, and other information seen from the worker's point of view.

- A = assessment Human services workers document their own analysis of the client's needs and progress at this point. The worker may describe a theoretical analysis as well.

- P = plan Specific interventions are presented here along with the reason for said plan. This may include referrals, medications, and other interventions described earlier in this chapter. Figure 8.8 provides an example of a progress report written from the SOAP model.

Keep in mind that many agencies provide their own forms for documentation. Human services workers are typically trained on how to complete required paperwork.

Mother's Name: <u>Jane Doe</u>

Minor's names: <u>Johnny Doe, 5/13/95; Chelsea Doe, 8/6/98; Heather Doe, 10/23/2002</u>

Date of alleged abuse/neglect: <u>04/05/2005–04/05/2006</u>

Name of alleged perpetrator: <u>James Doe</u>

Description of <u>abuse: Chelsea Doe claims that from approximately April 2005 until April of 2006 her father, James fondled her genital area every day after school. She claims that her mother was working during these abusive episodes and that he would take her into his room and abuse her on her parent's bed. Johnny denies that he was ever molested. After a careful examination of Heather, it does not appear that she was victimized either.</u>

Case plan: <u>James Doe must move out of the family home and lose all custody and visitation rights with all three minors until such time that all case plan requirements are fulfilled. James must participate in group therapy at Parent's United for a minimum of 1 year before any visitations are allowed. James must participate in individual therapy once per week for one year. James will enroll in a 16-week parenting class. James may not talk with the children by phone until such time that the children's counselors state that it would be appropriate.</u>
<u>   Jane Doe may maintain custody of all three minors if she fulfills all conditions of this case plan. Jane may not allow James to enter the family home. Jane must attend an educational and support group for non-perpetrating parents approved by CPS. Jane must participate in family counseling with her children. Jane must ensure her children attend individual therapy as recommended by their counselors.</u>
<u>   Chelsea Doe must participate in individual therapy as long as recommended by her counselor. She must see a therapist who specializes in the treatment of child sexual abuse. Chelsea will participate in family counseling as recommended by the counselor.</u>
<u>   Johnny Doe will be seen by a therapist for an evaluation to ascertain whether he needs individual therapy. He will participate in family therapy as needed.</u>
<u>   Heather Doe will participate in counseling if she begins to show any signs of having been molested or exhibits any other emotional problems.</u>
<u>   This case plan will remain in effect for the next year at which time it will be reviewed and revised.</u>

Figure 8.7 Child Protective Services Case Plan

Clinician: <u>Dr. Kristi Kanel, MFT</u>

Client: <u>John Doe</u>

Date of service: <u>05/16/06</u>

Type of Service: <u>Individual therapy</u>

S: <u>Client complains of feeling very sad this week. He is having</u>
<u>difficulty letting go of his wife. He can't think about anything</u>
<u>else but her leaving him. He says he alternates between being sad</u>
<u>and enraged. He calls her everyday, but she doesn't wish to talk</u>
<u>with him. He says his work performance is affected. He speaks</u>
<u>exclusively about his wife and his feelings of loneliness without</u>
<u>her. He denies feelings suicidal and has no plan to do anything</u>
<u>self-destructive. He is devoted to his children.</u>

O: <u>Client is teary while he speaks. His eyes look very tired and</u>
<u>he speaks slowly. His affect is congruent with the content of his</u>
<u>verbalizations.</u>

A: <u>Client continues to grieve the loss of his wife. His denial</u>
<u>about the loss is lifting, and so he is more in touch with sadness</u>
<u>and anger.</u>

P: <u>Client should continue taking the antidepressant medication</u>
<u>prescribed by his physician. Client will continue with weekly</u>
<u>counseling focusing on leaning how to adjust to life without his wife</u>
<u>and how to put his energy into being a father. Will consider referral</u>
<u>to a support group.</u>

Figure 8.8 Example of a Progress Note

Report Writing

Writing formal **reports** is an important skill for human services workers in all agencies. Some reports will be written for reviews by judges. Others will be written to collaborating human services workers to enhance multidisciplinary team work. Written reports should be organized under specific headings and be written in neutral and succinct language. Many human services students have been trained to write formal essays in college. This essay format is not typically how reports are written, however. While there is much variance in how a report should be written, there are some general rules about how to proceed. Hollis and Donn (1980) have developed a framework for a variety of reports that human services workers generally write. Of course, there is not just one way to write a report. How and what is written will depend on the purpose of the report from the writer's point of view as well as the purpose from the recipient of the report's point of view. Some of the purposes for writing reports they list include:

1. requesting assistance from another person
2. receiving a request from another person
3. making referrals
4. developing conjoint and consultative reports
5. adding information to existing records
6. obtaining objective data
7. obtaining objective data plus interpretations
8. obtaining diagnostic information
9. obtaining recommendations
10. obtaining progress report
11. obtaining preliminary report
12. recording baseline information
13. summarizing psychological support information
14. reporting research studies
15. reporting for legal purposes
16. periodic summary reports
17. agency reports associated with professional activities
18. special reports (may be associated with grant writing or funding issues) (Hollis & Dunn, 1980, pp. 6–15).

The format for a report varies, but it should generally be written in an objective manner with little embellishment. In other words, reports should not look like literary works. They are correspondences constructed to provide specific information. Many reports are written with the purpose of providing the receiver a recommendation about the client. At times a psychologist may write a report to recommend that a parent maintain or lose custody of a child. Sometimes, mental health clinicians write reports to probation officers and the court to recommend that a client remain on probation, go to prison, or be released. Some reports are written to help school officials develop a treatment plan for a learning-disabled child. Figure 8.9 provides some typical topics for consideration in making a recommendation report.

CRITICAL THINKING / SELF-REFLECTION CORNER

- Why are detailed progress notes and treatment/case plans vital to the provision of human services?

- What are your initial reactions to the idea of report writing?

- How is a report written by a human services worker similar and different from a typical book report?

Identifying Data:
   Identification of person to whom report is sent
   Identification of person about whom report is written
   Identification of person writing report
   Report Title
   Date of examination(s)

Behavioral Symptoms and Characteristics:
   Symptoms observed directly by the therapist
   Symptoms reported by others
   Symptoms reported directly by client
   Client's relationship to the environment

Other Characteristics:
   Physical characteristics of the client
   Organic concomitants of the disorder

Summary

Diagnosis

Recommendations:
   Environmental changes
   Treatment Procedures

Anticipated length of treatment

Prognosis
   With the recommendations followed as given in the report
   Without treatment

Figure 8.9 Topics Included in Recommendation Reports

Chapter Summary

When an initial contact is made between a client and a human services worker, the worker must assess the needs of client to decide on proper interventions. Human services practice may be conducted at the micro (individual intervention), mezzo (group and family intervention), or macro (community and societal intervention) level. At times, the worker, alone, provides the interventions. At other times, a variety of human services workers all work together to meet multiple needs of the client.

There are a variety of human services interventions including outpatient clinics, residential facilities, self-help and support groups, and medications. HMOs are self-sufficient agencies that provide services at the micro and mezzo levels, work from a multidisciplinary team approach, and contain all of the above-mentioned services within their system. This allows for continuity of care and economic efficiency. The intervention strategy is dependent on how severe and chronic the problems are for the client. Primary interventions aim to prevent problems, secondary interventions focus on solving a problem as soon as possible, and tertiary intervention emphasize helping people with longstanding problems to function in the best way that they are able. Additionally, human services workers must help clients prioritize their needs. Crisis intervention and suicide assessment often play a vital role in helping clients whether it be to help with day to day stress or to deal with major disasters, such as Hurricane Katrina. Human services workers must also be competent at documenting their intervention plans and progress with clients. At times, workers must submit reports that provide information to other human services workers and others involved with a client or the agency.

Suggested Applied Activities

1. Pair up, and have one student role-play a client who is either a low-risk, middle-risk, or high-risk suicidal client and the other student role-playing some type of human services worker. Using Table 8.1, practice assessing for suicidal ideation, plan, etc. Try to develop an intervention based on the assessed risk level. Switch roles and have the new client role-play a different risk level. What were some of the difficulties that the human services worker faced in doing this task?

_____

_____

_____

_____

_____

_____

_____

2. Watch a movie or television show. Select a character who might be seen by a human services worker because of emotional problems, poverty, child abuse, domestic violence, criminality, substance abuse, and the like. Write out a "mock" treatment or case plan for the character.

_____

_____

_____

_____

_____

_____

Chapter Review Questions

1. What are the basic steps in conducting a suicide assessment?

   _____

   _____

2. What are the appropriate interventions for a low-, middle-, and high-risk suicidal client?

   _____

   _____

3. What does the acronym HMO stand for?

   _____

   _____

4. Name three types of written reports that human services workers must often submit or maintain in a client's chart.

   _____

   _____

5. What types of situations are dealt with when conducting trauma response?

   _____

   _____

6. To develop appropriate interventions, human services workers must conduct an _____ .

7. What is the nature of a 12-step program?

   _____

   _____

8. Who might live in a halfway house?

   _____

   _____

9. What type of clients might benefit from hospitalization?

_____

_____

10. What is the purpose of crisis intervention?

_____

Glossary of Terms

ABC model of crisis intervention is a three-stage model in which workers first attempt to develop rapport through basic attending skills (A), identify the problem and offer new ways of thinking about the situation (B), and offer coping strategies (C).

Assessment is a process in which human services workers interview a client or the client's family to gather information about the needs of the client. The purpose of an assessment is to determine what intervention strategies should be implemented.

Board-and-care homes are private homes that usually house about 6 residents who are disabled physically or mentally. The operators of the homes receive money from each resident. Residents typically receive government support because of their disability. The homes distribute medications, provide food, and supervision, and assist with transportation needs.

Case plan is a written document that specifies the problems assessed that need addressing and intervention plans.

Chronic refers to a problem that has been going on for many years, it is said to be a chronic condition.

Collaboration occurs when two or more human services workers discuss and develop intervention strategies for the same client or for the implementation of a program.

Crisis intervention is a type of intervention in which the worker attempts to help a client return to a normal level of functioning by offering adaptive coping strategies to manage a stressful situation and by helping the client perceive the situation in a more manageable way.

D.A.R.E. (Drug Awareness Resistance Education) is a primary prevention program designed by local law enforcement to help elementary children stay away from drugs.

Determination is the stage of suicide assessment in which a worker establishes how firmly decided a client is to commit suicide, and if a decision is not firm, what can be done to keep a client from harm.

Health maintenance organization (HMO) is a privately funded agency in which medical, psychological, optical, and even dental needs may be serviced through a family's insurance plan.

Inpatient treatment usually refers to a hospital setting where clients reside and receive various treatments, such as group therapy, medication monitoring, and individual therapy. Because of the high cost of a hospital stay, this type of treatment is usually reserved only for people who are a danger to others or to themselves.

Intake is a first-assessment interview that establishes what the client's needs are and possible interventions.

Intake worker is a human services worker who primarily conducts an initial assessment of a client and then decides on how to best devise an intervention plan

Means (of suicide) refers to the method a client plans on using to commit suicide, such as a gun, pills, or a razor blade.

Medication refers to any psychotropic drug prescribed to stabilize a client's mood, reduce anxiety, manage impulsive behaviors, or lessen psychotic symptoms.

Mezzo is a level of intervention that focuses on working with groups and families.

Micro is a level of intervention that deals with individuals.

No-suicide contract can be either a verbal or written agreement between a client and a worker that has a client promise not to attempt suicide before speaking with the worker.

Outpatient is a type of intervention in which clients receive treatment at an agency or in an office. This is most suited for people who can function in society appropriately.

Partial hospitalization, daycare, and day treatment are programs for clients who don't need to live in a hospital but who benefit from group therapy and individual therapy for several hours a day at a hospital.

Plan (to commit suicide) is how a person intends to commit suicide.

Primary prevention is an intervention used early on to prevent a problem from occurring, usually in the form of education to at-risk groups.

Prognosis refers to the potential outcome of a problem—the chances of a problem being resolved satisfactorily or unsatisfactorily.

Progress notes are the written summary of a session in which a worker officially documents the services provided.

Project Head Start is an early-intervention enrichment program for preschool children usually from low-income families.

Reports are written for various purposes by human services workers to communicate a variety of aspects of a client's situation.

Residential facilities usually house about 8 to 20 people, all of whom are dealing with a common issue or problem, such as parolees, drug addicts, or battered women. Counselors, case workers, psychiatrists, and employment advocates usually work with these clients to help them transition back into society.

Secondary intervention is a type of intervention that attempts to treat emergency situations and problems that are not chronic. The aim is to prevent a client's problem from becoming chronic.

Scared Straight is a primary prevention program for at-risk teens that includes having them experience prison life and hear inmates talk about their lives in jail.

SOAP is a method of writing progress notes in which a worker documents the subjective statements of the client, the objective observations of the worker, the worker's assessment of the client's needs, and the plan of action.

Suicidal ideation refers to thoughts someone has about committing suicide.

Suicide assessment is a structured process of determining how serious a client is about committing suicide.

Suicide risk includes three levels, low, middle, and high risk. Low risk are clients who have thought about suicide but have no plans or means to carry out a plan. Middle risk are clients who have thought about suicide, have a plan, and the means. High risk are clients who have thoughts of suicide, a plan, the means, and intend on going through with the suicide.

Support groups are typically led by counselors and focus on helping group members increase self-esteem and feelings of empowerment and decrease feelings of social isolation.

Tertiary interventions are aimed at helping people adapt to their longstanding problems. People with chronic problems often need some form of intervention throughout their lives.

Triage is a method of assessing and prioritizing a client's needs and problems.

Twelve-step programs are groups that use the 12-step approach to recovery, of which Alcoholics Anonymous was the first. These groups seem to be one of the most effective methods for people with addictions to maintain their sobriety. They are considered mutual self-help groups and are not led by professional counselors.

Voluntary or involuntary hospitalization is recommended for clients who are a danger to themselves or to others. When a client refuses to go voluntarily, the involuntary hospitalization is usually the only option.

Case Presentation and Exit Quiz

General Description and Demographics

Jim is an 18-year-old male who is single and living with his parents. Jim has never held a job but has graduated from high school. During the summer after graduation, he began having feelings of overwhelming anxiety and depression. He told his parents that he felt people were out to hurt him and were always talking about him. Jim stopped leaving the house and mostly stayed in his room watching television. When he did come out to eat, he would usually talk about a buzzing sound in his room and that his television was broadcasting special messages to him. Jim told his mother that he sometimes wants to kill himself because he can't stand being so depressed.

Jim's mother arranges for Jim to talk to their longtime family physician, Dr. Rogers. Jim and his mother tell Dr. Rogers about Jim's complaints, which he's had for the past three months. Dr. Rogers refers Jim to a colleague of his, Dr. Jones, who is a psychiatrist.

Dr. Jones meets with Jim and his mother. Dr. Jones inquires about Jim's feelings of wanting to kill himself. Jim says that he has a plan to do it but does not have the means. Jim says that he hears a voice telling him that he would feel better if he could just shoot himself with a silver bullet because that would get rid of the demons inside him. Jim, however, doesn't have a gun or access to one. Jim tells the doctor that if could just feel better, he wouldn't want to kill himself.

Jim denies using any drugs or alcohol. He has no friends and no hobbies. He is beginning to argue with his father over just about everything. Jim yells sometimes but doesn't remember the fights. Jim is afraid that something is wrong with him, but he doesn't know what it could be. Dr. Jones discovers that Jim began hearing voices two years ago, but Jim never told anyone.

Dr. Jones's Treatment Plan

Dr. Jones prescribes Haldol, an antipsychotic medication, and suggests that Jim start taking it immediately. He also refers Jim to a social worker who works at the same HMO as Dr. Jones. The social worker will consult with Dr. Jones about how to proceed.

Assessment by the Social Worker

John Madison, a licensed clinical social worker, meets with Jim and his mother. John discusses Jim's history with them. John also asks about Jim's social relationships, school performance, suicidal feelings and history of suicidal ideation, and Jim's symptoms and complaints. John writes up his session as follows:

Social Worker's Progress Notes

Jim is an 18-year-old male who complains of depression, anxiety, and loneliness. For the past two years, he has been hearing voices, which have gotten stronger the summer after he graduated from high school. He says the voices tell him that to feel better he should shoot himself with a silver bullet to rid himself of the demon inside. Jim denies having access to a gun and seems motivated to feel better. He reports various delusions, such as feeling like the television is talking directly to him. He also experiences delusions of reference, such as believing that everyone is talking about him when he goes out in public. Jim has been unable to work because of his anxiety and depression. He has begun to fight frequently with his father, but doesn't remember doing so.

Jim was cooperative during the interview, but lacked emotional expression or humor. He was anxious and at times expressed himself in a confused, disorganized manner.

Jim is showing symptoms of paranoid schizophrenia. Although Jim has some stress in his life, such as graduating from school and having no job or money for himself, these stresses do not appear to be causing his symptoms.

Jim will continue taking the Haldol prescribed by Dr. Jones. I will refer Jim to the day-treatment center at St. Joseph's Hospital, which is covered by his medical insurance. I will oversee his treatment there and serve as case manager while he attends various support groups, educational groups, employment training groups, and socialization groups.

Symptoms	Treatment Plan	Duration
hearing voices, delusional	medication prescribed by Dr. Jones	indefinitely
depression	case management, medication socialization groups at day treatment	indefinitely 6 months to 1 year

Symptoms	Treatment Plan	Duration
suicidal ideation	case management, medication	indefinitely
	crisis intervention, case management	6 months to 1 year
bored, inactive	various groups at day treatment	as needed

John Madison's Treatment Plan

Symptoms	Treatment Plan	Duration
hearing voices, delusional	medication prescribed by Dr. Jones	indefinitely
depression	case management, medication	indefinitely
	socialization groups at day treatment	6 months to 1 year
suicidal ideation	case management, medication	indefinitely
	crisis intervention, case management	as needed
bored, inactive	various groups at day treatment	6 months to 1 year

Exit Quiz

1. At this stage in Jim's life, his schizophrenic symptoms can be considered
   a. chronic
   b. severe
   c. unmanageable
   d. all of the above

2. The treatment plans designed by all of the workers fall into which category?
   a. primary prevention
   b. secondary prevention
   c. tertiary prevention
   d. none of the above

3. Jim's suicidal risk is most likely
   a. low
   b. high
   c. middle
   d. no risk at all

4. When John Madison, writes that Jim was cooperative during the interview but lacked emotional expression or humor, which part of the SOAP method of writing notes was this ?
   a. subjective
   b. objective
   c. assessment
   d. plan

5. When John writes that Jim's symptoms of schizophrenia are probably not related to stress, John was addressing which part of the SOAP model?
   a. subjective
   b. objective
   c. assessment
   d. plan

6. When John describes Jim as saying that the voices tell him that to feel better, he should shoot himself with a silver bullet, which part of the SOAP model is he addressing?
   a. subjective
   b. objective
   c. assessment
   d. plan

7. According to John's treatment plan, which statement is most accurate?
   a. Jim will live in the day-treatment center for 1 year
   b. Jim will attend outpatient psychotherapy
   c. Jim will live with his parents while attending groups during the day
   d. None of the above

Exit Quiz Answers

1. b	4. b	7. c
2. c	5. c	
3. b	6. a	

CHAPTER 9

Human Services Delivery to Client Populations

Introduction

Generalist human services workers are capable of designing and implementing treatment plans for many client populations because of their knowledge of people's many needs and issues, and of the resources available to meet their clients' needs. Chapter 7 provides detailed discussions of the history, prevalence, needs, and issues of many client populations. Chapter 8 describes the many general assessment and intervention options available for human services professionals. Information in Chapter 7 and Chapter 8 is used in this chapter to examine how specific human services interventions relate to specific populations. Human services delivery for these populations are described for emergency situations, situations at the secondary and tertiary levels of intervention, and at the primary prevention level of intervention.

Human Services Delivery to the Poor

Emergency Situations and Interventions

The emergency situations faced by people living in poverty have to do with basic needs, such as food, water, safe shelter, and emergency medical assistance. Social services systems usually offer emergency food stamps and emergency medical care to people who would die or become seriously ill without them. Many hospital emergency rooms will assess a patient's eligibility for **indigent** (services for the poor) medical services. Most hospitals will not turn away critically ill patients because they do not have insurance or money. State and federal taxes fund these programs.

In addition to government-funded programs, many churches provide meals to those in dire need. Other nonprofit agencies provide emergency shelter and food for homeless people. Without these homeless shelters, many poor people would starve to death or die from exposure to harsh weather conditions.

Secondary Intervention

These interventions assist people in a temporary crisis. For instance, people who suddenly lose their jobs. They may have enough money for food, shelter, and medical care for only 30 days. Although these are not emergency situations, providing assistance to these people as soon as possible can prevent additional problems. They may need supportive counseling that encourages them to "hang in there" and provides resources that may help find new employment. This approach works best with people who have previously been able to support themselves but are now going through difficulties.

Some homeless shelters are now extending the number of days people can stay because of the difficulties brought about by the current economy. These shelters offer job training and group counseling, as well as food and shelter. Residents are motivated to return to autonomous living in society because they have previously supported themselves and have many coping skills and the confidence to return to that level of functioning.

Tertiary Intervention

Some people live in ongoing poverty and the likelihood of their ever being able to support themselves financially without assistance is low. They may have been raised in homes in which the mother received financial assistance from the government. In these cases, the medical care was probably also subsidized by the government. Additionally, they probably received food stamps and were part of the government school lunch program. They may have even lived in low-income housing. It might be possible that the mother may have never worked outside the home or had any intention of ever working. Being raised in conditions such as these often leads to cycles of living in poverty and depending on welfare. The mindset is one of entitlement to government assistance and accepting that they have no other way to survive. Dependence on the system to support the family is not considered negative, but rather a way of life.

The original welfare program, **AID to Families with Dependent Children** (AFDC), has been significantly changed since its inception in the 1960s. The 1996 Welfare Reform Act signed into legislation by the Clinton administration required that welfare recipients attend college, trade school, or seek employment as part of the condition of receiving government financial assistance. This Welfare to Work program was an attempt to decrease the cycle of welfare and encourage people to support themselves and their families. When AFDC was first established, families received financial assistance as long as they had minor children at home and received a set dollar amount for each child. The government fully funded many households, some for as many as 20 years sometimes. This com-

True Stories From Human Service Workers

Secondary Intervention at a Homeless Shelter

Workers in homeless shelters focus largely on the here and now, rather than on past difficulties. Wise Place, a homeless shelter in southern California, keeps the focus on crisis intervention for people going through tough times.

Example: Cindy Snelling, a counselor and generalist practitioner at Wise Place, says that "When counseling the clients, cognitive theories and techniques are used the most. The focus is on the here and now and on helping them figure out how to move forward."

plete financial reliance on the government created a population who developed a sense of learned helplessness. It was hoped that assisting these people to get jobs would increase their self-esteem and desire to support themselves.

Currently, these recipients may still receive financial assistance but only for a few years while the mother seeks employment and job training. Also, the amount of money that any family may receive is limited to a predetermined amount. In other words, recipients do not now receive additional funds for every child they have. This program is only a beginning in changing this cycle of poverty that many people have fallen into. Although these recipients may not receive financial assistance indefinitely, they often rely on government-funded programs, such as free school lunches, food stamps, and medical care to help subsidize any income they earn. Unfortunately, even though they do work, they are often underpaid and cannot afford basic care for their children.

Primary Prevention

A few programs have been developed that work with children and teens to make sure they feel prepared to enter the job market, manage money, and take care of themselves throughout life. As early as 6th grade, some children are learning how to invest money, how to manage a checking account, why saving money is important, and how to use credit wisely. Many high schools offer courses that focus on family life and independent living.

Perhaps the most common types of programs that aim at preventing poverty are those that focus on encouraging adolescents to complete high school and attend college. Education can have a huge impact on income. Primary prevention education with teenagers who are about to become adults can make them realize that finishing high school, getting adequate job skills training, and even going on to higher education can get them out of the trap of poverty that their parents found themselves in. This idea of economic mobility in the United States is strongly believed to be based on attaining marketable training and higher education.

Human Services Delivery in Child Abuse Situations

Emergency Situations and Interventions

When a case of child abuse is reported to the police or **child protective services,** an emergency response system takes immediate action. The first step is to assess whether a child is in immediate danger. Such factors as the age and location of a child and the type of abuse determine how soon an emergency worker responds to any given case. Typically, any type of abuse involving infants receives priority status since they are the most helpless of all minors. On the other hand, older adolescents are considered to be more capable of self-care and may be last to receive emergency assessment and intervention.

Any minor that is assessed to be in need of immediate medical care, food, shelter, clothing or supervision receives emergency services. They are provided with all of these needs either by being placed in a government-funded emergency shelter, or by being given treatment in a hospital emergency room, or by being given food and clothing. If a social worker assesses that a child would be in danger by remaining with a parent or guardian, that child will be removed from the home and put in a temporary emergency shelter run by the government. The child remains under the care of the state until other arrangements are made that can assure the safe care of the minor. Relatives may be a good resource to turn to in emergency cases.

The same is true if a child is at risk of being physically or sexually abused. If a social worker assesses that another adult in the home cannot protect a child from an abuser, the child will be removed from the home and put in a state-funded emergency shelter. The age of a child and the severity of the abuse increase the likelihood of a child being removed. Children who have been and continue to be at risk of sexual abuse are often provided with special services from social workers, counselors, attorneys, and law enforcement who all specialize in dealing with sexual abuse emergency situations. The child is interviewed in the presence of all behind a one-way mirror in an attempt to reduce the trauma of being interviewed. This helps reduce problems when it comes time to try the case in court. Also, emergency medical care and psychological intervention are available at these agencies.

The primary goal of emergency care for children who are abused is to ensure no further abuse will take place and that the child's physical and emotional well-being are taken care of in hopes of preventing deterioration in functioning. Additionally, basic needs for survival must also be provided.

Secondary Intervention

Once a child's safety and basic needs are assured, the focus turns to the psychological trauma. Counseling for children and their parents may be provided to assist in dealing with the possible break up of the family unit. Safe reunification is the goal in most cases. Even when children are not removed from their homes, family or individual counseling may help families express feelings, fears, and learn more appropriate coping and communication skills. Children who are abused often benefit from play therapy that encourages them to color, paint, play with clay, or use dolls to act out their experiences. Play therapy is effective because it is an easy way for children to express themselves, and they feel most comfortable with play objects in hand while talking about traumatic situations.

Parents who are first-time offenders are often referred to parenting classes in which they learn about normal child development and appropriate expectations, as well as effective disciplinary methods. If drug or alcohol abuse is an issue, parents are referred to drug and alcohol awareness classes or even a twelve-step program. Sometimes, parents may attend support groups or even more confrontational groups where they can openly express their feelings about the system and offending or nonoffending parents, and where they can also discuss how their own childhood experiences have affected their own parenting abilities. Individual counseling may also be useful for these parents and children.

The goal of the counseling and educational groups is to teach new coping skills, assist the children and parents to express their feelings and better understand why the abuse occurred, and to prevent any further abuse from occurring. Sometimes children remain in the home while crisis intervention and counseling is provided, while other children live with relatives or in group or foster homes until treatment is completed. The duration of treatment for isolated incidents of abuse may range from six weeks to one year.

Tertiary Intervention

Sadly, some parents have treated their children abusively for many years and require longer-term services. Whether these parents' drug and alcohol addictions or serious emotional problems have caused this abuse, they cannot seem to care for their children properly, despite receiving help from various social services agencies. These cases need ongoing monitoring and case plans, which sometimes last for more than five years. This often means frequent hearings with a judge and many chances to improve in their parenting abilities. Some people just can't seem to pull it together, no matter how many services they receive.

Some need to be involved indefinitely in twelve-step groups, such as AA. Others need to participate in support groups, such as Parents United, Parents Anonymous, and other groups designed that help parents stop their abusive behavior. At some point, however, many of these parents lose custody of their children, who are either given up for adoption, placed in foster or group homes until they turn 18, or live with relatives while their parents are only permitted supervised visits with them.

Group homes provide counseling services for the children and usually implement a program based on the principles of behavior modification in an attempt to reinforce and teach coping skills and eliminate negative behaviors. Children raised in chronically abusive conditions have many emotional and behavioral disorders and need regular therapy and sometimes medication to manage uncontrollable feelings of rage, fear, and depression. They are at high risk for suicidal behavior, self-mutilation, and drug abuse. Those children placed in foster homes or adopted out must also receive services to help adjust to their new family and resolve feelings they hold toward their own parents. The trauma of being chronically abused as a child often follows the person well into adulthood, and the person often needs ongoing therapy as an adult. Support groups, such as Incest Survivors Anonymous (ISA) and Adult Children of Alcoholics (ACA), offer these people ongoing support throughout their lives. The emotional consequences of chronic abuse can often take 20 years or longer to overcome, even with the help of effective therapists. Because therapy can be costly, it is vital to let clients know about low-cost or no-cost resources available at nonprofit agencies and at twelve-step groups.

Primary Prevention

On a more optimistic note, many programs are designed to prevent abuse from occurring in the first place. At-risk groups are targeted and provided with assistance in hopes of giving them skills and resources that will increase chances for successful parenting. At-risk groups, such as single mothers, pregnant teens, and low-income families, may receive parenting education, financial assistance, and support for housing, child care, and medical care. Hotlines have been developed that allow parents to call and vent frustrations in hopes that this will prevent them from acting out these feelings on their children.

Children also receive services that attempt to prevent abuse from occurring. It might be education at the elementary school level in which children are taught about appropriate touching, or it might be at the high school level where teens are taught about proper parenting techniques. Pregnant teens and new teen mothers are also provided with primary prevention services in an effort to reduce the risk of abuse occurring. Many programs teach these teen mothers how to care for a baby before and after birth and how to use resources in their community. Having access to child care, medical care, and completing high school is important for these teen mothers. Helping them to become self-sufficient by encouraging them to complete school so they can be competitive in the job market will reduce their stress. Lowered stress reduces the tendency to engage in abusive behaviors with children. Being able to work and support herself and the child will also reduce the likelihood of the child being neglected.

The overall goal of primary prevention is to target at-risk groups, teach them about child abuse, how to prevent it, and how to manage stress effectively.

Human Services Delivery to the Elderly

Emergency Situations and Interventions

Because many elderly people need help caring for themselves, many programs provide services that meet immediate needs for protection, shelter, food, and medical care. Not all elderly people are unable to work or provide for themselves, but when aged people have Alzheimer's disease and other forms of **dementia,** are frail, or suddenly become ill, public and nonprofit agencies step in to make sure they are safe and are not being abused or neglected. Many elderly people with Alzheimer's disease may wander outside their homes, putting themselves in unsafe situations. They may need immediate hospitalization or supervision in a daycare center until their behavior can be better managed.

Most government-funded social services agencies include both Children's Services and **Adult Services.** These adult services provide emergency care for the elderly and disabled adults who cannot take care of themselves and who do not have family to help them. Social workers and nurses often visit elderly people at their homes to ensure their needs are met when it comes to their attention that an elderly person may not be eating, is not managing an illness appropriately, or if basic hygiene and sanitation conditions are not adequate. Immediate intervention is provided to ensure that the elderly person's basic needs are met. Social workers may transport the person to a hospital, see to it that food is brought to him or her, or hire someone to clean up the home.

Sometimes elderly are subject to being abused physically, sexually, financially, or neglected in institutions. Adult Services serves as a watchdog over such institutions and responds immediately when any abuse is reported. Adult Services also responds when an elderly person has been abused by family members or acquaintances as well.

The goal of emergency services for the elderly is to ensure that such basic needs as food, shelter, clothing, medical care, safety, and sanitary living conditions are available.

Secondary Intervention

Some elderly people may have their basic needs met but need immediate assistance. These individuals may have fairly good support systems, such as adult children who help care for them. Often, these adult children enter into crisis states themselves because their caretaking responsibilities have become overwhelming. Many programs, such as the Alzheimer Association, have been created to assist caretakers. Counselors at this agency come to a client's home and work with the elderly person on various cognitive and recreational skills, giving the caretaker a much-needed break.

Sometimes the crisis is financial. The elderly person and/or the children often feel overwhelmed with medical expenses or just daily living expenses. People who retire or can no longer work must survive on a limited income. This can be scary. Lifestyles must change, and counseling can help people adjust to these new changes. It can be reframed as a normal transition in the life cycle that everyone goes through, and counselors can assure a person that many resources are available to help. Human services workers often serve as advocates for the elderly, helping them access pension money, social security benefits, and sometimes life insurance benefits after a spouse dies. They may also be assisted in getting federally funded medical insurance, such as Medicare, which pays for most medical care and medications.

Tertiary Intervention

Many elderly people can live independently throughout their lives. They are physically and mentally healthy and have sufficient social supports to live on their own. Some elderly, however, cannot manage on their own because they are terminally ill, have cognitive impairments related to Alzheimer's disease or other dementias, or have difficulty getting around and may require a wheelchair. These individuals may need either professional or nonprofessional nursing support indefinitely, which may be provided in their own homes.

More often, however, the needs of elderly people are too extensive and can be met only in a residential facility designed to assist seniors. These facilities range from total care institutions for people who are very ill and disabled to assisted-living apartments for seniors who need help occasionally. The decision to have one's parent live in a facility is often emotionally difficult for adult children who often feel guilty because they feel they should be able to take care of their parents. Unfortunately, most children must work full time and are busy raising their own children and simply cannot take proper care of very ill and needy parents. Social workers and counselors can help these children understand that sometimes their parents are safer in one of these facilities than in their own home. They can be reassured that their parents may prefer to be around others of the same age.

Primary Prevention

Almost every city has a well-established senior center operating on a regular basis. These centers have proven to be very helpful in keeping the elderly physically active, involved in the community, educated about nutrition and good health, socially adept, and emotionally healthier than if they merely stayed at home by themselves. By participating in various groups, such as music appreciation, tai chi, crafts, reminiscent activities, and tax-education classes, these seniors are keeping their minds active, which lessens the likelihood of cognitive impairment. Social interaction can help prevent depression. Being educated about taxes and other financial situations can prevent financial crises.

These centers also provide a place to eat a healthy meal with others, which can help prevent malnutrition. Some of these centers also have programs for seniors who want to volunteer at various agencies. Such programs improve self-esteem and help seniors feel that they are contributing to society.

The overall goal of senior centers is to keep seniors active and healthy for as long as possible. Healthy stimulation and social interaction seem to assist in maintaining good health.

Human Services Delivery to the Disabled

Emergency Situations and Interventions

People with physical disabilities may be more prone to crisis situations (Doyle, in Kanel, 2007) and more likely to need emergency care because these various disabilities often make it more difficult to function, create conditions more conducive to accidents, and have an unpredictable quality to them. Fortunately, people with recognized disabilities do not have much difficulty receiving medical care. Government funding for such individuals is readily available.

As with the elderly, individuals with disabilities may be vulnerable to abuse and neglect. Government agencies at the county, state and federal levels have been created to take care of these situations. Even though the **Americans with Disabilities Act** (ADA) was passed in 1992, those with disabilities still have difficulty receiving funding for human services. Although emergency services are usually easy to access, some of the primary prevention services may not be as easy to access.

Secondary Intervention

The goal of secondary intervention with individuals who are disabled is not to cure them of their disability, but to manage crises related to the disability. Many of the crisis situations encountered by the disabled population have to do with inadequate knowledge and understanding of a particular individual's disability and failure to establish or keep in place the necessary support systems (Doyle, in Kanel, 2007). As with all crisis intervention, effective treatment of individuals with disabilities is rooted in a system of comprehensive collaboration among various professionals. Additionally, human services workers must be knowledgeable of the many resources available to help them with legal concerns, medical needs, and other needs related to the disability. Societal stigma against this population, discrimination, and embarrassment about dependency are often components of a crisis state for individuals with disabilities and their families. Mental health counselors, both professional and nonprofessional may serve as a needed support system for a person with a disability. Many people with disabilities are capable of using regular mental health treatment. They deserve meaningful intervention and attention, not to be stigmatized or patronized.

Secondary intervention might include advocacy to receive equal services and treatment at work, school, or at an agency. This requires the human services worker to be knowledgeable about laws and rights.

For example, public school systems, on parents' request, must test any child for learning disabilities, and, if a child has a learning disability, the school must provide the intervention that a child with that disability requires. Some parents might seek the assistance of a counselor for this child, not knowing that the school system should be providing services. In such instances, the counselor should act as an advocate for this child to receive the benefits mandated by federal legislation.

Tertiary Intervention

Because many disabilities cannot be repaired or significantly changed, much of the intervention for this population is tertiary in nature. That is, the function of intervention is to provide a healthy and as normal a quality of life as possible for the disabled person. Keeping a person functioning in mainstream society as much as possible is the aim. Some students (those suffering from dyslexia or attention-deficit hyperactivity disorder [ADHD]) may be able to manage a mainstream class for most of the day, while attending a special resources class for certain subjects. Others may have to attend a special school for students with disabilities, such as the Braille Institute for the Blind or a special school for autistic children. No matter where the child attends school, the goal is to provide as normal an experience as the one students without disabilities receive at school.

Other people with disabilities may have to reside indefinitely in board-and-care homes or residential facilities, such as hospitals or group homes. Their disability may be so severe (profound mental retardation, for instance) that it prevents them from meaningful interaction with society. Permanent hospitalization or institutionalization is only considered as a last resort, however. Many previously institutionalized disabled people can now live in board-and-care homes or in private homes with their families, attend special programs in the community for individuals who are disabled where they go on field trips with trained human services workers. They may even participate regularly in other social activities, such as cooking, singing, dancing, and arts and crafts. These outpatient programs give them a more normal life and a higher quality of existence.

Most people with disabilities receiving tertiary intervention have case managers whose job it is to assess the person's needs and connect the person with many community resources. These case managers must know how to use the laws designed to provide a better life for them as well.

Primary Prevention

Preventing certain disabilities from occurring may be possible. Some disabilities result from genetic abnormalities. Much research is currently focusing on hereditary disabilities and methods to detect the genes that pass on those traits. Parents who know they may pass on a disability might be able to take medication or get other types of treatment that may slow or even prevent a disability altogether. Some might even opt not to carry the pregnancy to full term.

Other disabilities result from taking certain chemicals, drugs, or alcohol during pregnancy. For example, in the 1940s and 1950s, physicians were treating severe morning sickness with a new drug, thalidomide. This drug created severe birth defects in babies born to mothers who took the medication. So banning the drug for pregnant women prevented further thalidomide-related birth defects. Another preventable birth defect is fetal alcohol syndrome, which is caused by a mother's heavy alcohol use during pregnancy. Prior to the 1970s, pregnant women regularly consumed wine and other alcohol throughout their pregnancies. Studies have since shown women who drank heavily during pregnancy gave birth to children who were mentally slow and behaviorally challenged. As a result, alcohol consumption during pregnancy is strongly discouraged, which has lessened the incidence of fetal alcohol syndrome.

In general, educating pregnant teenagers early on about the effects drugs and alcohol can have on their unborn babies is the best preventive way to intervene. Despite all precautions, however, some babies are born with disabilities, the causes of which have yet to be identified. The best that can be done is to detect the disability early in a child's life so treatment can begin. For example, the sooner a child who is blind learns Braille and how to use a guide dog, the better the quality of life. The same holds true for children who are deaf or autistic. Early intervention can prevent a lifetime of crises and tertiary institutionalization.

Human Services Delivery in Domestic Violence Situations

Emergency Situations and Interventions

Domestic violence is the leading cause of injury to women between the ages of 15 and 44 in the United States (Committee on the Judiciary United States Senate, 102nd Congress, 1992). In the United States, more than three women are murdered every day by their husbands or boyfriends (Bureau of Justice Statistics Crime Data Brief, 2003). Domestic violence is the leading cause of women's emergency room visits in the United States and one of the leading causes of death. Not only are women at risk for injury, but their children may be in danger as well. There is a strong connection between spousal abuse and child abuse (Bancroft & Silverman, 2003; Bowker, Arbitell, & McFerron, 1988; Langford, Isaac, & Kabat, 1999). When physical or sexual abuse causes someone in a family to be injured, a possible emergency situation exists.

Hospital emergency rooms are well equipped, and the staff is well trained on how to treat women and children who have been battered. Recent legislation made it a requirement for physicians, nurses, chiropractors, and dentists to report suspected cases of spousal abuse to the police because the incidents of domestic violence are so frequent. It was hoped that this would be one way to prevent further abuse from occurring.

Often, domestic violence occurs at night. Many women leave home with their children and nothing but the clothes on their backs to escape a life-threatening situation. **Battered women's shelters** have emergency services available to help these women and children. When an abused woman calls the 24-hour hotline affiliated with a battered women's shelter, an assessment is made to determine if it is an emergency situation, then the woman and her children either drive to a location to meet a worker from the shelter, or she is told to go to an emergency room. She may be admitted to the shelter that day or evening, or she may be given vouchers to stay at a local motel until a shelter has a bed for her.

The goal of emergency services for women and children who have been battered is first, to ensure that injuries are dealt with by medical personnel, second, to ensure that she is no longer at risk of being injured that day or evening, and third, to provide a safe shelter for her and the children where the batterer cannot gain access. All battered women's shelters have confidential locations. In fact, it is a felony to disclose the location of one. This ensures the safety of these women and their children, all of whom are in danger of being killed within the first 72 hours after they leave home.

In addition to safe shelter, other emergency services provided at the shelters include food, child care, sanitary sleeping arrangements, and clothing. Legal advice is also provided. The woman who was battered may wish to petition for a **temporary restraining order** as extra protection from her batterer. Most district attorneys' offices connected to local courts have a special department that deals specifically with domestic violence. Trained advocates and counselors provide emergency legal assistance that may include filing for child custody, emergency financial assistance, and filing for divorce.

Secondary Intervention

Not all women seeking services related to domestic violence are in emergency situations. They may need assistance from the district attorney's office regarding filing for a restraining order. They may need guidance from legal aid about how to file for divorce and seek child custody. They may need temporary financial assistance from social services. These women sometimes have access to resources to tide them over until the system kicks in with its help.

Example: A 62-year-old woman visited her physician for a routine medical exam. The doctor noticed bruises on her neck and ribs, as well as a black eye. He found out that she had been battered by her husband. He told her not to go home. He filed a report and recommended she drive to a neighboring county to stay with her grown daughter. This woman had money in her purse, a car, and a place to go. She stayed with her daughter that night, returned to her home court the next day, filed a restraining order, and set up a date to return and deal with money issues. The advocate at the court recommended she schedule an appointment with a therapist to talk about her feelings and develop a plan. She participated in crisis intervention with the therapist. Although she needed immediate services, this situation is not exactly an emergency. She had a place to go, money, food, and access to legal assistance.

Much of the secondary intervention provided for this client was aimed at educating her about the **battering cycle** so she could make choices that would be in her best interest. Many battered women benefit from understanding the cyclical nature of domestic violence. In the beginning, a woman and man get along fine and are in a so-called honeymoon phase. Over time, however, normal tensions and stress arise. Batterers lack communication skills and coping abilities, which creates high levels of tension and makes the woman feel she must "walk on eggshells" in an effort to avoid an argument or a tirade. Unfortunately, for these men, the explosive stage is inevitable and is accompanied by verbal abuse, physical abuse, or sexual abuse. At this stage, the woman is most likely to seek help. She is vulnerable, injured, and scared. During this crisis state, she is usually more receptive to crisis intervention by counselors and law enforcement. If she doesn't get help during this phase, she may easily return to the honeymoon phase, and the cycle continues.

Most battered women's shelters operate on a 45-day model. This is considered sufficient time to help a woman deal with her feelings of rage, fear, and shame; secure employment, apply for financial assistance, file for divorce, restraining order, and child custody; or enroll in job training courses. If the problem is not a chronic, long-standing one, most women benefit from secondary intervention and function well in society. The hope is that they will not continue in a relationship with a batterer nor start a new relationship with an abusive person.

Tertiary Intervention

Some women have lived in ongoing abusive relationships for many years. They have participated in treatment, even filed for divorce or restraining orders, but return to the abusive partner. Many times these women have developed battered woman's syndrome (discussed in Chapter 7). They may need long-term therapy or case management to assist them in finding relationships that are not abusive. They may live in poverty, be disabled, or may have been raised in an abusive home. These factors make it difficult to stay out of abusive situations. They may not have the material, psychological, or social resources to cope with daily stress on their own and so they tolerate abuse. This type of woman may benefit from support groups, medication, or educational groups.

Human services workers must manage their own frustrations with these women who often return to their batterer or refuse to leave him in the first place. They need emotional support and understanding about why they stay, which is usually because they fear being alone, being killed, taking their children away from their father, and being labeled by society. It might take 5 to 10 years for a woman to finally leave an abusive relationship. She may have needed counseling for 10 years to learn that she can function on her own and that she will have support should she leave.

Primary Prevention

As with all the other problems discussed, preventing abuse is by far the most desirable form of intervention. Many programs exist in which human services workers visit high schools and conduct education about domestic violence. Teens are taught about the battering cycle, how to detect a high-risk abusive person, how to assert themselves, and how to communicate and create a healthy relationship. Dating violence is very prevalent, and teens are taught that they don't have to endure it.

Human Services Delivery
in Sexual Assault Situations

Emergency Situations and Interventions

Most communities have created sexual assault victim services, either through nonprofit organizations or through existing justice centers. The sexual assault centers provide 24-hour hotline services staffed by trained volunteers, and supervised by licensed counselors. They often work collaboratively with law enforcement officials when the victim wishes to press charges against her assailant. The advocates at these sexual assault centers often accompany the sexually assaulted victim to the hospital after the assault and stay by her side during the rape evidence exam as a support person. Victims often need emergency medical care for injuries sustained during the rape.

In addition to hospital exams, victims of sexual assault need to be in a safe location, such as a friend's or relative's home, a hotel, or a shelter. They may need food and clothing as well, depending on how the assault occurred. During the first 72 hours following the rape, advocates from sexual assault centers conduct follow-up visits as this is when the victim is most vulnerable to psychological shock.

Secondary Intervention

After the immediate medical and legal emergencies have been addressed, the victim needs crisis intervention. She usually benefits from treatment that focuses on transitioning her from seeing herself as a victim to seeing herself as a survivor. Both in individual and group counseling, she should be educated about the prevalence of sexual assault and the dynamics of rapists. The goal is to help her see that she is not to blame nor is she damaged.

Family members may also benefit from crisis intervention to help them cope with the victim's crisis state. She may be disorganized for a while until she can assimilate the trauma as part of her life.

In addition to counseling, sexual assault victims can benefit from advocates who accompany them to court proceedings and other agencies. After being raped, a victim often feels like she is in a daze and has difficulty communicating with people. It is very helpful to have someone by her side that understands what she has gone through.

Tertiary Intervention

Some victims of sexual assault do not seek professional services after the assault. They may not report the rape to law enforcement. In fact, most rapes probably go

True Stories From Human Service Workers

Crisis Intervention with Sexual Assault Survivors

At first, many rape survivors are hesitant to attend support groups. Their immediate state of crisis often prevents them from feeling comfortable being around others and talking about their assault.

Example 1: Kara Hay, a counselor at a sexual assault center in Orange County, CA, says, "Group therapy is vital to the recovery of many victims. Hearing others' stories and sharing their own stories with others helps them realize that they do not have to go through the pain alone. They realize that the heinous crime that was perpetrated against them does not have to be a secret, and they can live full and happy lives despite the awful ordeal."

Example 2: According to Brande Titis, supervisor of client services at a sexual assault center based within the Community Services Program in Santa Ana, CA, "We use the crisis intervention model because of its efficiency. It is the only model in which we have been properly trained. Our volunteers respond to hotline and hospital calls 24 hours a day, conduct follow up visits within 72 hours with all clients. Advocates accompany clients to hospitals, law enforcement agencies, district attorneys' offices, court proceedings and other agencies."

This agency's ability to provide all of these services helps decrease the risk of the victim feeling alone. According to crisis theory and the secondary intervention model, by providing services that meet victims' various and most urgent needs in a timely manner, the agency is helping clients remain functioning in as normal a manner as possible.

unreported since date rape is one of the most prevalent forms of rape, and many women simply do not realize that they have been raped when it was done by an acquaintance. Additionally, some victims fail to seek help because of shame, fear, social pressure not to deal with the assault, or lack of knowledge about how to use resources.

After a sexual assault, some victims are able to function at minimally acceptable levels. They do this by using psychological defense mechanisms, such as denial, repression, rationalization, and self-blame. The trauma can sometimes be forgotten for several years. Some victims never tell anyone that they were raped. When a victim waits many years before seeking help, she has usually been suffering from **post-traumatic stress disorder** (PTSD). Long-term therapy is needed to help her open up about the event that she has spent years trying to forget. The anxiety, nightmares, sleeplessness, numbness, and hypervigilance she experiences are indicative of PTSD. She will most likely need many years of individual, marital, and/or group therapy to work through the trauma and be relieved of these symptoms. The longer a victim waits to seek help, the longer her treatment will be. She has learned coping skills to survive that may have hindered her social relationships, work and academic functioning, and her ability to feel spontaneous joy and comfort in the world.

Primary Prevention

Some high schools offer guest speakers to their students who visit campuses and provide educational talks about sexual assault, in particular, date rape and drug-induced rape, which can happen when a drug (such as rohypnol, often called "roofies") is slipped into someone's drink. These educational programs aim to encourage young women to assert themselves with men, say no, make a fuss if someone tries to rape them, pay attention to possible clues that someone might be untrustworthy, not put themselves in risky situations, and to learn self-defense techniques.

College campuses also provide many opportunities for students to learn about rape prevention through various workshops and support groups in which men and women can address sexual assault issues.

Human Services Delivery in Correctional System Situations

Emergency Situations and Interventions

When people get arrested, it usually creates a feeling of emergency for the person arrested and significant others. The legal system handles what happens after the arrest. Either the person stays in jail or gets out on bail. The person either hires an attorney, or gets one appointed to him or her by the court system. Human services workers are not generally involved in this aspect of intervention.

Secondary Intervention

Human services workers, however, do become involved once the preliminary interventions have been completed. Many people who break the law by committing burglary, murder, assault, forgery, and theft go to some type of correctional facility. Human services workers play a larger role in working with first-time offenders and juveniles than with people who have long histories of criminal behavior.

Human services workers are also involved with "family" crimes, such as domestic violence and child abuse. Social workers, therapists, and probation officers, among others, must work collaboratively on these family crimes. These offenders rarely go to prison. The court system and society holds conflicting views on these offenses. It is hard to decide whether these crimes result from emotional disorders, or from bad choices and greed, the cause of so many other crimes. Think back to the inventory you took in Chapter 6. You may also have had ambivalent feelings and reactions toward these perpetrators. These offenders rarely go to prison because society prefers to keep families together when possible. Also, the perpetrator is often the sole bread winner of the family, and so keeping him or her out of prison may help keep a family out of the welfare system.

So if they don't go to prison, what interventions are available? Probation is one common intervention for first-time offenders and juveniles. Probation can be formal or informal. People on formal probation must visit their probation officer about once a month. Probation officers serve as case managers, working with offenders to ensure they are functioning within the law, attending any required counseling or twelve-step groups, and are not associating with the wrong people. As long as offenders comply with the rules of their probation, they do not have to do additional time in a correctional facility. If they break those rules, then incarceration may be inevitable.

Many people involved in crimes related to substance abuse, such as drunk driving, possession of drugs, and public intoxication, may be referred to **diversion programs.** These programs usually consist of drug awareness and drug education groups, individual and family counseling, and community service. The offenders eligible for diversion programs are not usually chronic drug addicts because addicts usually need more intense treatment. However, juveniles and recreational/social drug users may benefit from these programs.

Perpetrators of domestic violence are often sent to mandatory, structured treatment programs for batterers. These programs last between six months and two years and include anger-management groups, individual therapy, drug and alcohol counseling, twelve-step programs, and parenting classes. If a perpetrator has a long history of arrests for spousal abuse, he may have to be incarcerated.

Perpetrators of child abuse receive intervention plans from child protective services. A social worker assigned to a case serves as its case manager and develops a plan appropriate for the offense. Perpetrators of severe child abuse and neglect go to prison; however, first-time offenders convicted of abuse that was not life threatening may be referred to parenting classes, twelve-step groups, individual therapy, and family counseling. The case manager monitors the completion of the case plan and works toward reunifying a family if it is safe for the children.

When a family member sexually abuses a child, intervention is usually geared more toward counseling and reunification than punishment. Strangers who sexually abuse children are more likely to be incarcerated, though not for very long. Perpetrators of incest may be given probation that includes mandatory involvement in group therapy and individual counseling. If, however, these offenders have a longstanding history of child molestation, they may be given significant jail time.

As with all secondary interventions, the goal is to prevent any further offending behaviors. Sometimes crisis intervention is enough, but many problems need more intense psychotherapy and group therapy.

Tertiary Intervention

People who commit serious crimes, such as murder, kidnapping, armed robbery, drug distribution, and the like, are usually incarcerated. Sometimes the incarceration is to punish, other times it is to protect society. Even some of the family crimes and substance abuse crimes mentioned above receive incarceration sentences from judges. When crimes are not considered to be a crime against another person, such as petty theft, forgery, drug use and possession, offenders may be allowed to serve part of their sentences at a halfway house. These halfway houses provide employment training and counseling, group therapy, twelve-step groups, and personal counseling. The offenders learn to function in society as a law abiding citizen, something they may have never done before. Sometimes, these chronic criminals need daily support to help them avoid involvement with the criminal justice system.

Primary Prevention

As mentioned in Chapter 8 a famous example of a primary prevention program in the area of crime is the Scared Straight program. At-risk juveniles are either taken to prison, or prisoners visit these juveniles at an agency. The convicts tell the scary truth about incarceration to these youths. A similar program involves having at-risk youth participate for a brief time at a boot camp, a sort of mock prison facility where they must adhere to very strict rules.

CRITICAL THINKING / SELF-REFLECTION CORNER

- Should all people who commit crimes go to prison?

- How should society decide who should go to prison and who should receive counseling and educational courses?

- Do you think child abusers, rapists, and spousal abusers should receive the same consequences as other criminals? Why or why not?

- Do you think probation is a good idea?

- What other interventions do you think should be imposed on first-time offenders?

Human Services Delivery in Substance Abuse Situations

Emergency Situations and Interventions

Substance abuse emergencies may be either life-threatening emergencies or legal emergencies. Life-threatening emergencies, such as suicide attempts, heart attacks, strokes, or overdoses, must be treated in a medical hospital. An illness or injury must be managed and stabilized before any other treatment for substance abuse begins.

When substance abusers are arrested for drug possession, driving under the influence of alcohol or an illegal substance, or any other illegal drug-related crime, they need immediate assistance.

Once a person has been cleared medically and legal issues have been managed, workers can begin to work with a person on their abuse of drugs or alcohol.

Secondary Intervention

Brief intervention for alcohol-related problems may be effective for those who are not alcohol dependent. That is, they report drinking at levels that may be risky but have not yet created serious medical or legal problems in their lives. The goal of this type of brief intervention may be to reduce drinking to moderate levels. If the drinker is alcohol-dependent, the goal would be **abstinence.** Treatment for alcohol-dependency is discussed under tertiary intervention.

Common elements of brief intervention include the following:

1. providing information about health risks associated with heavy drinking
2. emphasizing that it's the patient's own responsibility and decision to drink
3. advising on how to reduce or stop drinking and how to engage in "low-risk" drinking
4. providing strategies to reduce drinking, such as pacing one's drinking, sipping, and so forth
5. using an empathic counseling style
6. encouraging patients to rely on their own resources to bring about change and to be optimistic about their ability to change (National Institute on Alcohol Abuse and Alcoholism, 1999)

Short-term counseling and crisis intervention may also be appropriate and effective for some drug users, especially if they have just begun to abuse drugs. In particular, adolescents may benefit from brief intervention if they haven't yet developed a lifestyle in which drug use has become the focal point. These drug users may simply need drug education classes, family therapy, or supportive counseling. The focus of these interventions should be on how to return to their previous level of functioning prior to drug use. The drug user might be encouraged to become involved in productive recreational activities, to rekindle friendships that may have been damaged by drug use, and to increase satisfaction from work or school. Sometimes, the drug use is an attempt to cope with other life problems. Counselors can often help drug users express feelings and talk about problems and learn ways to cope with them without resorting to drug use.

Some people who abuse drugs and alcohol may also benefit from **twelve-step facilitation.** While it may be true that a person who is addicted and physically dependent on drugs or alcohol may need to participate in a twelve-step group indefinitely, some might benefit from a twelve-step group for a brief time. They may need the support of the group to help them shift their social world into one that doesn't include drug use. A twelve-step group for some people can be used as a transitional social world until they have a healthy stable social world developed in their own life.

"Twelve-step facilitation (TSF) consists of a brief, structured, and manual-driven approach to facilitating early recovery from alcohol abuse/alcoholism and other drug abuse/addiction. It is intended to be implemented on an individual basis in 12 to 15 sessions and is based on behavioral, spiritual, and cognitive principles that form the core of twelve-step fellowships such as AA. TSF is suitable for problem drinkers and other drug users and for those who are alcohol or drug dependent" (Nowinski, 2000). The goal of TSF is to facilitate the acceptance of the need for abstinence from alcohol and other drugs and the willingness to participate actively in a twelve-step fellowship as a means of sustaining sobriety. After a few months of twelve-step group participation, some users who are not physically addicted to alcohol or drugs may be able to use alcohol or drugs moderately and still function appropriately in society. However, some people who have had chronic drug and alcohol problems cannot ever drink or use drugs at all and may need to be involved with a twelve-step group indefinitely. We turn to those chronic abusers next.

Tertiary Intervention

For individuals who drink or use drugs chronically, the goal is complete abstinence. During the TSF process, a counselor attempts to convince these clients that willpower alone is not sufficient to sustain sobriety. Instead, they must surrender to the group conscience of the twelve-step group and accept that a higher power is the locus of changing one's life. Clients remain in therapy for a few weeks after joining a twelve-step group. This allows clients to discuss with their therapist how they can best use the group, and a therapist can offer encouragement to continue going to the group. A TSF therapist also conducts a few sessions with significant others during this time.

Some individuals with drug and alcohol addictions need treatment beyond TSF and twelve-step groups. "No single treatment is appropriate for all individuals. Matching treatment settings, interventions, and services to each individual's particular problems and needs is critical to his or her ultimate success in returning to productive functioning in the family, workplace, and society" (National Institute on Drug Abuse, 2003).

Intervention for clients who abuse drugs and alcohol chronically may include such medications as methadone, LAAM, and naltrexone that help those addicted to opiates reduce their dependency on those types of drugs, as well as antidepressants, mood stabilizers, or neuroleptics that help treat mental disorders, such as depression, anxiety, bipolar, or psychosis, that may accompany drug and alcohol addiction. For those with severe physical addictions detoxification is often necessary. During a detoxification process, an addict may be given medication to ease the symptoms of withdrawal from an opiate, pain pills, alcohol, cocaine, or crystal methamphetamine. This may take three to five days. After a person is stabilized on medication, treatment can begin to focus on the psychological and social aspects of the addiction.

Medical detoxification safely manages the acute physical symptoms of withdrawal associated with stopping drug and alcohol use, but it is rarely sufficient in helping addicts achieve long-term abstinence (National Institute on Drug Abuse, 2003). Recovery from drug addiction can be a long-term process and frequently requires multiple episodes of treatment. Participation in twelve-step groups such as Alcoholics Anonymous (AA), Narcotics Anonymous (NA), or Cocaine Anonymous (CA) are usually considered necessary for long-term abstinence. These are usually attended both during and after formal treatment.

Formal treatment may be on an outpatient basis, such as individual psychotherapy or group therapy at a day-treatment center. Some people are in a long-term residential treatment program, often referred to as a **therapeutic community (TC),** which could last from six months to a year. The TC model focuses on resocialization of the individual and helping the person develop personal accountability and responsibility to live a socially productive life. This treatment may be highly structured and confrontational and includes cognitive behavioral therapy in which clients learn how to examine damaging beliefs, self-concepts, and patterns of behavior and to adopt new, more harmonious and constructive ways to interact with others. TCs may include employment training and drug testing as well. The residents at the TCs usually have very severe problems with drugs and alcohol as well as involvement with the criminal justice system and mental health problems.

Short-term residential programs follow the twelve-step approach and consist of three to six weeks of inpatient treatment, followed by extended outpatient therapy and ongoing participation in a twelve-step group. Relapse prevention, supportive expressive therapy, and education are all part of ongoing outpatient therapy models that serve as adjunct treatment to involvement in a twelve-step program.

Because drug and alcohol addictions are so complicated, long-term treatment is usually required. The goal is thorough modification of an addict's lifestyle, including social interactions, emotional expression, and ways of connecting with others. Patience and commitment are essential for human services workers who deal with this population.

Primary Prevention

As with all primary prevention programs, the goal is to educate at-risk people about the negative consequences of drug use and alcohol abuse. Students in elementary school participate in "red ribbon" week. They sign commitment contracts stating they won't use drugs, smoke cigarettes, or drink alcohol. Nancy Reagan's campaign during the 1980s told children to "just say no." Subsequent to the "just say no" campaign many local police departments in collaboration with elementary schools implemented the D.A.R.E. (Drug Awareness and Resistance Education) program in which the students were educated about drugs and alcohol and given strategies to avoid using drugs. Younger children were targeted because unfortunately by the time children enter Junior High School, they may have already tried drugs or alcohol. The earlier using drugs and alcohol can be prevented, the easier it may be to help people avoid becoming addicted.

Human Services for AIDS and HIV Clients

Emergency Situations and Interventions

Intervention with these clients becomes an emergency when someone contracts an illness that becomes life threatening because of their damaged immune system. Basic medical emergency care will then be necessary.

Another emergency situation related to patients with HIV and AIDS might be suicide attempts. Sometimes, when people discover that they are HIV-positive or have contracted a life-threatening disease that may lead to a lot of pain, they try to kill themselves rather than wait for the disease to kill them. Suicide prevention should be immediate and focus on reasons for living. People may need to be educated that HIV/AIDS is not necessarily a death sentence. Medication has done much to prolong the lives of people who have been diagnosed with the disease. They should be encouraged to focus on living as healthy a life as possible. If a person must be hospitalized after a suicide attempt, optimistic support groups should be attended. Here, a person infected with HIV can interact with other HIV-positive people who are living happy lives.

When people with AIDS attempt suicide because they are suffering physically or are worried about financial costs of an illness, they must be helped to see that medication can relieve their pain and also provided with resources that can help cover their medical expenses. Workers can also help people with HIV/AIDS understand that others have overcome opportunistic infections and have continued to live for years. New medical advances have greatly prolonged the lives of those with HIV/AIDS. Many times, family members participate in counseling sessions to share their feelings about the suicide attempt. Patients may decide life is worth living when they hear the sadness and loss their death causes family members to feel.

Secondary Intervention

Crisis intervention may be useful for some people dealing with HIV/AIDS issues. For instance, crisis intervention may be helpful for people who are fearful of being tested for HIV. These individuals may have engaged in risky behavior and are now afraid to find out the consequences of this behavior. These clients must be told that knowing whether they are infected may save their lives. If they are infected, they can begin taking anti-viral medications, practice healthy nutrition, practice safe sex, and participate in stress management and exercise. These behaviors may prolong their lives. If they aren't infected, they can use their fear as a motivator to ensure they practice safe sex in the future or eliminate possible infection in the future by not sharing needles if they are an IV-drug user.

Another type of person in crisis may be the one who has already tested positive for HIV. They need education about the virus and how to avoid spreading it as well as the differences between being HIV-positive and having AIDS. They also need to practice the healthy lifestyle behaviors mentioned above. These clients may also need assistance in disclosing their HIV status to loved ones. Sometimes they are rejected by family because they may be gay. Other times, they risk losing a loved one because they contracted the virus through infidelity or because they were a secret drug addict. They will need supportive crisis intervention to deal with these emotionally painful consequences. Optimistic support groups are excellent in helping them share common concerns and receive problem-solving advice. They also need to be referred for medical assistance and encouraged to comply with the sometimes burdensome process of taking medication (Magallon, 1987; Price, Omizo, & Hammitt, 1986; Slader, 1992).

The main goal of secondary intervention for those infected with HIV or those worried about getting tested for HIV is to help them realize that HIV is not a death sentence. They need education and emotional support while they learn to adjust to a new lifestyle.

Tertiary Intervention

Those who have been HIV-positive for several years often require only medication management to keep the virus from duplicating thereby destroying their immune system. However, at some point, they may start developing symptoms related to HIV. When these patients develop illnesses indicative of **AIDS-related complex (ARC),** they may need medical care beyond anti-viral medication. These illnesses include rawness in the mouth (thrush), flu and colds that don't subside, coughs, night sweats, and fever. This may make a person feel dirty and contaminated. They may isolate from others, have to apply for disability and cease employment, and need somebody to help them with daily living. The development of ARC may be seen as the precursor to developing AIDS. They might bounce back after a few weeks, and be able to live relatively healthy lives for a while. Unfortunately, another bout of illness may occur in a few months. They need support from groups or case workers while they adjust to not working and relying on others for assistance.

When people develop AIDS, they must grapple with life-threatening diseases and the real possibility of dying. It may not be immediate, but they should get legal counseling to prepare living trusts, wills, and other documents. They may need grief counseling as will their significant others. They may live in a hospice when the disease becomes terminal. Others live in and out of hospitals, set up nursing care at their own homes, or have significant others care for them. Case workers must provide supportive counseling and guidance for all. They can focus on how this can be a time to become closer as a family. If the person is feeling well enough, support group attendance may be helpful as well. Case managers and counselors should try to encourage AIDS patients to live as long as possible, comply with medication, be optimistic, enjoy life and create satisfying relationships with others.

Primary Prevention

Of course preventing HIV is better than having to treat it. Some high schools offer education about how to prevent sexually transmitted diseases (STDs). However, conservative political philosophy has influenced policies that would require schools to provide such programs and in some cases has limited and even prevented schools from offering this information. In fact, students need a parent's signature to participate in these educational courses, and some parents won't give permission for their children to attend. Additionally, most of these presentations cannot discuss the use of condoms as a means to prevent the spread of STDs. Instead, many simply push abstinence from sex as the only way to prevent pregnancy and STDs. However, some school nurses' offices do offer free condoms to students who ask for them.

Education at the college is more detailed and effective. Condoms are readily available at college health centers. They are also free and available at most public health centers as well. Some attempts have been made to offer drug addicts "bleach kits" so they could clean needles prior to sharing them. These programs, which started in the 1980s and 1990s, did not receive the political support needed for them to continue.

Since the spread of HIV is on the rise for heterosexuals, in particular Latina girls, more emphasis needs to be placed on primary prevention in this area. While abstinence does prevent the spread of HIV, it is not the only answer. Safe sex and treatment of drug addiction must also be addressed.

Human Services Delivery to At-Risk Adolescents

Emergency Situations and Interventions

Adolescents are prone to crises because they have most of the physical and intellectual capabilities of adults, yet lack the emotional maturity, appropriate judgment, and decision-making abilities of adults. They often act before they think, which can get them into emergency situations. Teen suicide rates are very high, second only to car accidents in terms of cause of death in teens (Wyman, 1982). They need immediate crisis intervention services after a suicide attempt once medical treatment has been completed.

In addition to the emergency situation of suicide, teens are also at risk for running away from home, becoming pregnant, and for being involved in gang violence and crime. Shelters for runaways offer teens a safe place to stay until they can be reunited with their families. Teens who seek out such shelters receive intensive crisis intervention services, group therapy, and basic needs, such as shelter, food, and medical care.

Teens who discover they are pregnant may also need emergency assistance, particularly if they're having medical problems, such as bleeding or pain. These young girls must be referred to knowledgeable and nonjudgmental medical professionals who can provide treatment for any medical problems, as well as prenatal care and education, and pregnancy termination services, if needed. A teen who is 10 to 12 weeks pregnant and wants to end her pregnancy also poses an emergency situation by needing an immediate abortion. Special clinics are available that provide emergency abortions, prenatal services, and adoption services. Trained counselors provide crisis intervention and educational intervention for teens pondering what to do about an unplanned pregnancy. Any female who is pregnant deserves to be informed about her rights to continue with the pregnancy, terminate the pregnancy, or use adoption services. If a teen decides to continue a pregnancy, she will need ongoing services that fall into secondary and tertiary intervention.

Gang involvement may also create a need for emergency intervention. Unfortunately, when teens join gangs, they put themselves and their families at risk for drive-by shootings and other forms of violence. Additionally, gang involvement makes youth at risk to be arrested for committing crimes, which creates the need for emergency response by parents. Both medical professionals and law enforcement usually handle these types of emergency response interventions.

Secondary Intervention

Many police departments have created gang units that specialize in minimizing the negative effects of gang involvement. They attempt to work with gang members and guide them into other activities. They may even attempt mediation between enemy gangs. Diversion programs are available that provide group educational classes for gang members who have not yet become chronic criminals. The goal is to get the member out of the gang lifestyle as soon as possible. After-school recreational teen centers are available in some communities. Gang members can participate in sports, job training, and other activities.

Intervention for runaway teens at this level includes family therapy, group counseling and individual therapy. The focus is on helping the family make changes that will assist the youth in being able to tolerate living at home. Sometimes, the parents need drug and alcohol counseling. The teen may also need help with drug and alcohol addictions. Teens who run away because they've been abused or because of the violence in their homes need help dealing with these issues as well, often with the aid of child protective services. Many mental health centers are available to provide these types of counseling services. Both community mental and behavioral health centers and nonprofit mental health centers are capable of helping with these problems.

As stated above, once a teen decides to continue with a pregnancy, she should participate in ongoing prenatal care with a physician. She may decide to put the baby up for adoption and can receive counseling and legal intervention through public adoption agencies and private and nonprofit agencies. All states have services for these situations at no cost to the pregnant teen. Many communities have homes for the pregnant teen until she gives birth, and sometimes for a period after birth. The goal is to ensure that the teen and her baby are taken care of properly and to provide parenting education. These residential facilities also hope to provide education to prevent future unplanned pregnancies.

Suicide prevention is really a mental health issue and will be discussed below. Teens who attempt suicide need counseling to help them deal with the situation that may have led to such desperate measures. If the situation can be changed, the teen may then return to normal functioning. If the problem is longstanding and the depression is chronic, they may need tertiary intervention.

Tertiary Intervention

For any longstanding depression, medication is an option. Teens, like adults, may need to take anti-depressants for an indefinite period of time to control severe depression. This may be the only way to inhibit suicidal thinking. In addition to medication, chronically suicidal and self-mutilating adolescents may need ongoing group therapy, individual therapy, or a twelve-step group. Mental health clinicians who specialize in these types of adolescent issues should also be contacted when possible.

Chronic runaways may be difficult to treat. They have often had a history of lack of boundaries in the home and don't respond easily to counseling. Because they have often been abused, neglected, or involved in delinquent behavior, such as ditching school regularly, they have developed a lifestyle that doesn't include structure. They may need to be placed in a state-funded group home where supervision is strong. Sometimes they become emancipated if they can work and take care of all their needs on their own. But some teens and their families may need ongoing intervention from family counselors and child protective services to assist in keeping the child safe. Sadly, some families spend years coping with teens who run away, return home, only to run away a few weeks later.

For those teens heavily involved in gang activities, intervention often includes revolving-door incarceration in juvenile hall. Attempts are made to teach these teens how to function outside the gang, how to deal with life stress, and how to express and manage feelings. Group counseling is probably their best chance at being helped during incarceration. It is especially helpful when former gang members visit and share their experiences. In addition to incarceration, programs exist that provide job training for former gang members. They may also have opportunities to earn a high school diploma through special programs. The focus of tertiary intervention programs is to help the teen stay out of the gang lifestyle and learn how to function as a "civilian." Sometimes, they may need to move to another city or state, or spend time in a teen "boot camp." Much of what happens to these gang members depends on the effort exerted by their parents. Some parents simply give up and let their child go his own way. Worse yet, are the parents who themselves are gang members and encourage their teens to continue involvement in the gang.

Primary Prevention

Educational programs have been developed that attempt to keep children from joining gangs. These programs usually begin in elementary school and are sometimes presented in junior high school, and less frequently offered in high schools.

Former gang members along with law enforcement may visit schools and discuss the consequences of gang affiliation.

Likewise, high school programs have been developed that attempt to show adolescents the consequences of pregnancy. Family life classes often have the teens carry around an egg for a few weeks without letting it drop, crack, or spoil. They have timers that go off indicating when they need to feed the egg, change it, and put it to sleep. Other prevention interventions include educational presentations about the use of birth control, and how abstinence can ensure that unplanned pregnancies won't occur. These usually don't happen until high school, however, and so teens younger than that are missing valuable information.

Prevention programs for teen suicide attempts, self-mutilation, and runaways are not always readily available. Perhaps society should spend time and money researching the need for these programs.

CRITICAL THINKING / SELF-REFLECTION CORNER

- Why should government taxes be spent on services designed to help people who seemingly choose to get into trouble, such as teens who get pregnant or join gangs, and people who use drugs?

- How would you eliminate the problem of unwanted teen pregnancy?

- What do you think should be done to completely eliminate gang violence?

- Should a school system be responsible for educating students about birth control and ways to prevent HIV/AIDS? Why or why not?

Human Services Delivery for Mental Illness and Emotional Disorders Situations

Emergency Situations and Interventions

Several emergency situations exist in the area of mental illness and emotional disorders. Sometimes depressed people attempt suicide. Psychotic people who have decompensated into a delusional state may be unable to care for themselves. Others may lose control of their anger and attempt to harm others. All of these situations require emergency response from mental health workers. Most communities have facilities and workers designated to evaluate these behaviors and to decide whether involuntary hospitalization is needed to ensure the safety of the individual or of others. These community workers are often members of a **psychiatric emergency team** (PET).

Local law enforcement workers often work closely with these mental health workers to ensure safe transportation of these people to protective environments. After medical issues have been resolved, counselors typically provide crisis intervention to help contain dangerous behaviors. Sometimes, people need medication to help calm them down. Unfortunately, some people need restraints to assist in stabilizing an emergency.

Secondary Intervention

If a person has not been assessed to be in immediate danger, crisis intervention is usually provided by mental health professionals and paraprofessionals. If the problem is not a longstanding one, the counselor will identify current life stresses, and hopefully be able to assist the client in resolving them. If a counselor cannot personally manage all the problems, then other human services workers may be called in to assist with resolving the problems. People who benefit from secondary intervention are usually suffering from an adjustment disorder or acute stress disorder caused by a severe trauma.

Tertiary Intervention

Many people suffer from longstanding mental illness and emotional disorders that require more than brief therapy and crisis intervention. Those with personality disorders usually need many years of intensive psychotherapy. They may also need to participate in group therapy and take medication to manage symptoms of depression and anxiety. Likewise, those suffering from eating disorders, obsessive-compulsive disorders, generalized anxiety, dissociative identity disorder, longstanding sexual perversion disorders, and many childhood disorders, such as ADHD, autism, and separation-anxiety disorder, need ongoing therapy and behavior management counseling. They also need medication to assist them in functioning.

People suffering from schizophrenia and bipolar disorders often need medication indefinitely as well as case management services provided by community mental health. When the disorder is very severe, they often live in board-and-care homes. Psychotic people are often hospitalized during severe psychotic breakdowns. They are stabilized and then returned to the board-and-care home. Some can live independently if they comply with medication treatment. They usually see a psychiatrist throughout their lives.

Primary Prevention

Unfortunately, few prevention programs are designed to stop people from developing emotional disorders because many of these disorders are either hereditary or result from dysfunctional family dynamics. School systems and government agencies are hesitant to interfere with how parents raise their children. They are even hesitant to talk about self-esteem in schools because this steps on the toes of the parents. As far as genetic counseling, there still isn't a specific test that clearly indicates which genes carry mental illness. Society needs to put more emphasis on preventing mental illness, but this may mean interfering with parental rights to parent as they see fit.

Chapter Summary

The various client populations discussed in this chapter have needs that range from being of an emergency quality to at-risk. The human services delivery system in our communities have evolved to meet these needs. Some clients may seek human services during a crisis. Others are in the throes of a medical or legal emergency. At times, services are aimed at preventing an at-risk group from having a problem. Clients with chronic problems often use human services regularly. Whatever the needs of a particular client, human services workers should be well-informed about all the available human services delivery approaches that are appropriate for their clients' needs.

Suggested Applied Activities

1. Visit one or two agencies. Ask a worker or coordinator of programs to tell you about the different types of services delivered through the agency. Try to categorize each service into primary, secondary, tertiary, or emergency intervention.

   _____

   _____

   _____

   _____

   _____

   _____

2. Browse through your local Rainbow Resources Directory or the web for a list of various human services delivery agencies in your community.

   _____

   _____

   _____

   _____

   _____

   _____

Chapter Review Questions

1. What situations might arise for the following clients that require emergency services?
   a. abused child

   _____

   _____

b. pregnant teen

_____

_____

c. substance abuser

_____

_____

d. person dealing with issues related to HIV

_____

_____

e. person suffering from schizophrenia

_____

_____

f. What are some treatment options for people dependent on alcohol?

_____

_____

2. What are some general principles in delivering human services to battered women?

_____

_____

3. Why might a support group be effective for a victim of sexual assault?

_____

_____

4. What might human services workers keep in mind when designing a case management plan for a first-time offender?

_____

_____

5. What primary prevention programs are available for issues related to child abuse, domestic violence, substance abuse, and AIDS?

_____

_____

6. What is a twelve-step facilitation?

_____

_____

7. What human services delivery programs are useful for the elderly?

_____

_____

Glossary of Terms

Abstinence is often recommended for people addicted to alcohol or drugs and eliminating completely the use of any drugs or alcohol.

Adult services, usually part of community social services, sends case workers to investigate suspected abuses of people who are elderly and disabled and provides basic needs when necessary.

Aid to Families with Dependent Children (AFDC) is an agency established in the 1960s to provide financial welfare for eligible families with children under the age of 18.

AIDS-related complex (ARC) is a stage of HIV/AIDS during which a person infected with HIV begins having bouts of fever, vomiting, and other flu-like symptoms, but has not yet developed full-blown AIDS.

Americans with Disabilities Act (ADA) that protects and preserves the rights of people with disabilities, especially in the workplace and within institutional settings.

Battered women's shelter is a residential facility where battered women and their children may live for about 45 days while they manage legal issues, finances, employment, and emotional difficulties.

Battering cycle is an ongoing pattern of behavior seen in couples involved in an abusive relationship during which a peaceful period of time, called the honeymoon, is inevitably followed by growing tensions and stress, often making the woman feel as if she must "walk on eggshells" to keep the peace. But ultimately the batterer's poor coping and communication skills explode into verbal abuse and physically violent behavior, which is then followed by the batterer expressing deep feelings of remorse and apology, to which the victim responds with forgiveness and the return of the honeymoon phase. Without intervention, this cycle not only continues, but with each revolution, the abuse also becomes more severe and potentially life threatening.

Child protective services is usually a department within a community social services agency that protects children from abuse, as well as works to detect, prevent, and stop abuse of children and where suspected cases of child abuse are reported.

Dementia is cognitive deterioration that causes people to lose their ability to concentrate and to organize their perceptions coherently; it is a symptom of Alzheimer's disease and other diseases that affect the brain.

Diversion programs are alternatives to incarceration and are typically affiliated with the criminal justice system. Instead of jail time, first-time and juvenile offenders are ordered to attend educational classes and group therapy to prevent further criminal behaviors.

Indigent people are extremely poor people who have no financial resources whatsoever.

Medical detoxification is a procedure conducted in a hospital by a physician that uses medication to help a person withdraw from alcohol or drug addiction.

Post-traumatic stress disorder (PTSD) is an emotional disorder that often occurs in reaction to a serious traumatic event, such as rape, assault, and other personal, violent attacks. Symptoms include hypervigilence, dissociation, nightmares, flashbacks, and depersonalization.

Psychiatric emergency team (PET) is a group of mental health professionals who evaluate the mental state of individuals to determine whether they need to be hospitalized involuntarily because they are a danger to themselves or others, or just gravely impaired.

Temporary restraining order is a legal document that a person who is in danger files against the person who poses the threat, such an abusive spouse or a stalker, ordering that person to avoid any contact with the victim or face criminal prosecution.

Therapeutic community TC is an inpatient treatment model for substance abusers that focus on resocialization and ongoing educational groups.

Twelve-step facilitation is a very structured approach in which a therapist focuses on encouraging a substance abuser to participate in a twelve-step group as the primary way to sustain abstinence

Case Presentation and Exit Quiz

General Description and Demographics

The Gomez family consists of five children, Leona age 22, Jimmy age 19, Johnny age 17, Leticia age 14, and Maria age 7. The father, Jaime, age 45, works full time as a machinist. The mother, Liliana, age 40, does not work outside of the home. Jaime's mother, Maria, age 68, lives with them. Jaime's father died many years ago. Jaime's parents moved to the U.S. mainland from Puerto Rico 35 years ago to start a family business. Jaime, Liliana, and their children were all born in the United States. When Liliana's parents were young, they also came to the mainland from Puerto Rico with their parents. Liliana's parents live in a neighboring city, and they all get together often. Maria is good friends with Liliana's mother, Sylvia.

Problems within the Family

Johnny has been involved in a local gang since he was 15. There have been drive-by shootings at his house recently. He owns several guns and participates fully in gang warfare. His parents have tried to make him give away his guns and want him to quit the gang. He refuses to move out and is often verbally abusive to his mother and father, and physically abusive to his father. Leona has had several arguments with Johnny and has called the police to have him taken away. He frequently steals things from the home to sell. His mother feels sorry for him and allows him back into live the house after he has been gone for about one week. She doesn't want to lose his love.

He started using crystal meth about six months ago and becomes more violent when he is high. Before he began using crystal meth, he only smoked pot. His parents do not know what to do. Johnny has been caught stealing money from his grandmother, Maria. She keeps all of her money under her mattress, and one time after she received her social security check, Johnny stole $600.

Liliana has been suffering from *los nervios* episodically. She saw her primary care physician through her husband's HMO medical plan. He prescribed an antidepressant for her. She still suffers from intense bouts of anxiety and rage. This began one month ago, after Johnny stole Maria's money. Liliana's anxiety is so severe that she is afraid to let her daughters leave the house.

In the past week, little Maria has been afraid to go to school. She complains of stomachaches in the morning. The school counselor referred her to a family therapist. Maria tells the therapist that her brother Jimmy sometimes makes her lie in bed with him and touch his private parts and sometimes he touches hers. Maria doesn't like it and is afraid to tell her mother.

Leticia has a new boyfriend who talked her into having sex at a party last month. She never had sex before, and they didn't use any birth control. Leticia is afraid that she may be pregnant because her period is late. Her boyfriend, who's 22 years old, tells her not to worry about it.

Jaime continues to work daily. He is aware of the problems at home, but is passive for the most part. He is satisfied with letting his wife take care of the children. He feels powerless to manage his sons and feels inadequate when communicating with his daughters. Jaime drinks beer every day after work, a habit he's had since he was 15. His drinking rarely prevents him from going to work, but his wife and daughters don't like being around him when he drinks. On Friday nights, after he gets paid, he goes to a local bar to drink. Jaime is depressed most of the time but accepts that he is not meant to be a happy man.

Exit Quiz

1. Which intervention level should be provided to deal with Johnny's gang involvement problems?
   a. primary prevention
   b. secondary prevention
   c. tertiary prevention
   d. emergency services

2. A factor that might hamper Johnny's ability to stay out of gang life might be
   a. his parent's approve of gang behaviors
   b. his father has given up trying to control Johnny's behaviors
   c. his mother secretly wants him to steal so she can have some of the money
   d. all of the above

3. An effective intervention for Johnny might be
   a. press charges for robbery and have him go to Juvenile Hall
   b. have the police come to the house and confiscate the guns
   c. send him to an out-of-state boot camp
   d. all of the above

4. Johnny's substance abuse might be helped by
   a. long-term rehabilitation at a hospital
   b. group counseling and family counseling
   c. residential treatment
   d. medical detoxification

5. When little Maria's family therapist heard about what her 19-year-old brother had been doing, she should
   a. call in the brother immediately and confront him
   b. tell Maria to go home and order him to stop
   c. call child protective services immediately
   d. all of the above

6. Jimmy might benefit from
   a. jail time
   b. personal counseling
   c. mandatory group therapy
   d. all of the above

7. When the family therapist heard that grandmother Maria had her social security check stolen, she should
   a. help her find a part-time job to earn the money back
   b. report this as financial abuse to Adult Protective Services
   c. tell Maria to open a checking account
   d. none of the above

8. Little Maria might benefit from which level of intervention?
   a. primary prevention
   b. secondary intervention
   c. tertiary intervention
   d. none of the above

9. Liliana's anxiety might best be treated with what level of intervention?
   a. primary prevention
   b. secondary intervention
   c. tertiary intervention
   d. none of the above

10. Who should receive individual counseling?
    a. little Maria
    b. Liliana
    c. Jaime
    d. all of the above

11. Leticia needs which level of intervention?
    a. emergency intervention
    b. secondary intervention
    c. tertiary intervention
    d. none of the above

12. Jaime's drinking problem might best be treated at which level?
    a. primary prevention
    b. secondary intervention
    c. tertiary intervention
    d. none of the above

Exit Quiz Answers

1. c	5. c	9. b
2. b	6. d	10. d
3. d	7. b	11. a
4. b	8. b	12. c

CHAPTER 10

Stress Management

Introduction

At this point in the semester, the reader may have already taken some exams and may be preparing term papers and other projects, which may have created a certain amount of **stress.** The material presented thus far may have created feelings of anxiety, anger, and sadness. The multitude of problems and needs that people have can be overwhelming and can lead to job **"burnout."** It happens to many people in most occupations. Human services workers may be particularly vulnerable to burnout because of emotional stress from trying to assist people who have many emotional and social problems for which they seek help.

CRITICAL THINKING / SELF-REFLECTION CORNER

Take a moment now to consider how some of the following questions relate to your own reactions thus far to the course material:

- How long could you continue working happily and peacefully at a shelter where most of your clients are women who come in with black eyes, broken bones, and serious lacerations?

- How would feel working day after day with children who have been sexually molested?

- How do you think you would be affected by frequently hearing people say that they can't quit using drugs even though it means losing custody of their children?

Don't be discouraged about your career path by the possibility of becoming stressed or angry in those situations. In fact, those reactions are normal responses to a very stressful job.

Before examining **stress management** techniques, a brief discussion of stress and burnout may be helpful. While this discussion focuses on stress at the workplace, it can be universally applicable, not only to students stressed out from exams and social pressures but also to clients whose problems are creating stress in their lives.

Stress and Burnout

What Is Stress?

Stress is a normal part of everyday life. Chang (2005) even suggested that stress is an inevitable consequence of pressure-laden jobs. People experience stress usually in situations that require more energy than they have. This energy may be physical, psychological, emotional, or intellectual. People become stressed in potentially threatening situations. Not all stress is bad, however;. stress can motivate people to grow, discover new abilities, and take new challenges. Stress becomes harmful only when it is constant and unrelenting.

When stressful situations persist without hope of resolution, they become overwhelming. People in such situations start to experience anxiety, depression, anger, and frustration. If these feelings continue, impairments in daily functioning can occur. An inability to cope with impaired functioning can bring about a crisis situation. People in a state of crisis often seek professional help. Not getting the appropriate help can lead to serious consequences, such as suicide, drug and alcohol abuse, or emotional withdrawal from life.

The good news is that most people can cope with a certain amount of stress on a daily basis; some even seek out stressful situations.

What Is Burnout?

Simply put, burnout is job-related anxiety and dissatisfaction that hampers people's abilities at work and in other areas of their lives. Physical illness, a short temper, impatience, and frustration are typical signs of burnout (Russo, 1980). Maslach and Jackson (1986) identified three symptoms of burnout:

- lack of personal accomplishment

- emotional exhaustion and depersonalization

- de-individuation of clients

They proposed that burnout is a reaction to chronic stress on the job. Vettor and Kosinski (2000) suggested that when human services workers have these symptoms, their attitude toward clients may become negative and cynical, and workers may be unable to provide clients with the support they need. Pines and Maslach (1978, p. 224) have defined burnout as "a syndrome of physical and emotional exhaustion involving the development of negative self-concept, negative job attitudes, and a loss of concern and feelings for clients."

The causes of burnout are many and varied. Working in human services may increase the likelihood of burnout because workers often experience conflicts between the ideal and the real. Human services workers go into the field to help others, but when resources are unavailable, the agencies for which they work are unsupportive, and clients are unmotivated to receive help, workers experience a sense of "what's the use?" Burnout may be a defense against feelings of helplessness.

Human services workers may find it emotionally taxing to deal with populations who resent them, with limited capabilities to help themselves, and with performing tedious bureaucratic tasks daily with little positive feedback from authority figures (Gomez & Michaelis, 1995). It may also be emotionally taxing for human services workers to be faced with ongoing conflicts between their personal values and knowledge of the right thing to do and the norms of the organization (Russo, 1980).

Norms are the unwritten rules and guidelines that are understood and followed by the members of an organization. It may be difficult to believe, but some organizational norms may include behaviors that many consider to be morally wrong or at least incompetent. An easy example to illustrate this are the norms in prisons that allow guards to be physically brutal with inmates. Most people think this is wrong, and in the beginning, the guards probably thought it was bad. As time goes on, however, many workers slip into previously unacceptable behaviors because the norms of the institution encourage them. Another example might be the norm of arriving to work on time. In some agencies there is an understanding that workers may arrive 30 minutes late with no repercussions. To a new worker, this feels unfair. One can understand that a typical response would be to simply start coming in late so as not to experience feelings of resentment toward those who seem to "get away" with it.

Other conflicts may occur while working for human services agencies as well. Personality conflicts with supervisors and coworkers can be a precipitator of burnout and stress, especially if a worker receives no support from anyone. Cliques and factions are natural when groups of people interact regularly, and of course most people tend to gravitate toward those who are most like them. When there is no one around with whom a worker can relate, burnout may occur. In addition to personality conflicts, outright competition and professional jealousy may occur. It's bad enough to have to deal with clients who have a multitude of personal needs, but having to deal with coworkers and supervisors with emotional problems creates added stress on the job. When coworkers are insecure, paranoid, and who feel threatened, the risk of becoming burned out is high. In a job where the undercurrent is anxiety and diminished loyalty and commitment to workers, **morale** is eroded. Chaotic and dysfunctional work environments where individuals are devalued and discounted lead to physical and mental exhaustion in employees (Anonymous, 2005).

In addition to stress from organizational demands and coworker behaviors, human services workers may be at risk for burnout because many times, they are not able to help in the way they want to help. It is difficult to accept that some clients may not get better, change, and live happy, productive lives. They may die, get killed, or remain nonfunctional despite the best efforts of human services workers. Burnout may occur when the helping professional evaluates him or herself negatively when assessing work done with clients (Vettor & Kosinski, 2000).

The Impact of Stress and Burnout

Just as the causes of burnout and stress are many and varied, so too are the symptoms and behaviors manifested as a result of burnout and stress. Burnout usually manifests in physical symptoms, cognitive and emotional impairments, social deterioration, behavioral impairments, and impairments on the job.

Physical Symptoms

Humans are hard-wired to react to stressful situations with a fright-or-flight response in which the two hormones adrenalin and cortisol are produced. Overproduction of these two hormones can cause long-term damage to health (Anonymous, 2005). Many workers suffering from burnout complain of physical problems, such as dizziness, nausea, headaches, fatigue, heart palpitations, shortness of breath, or ulcers, high blood pressure, and other psychosomatic illnesses (Sparks, Simon, Katon, Altman, Ayars, & Johnson, 1990). Stress is increasingly appearing as a diagnosis on medical certificates as physicians now think that overall health will be improved by the reduction of stress levels. The Health and Safety Executive in the United Kingdom (Goldman & Lewis, 2005) commissioned a study on the effect work stress had on the development of musculoskeletal disorders that found that individuals under stress at work are prone to illness.

Cognitive and Emotional Symptoms

An inability to concentrate and memory loss are both **cognitive symptoms** of burnout. Two common **emotional symptoms** are depression and panic disorders (Sparks et al., 1990). Many see no hope for things getting better, and others perceive themselves as inadequate and incompetent. People who have had traumatic experiences on the job may show signs of post-traumatic stress disorder.

Example: A woman worked for Triple A, a well-known road assistance agency. One day her supervisor yelled at her and berated her in front of a customer. This was typical of her supervisor's management style. The woman broke down and sobbed for a few minutes. Then she became unable to speak. She was so traumatized that she sought the help of a therapist. The woman experienced nightmares, was hypervigilant, and re-experienced the trauma in her mind repeatedly. An interesting symptom was her inability to speak English after the trauma. She began thinking and speaking Swedish, which was her first language. She had apparently regressed to a childlike state to cope with the work trauma.

Social Deterioration

Social withdrawal and poor family relationships are also reported to exist when someone has experienced burnout (Freudenberger, 1975; Maslach & Jackson, 1986). A normally pleasant person may become tense and impatient with people including the public and loved ones. Individuals may not feel like interacting with their children, their spouses, or friends. They may interact in a numb state with very little emotional connection. All of these behaviors are signs of **social deterioration.**

Behavioral Deterioration

Some people who experience burnout may increase their drug and alcohol consumption. This increase in substance use may be a form of self-medication to relieve feelings of anxiety and depression. Others have difficulty in sleeping, eating, and performing other normal activities of daily living. When the **behavioral deterioration** of daily living is severe, individuals may apply for workman's compensation or disability to compensate them financially during the time when they cannot work.

Impairments in Work Performance

All of the previously mentioned symptoms and behaviors affect an individual's ability to perform his or her job adequately. Human services workers are particularly susceptible to having their work performance affected because of the human-to-human contact usually required on the job. When a worker merely sits behind a desk and does paperwork, it may be easier to hide burnout symptoms than when a worker must listen patiently to other people's problems.

Absenteeism, tardiness, and lowered productivity often occur when workers are burned out. One company reported that 44 percent of those surveyed said that they lose at least an hour of productivity a day because of stress, whereas 47 percent estimated that in the course of a year, they had been at work anywhere from one to four days when they were too stressed out to be effective (Chang, 2005). In a 2001 study of community crisis workers (Kanel, 2007), 45 percent stated feeling angry at the system when working with someone in crisis, and 52 percent said they think of quitting their job between one and five times a month!

Table 10.1 categorizes the various types, causes, and symptoms of burnout.

Table 10.1 Burnout: Definitions, Causes, and Symptoms

Definitions	Causes	Symptoms
anxiety and unhappiness at work that affects job performance and other areas of life	conflicts between ideals and reality	physical: diseases and physical problems such as dizziness, heart palpitations, fatigue and high blood pressure
lack of personal accomplishment	lack of resources available to help clients	cognitive impairments: poor concentration and memory
emotional exhaustion	lack of company support and very little positive feedback from authority figures	emotional impairments: feelings of helplessness, depression, panic, low self-esteem
depersonalization	lack of client motivation and limited capabilities to receive help and help themselves	social deterioration: impairments with coworkers, clients, family, and friends
de-individuation of clients	dealing with resentful clients	behavioral deterioration: activities of daily living change such as sleeping, eating, increased substance abuse
negative self-concept	dealing with tedious bureaucratic tasks	impairments in work performance: absenteeism, tardiness, lower productivity
negative job attitudes	conflicts between personal values and organizational norms	
loss of concern and feelings for clients	competitions and jealousy among coworkers	
physical exhaustion	negative self-evaluation of work done with clients	

CRITICAL THINKING / SELF-REFLECTION CORNER

Before moving on to the next section, examine your responses to the following questions to assess your own levels of burnout and stress.

- Have you ever felt like you didn't want to go to work? Why? Are you tired, bored, scared, or preoccupied with something else?

- Have you felt like you didn't want to go to class? (Don't worry, about answering honestly. Even professors sometimes don't want to go to class and teach!) Why? Is the teacher boring; is the material irrelevant, do you have something else on your mind?

- How is your functioning with your friends and family just before a midterm or final exam?

- Do you often feel worried before an exam?

- Do you worry when a paper or project is due?

- Do you believe you study enough? If not, why not?

- Do you blame your feelings on others, like the teacher, the boss, or your parents?

- What do you think are some effective ways to manage stress?

- What have you done to try to feel differently in some of the above situations?

Now that you have had a chance to think about your own burnout and stress, let's take a look at how to manage these situations. These suggestions may come in very handy at this point in the semester and at your job. Share these ideas with coworkers, supervisors, family, friends, and clients as well.

Managing Stress and Burnout

A 2001 study of community workers who regularly assist people in crisis suggests that talking with coworkers about one's stress helps relieve its emotional consequences (Kanel, 2007). Of the 67 workers surveyed, 80 percent stated that they talk with coworkers when feeling emotionally stressed after working with people in crisis. This is a great solution for work stress if there are supportive coworkers at the workplace. It may not be a practical solution if coworkers are competitive and when conflict is high among coworkers. In fact, the work environment itself may be the very source of stress. Stress may result from coworker conflict as well as unsupportive supervisors and conflicts with organizational norms. Of course, if a work environment is extremely dysfunctional and oppressive, people might consider quitting as a way to reduce work stress. Unfortunately, not everyone has that luxury. People usually need their jobs to pay bills, eat, and take care of family needs. So, while it would be great if we could all just leave when the work environment, coworkers, or supervisors became unbearable, quitting isn't necessarily the most practical solution. At some point, learning the coping skills necessary to manage the normal, daily stresses in almost all work settings is essential.

The best solution for work stress is to teach managers how to create stress-free work environments and how to interact with staff members in ways that make them feel supported and appreciated. Then all employees could be instructed and coached on how to communicate with one another so that no one feels hurt or inadequate. If everyone learned to cooperate and get along, work would be wonderful. Does this sound realistic to you? Of course not. That doesn't mean that some of these things can't be increased. In fact many companies offer in-service training, staff retreats, and workshops to improve employee morale and increase competence among those who supervise.

While individual counseling for employees who are stressed may be temporarily helpful, if the company doesn't deal with the root causes of the stress, counseling is "like cleaning up the fish in a pond but then putting them back in the dirty water" (Mendoza, 2005, p. 2). Not every organization offers stress-management training or even effective managerial training about how to help employees who are stressed. Managers may be aware that employees are stressed but may feel incapable of implementing strategies to deal with workplace stress. Some may even view workplace stress and stress management as simply a current trend that need not be taken seriously (Mendoza, 2005).

A Four-Pronged Approach to Managing Stress

- recognize your own problem areas

- work on your own problem areas

- improve interpersonal communication

- maintain a sense of humor

After reviewing the details of the four stress-management strategies that follow, take a look at the worksheet in the "Suggested Applied Activities" section, which may be useful during times of stress.

Recognize Your Own Problem Areas

Before deciding to quit a stressful job, individuals should examine their own part in any problems at work. (Students can do the same for stressful situations at school.) Most stress-management strategies focus on perceptions of the problems and ways to change those perceptions. This approach is helpful because it gives people control of their own thoughts, whereas it is much harder to be in control of others' behaviors. The cognitive-behavioral therapy approaches have been instrumental in helping people learn how to rethink their situations so they can deal with them more easily. The basic philosophy behind these approaches is that the situations themselves do not make us feel bad, rather it is our perceptions of them that lead to negative such feelings as anger, depression, and anxiety. In the first century A.D., the Greek philosopher Epictetus said, "People are disturbed not by things, but by the view which they take of them" (cited in Ellis, 2001, p. 16). Since then, cognitive theory has become a major force in counseling and stress management.

Ellis's rational emotive behavioral therapy model (discussed in Chapter 5) is simple and easy to implement: When trying to change personal perceptions and reduce stress, consider using the following five steps:

1. Identify irrational, ineffective thinking.
2. Examine whether these thoughts have been beneficial in the past.
3. Identify alternate thoughts that are more realistic, more rational, and based on facts.
4. Make an effort to say these more rational thoughts when feeling badly.
5. Evaluate whether these new thoughts have improved stress levels (Ellis, 1962).

What follows are some common types of **irrational and self-defeating thoughts.** These thoughts may be self-imposed or may come from others. Regardless of their source, it's important to eliminate them and to start thinking more realistically.

SELF-CRITICAL THOUGHTS

People in stressful situations often resort to **self-critical thoughts,** such as calling themselves stupid, ugly, fat, worthless, inadequate, and so forth. It's bad enough to deal with stress without adding labels like these. If people can just stop calling themselves bad names, they might be able to focus on resolving the stressful situation. When people calls themselves one of those names they're going to feel horrible, which makes it more difficult to cope with the demands of daily life. Over time, stress builds, and people become burned out. The trick is to stop that inner, name-calling voice and realize that no one is perfect. Once people accept that mistakes are inevitable and don't make them horrible people, they can join real life. Mistakes, instead, might be thought of as a way to learn about what to avoid and what to improve on next time. That can be hard to do if people view their mistakes as just additional evidence of their stupidity. Likewise, losing weight can be made more difficult when people think of themselves as being a "fat pig," "ugly," or "disgusting." These words make people feel bad about themselves, which can sabotage their positive intentions, such as eating sensibly and exercising.

CRITICAL THOUGHTS ABOUT OTHERS

Self-criticism is as self-defeating as criticizing others is. Just as some people tend to blame themselves when things go wrong, other people look for others to blame when something goes wrong. Blaming leads to feelings of anger and resentment. These feelings are not conducive to solving problems and feeling happy. Ellis (1962) proposed that no human being should ever be blamed for anything he does, and that it is the therapist's job to help rid people of thoughts in which they blame themselves, others, or fate and the universe.

Irrational Thoughts Many times people tell themselves that they just can't stand it if things don't go the way they want them to go. They tend to exaggerate the gravity of certain situations and blow them out of proportion. Doing this tends to make people feel anxious or enraged. A typical example might be when a driver cuts someone off on the road. He or she may be telling him or herself, "How dare he do this to me! I will not let this rest! I cannot stand it when people are rude to me!" The rational counterpart would be, "I sure don't like it when people drive dangerously, and accidents are likely when people take chances. I would prefer that people consider me when they drive."

Another example might be when someone doesn't get hired for a job, or a student scores poorly on an exam. Thoughts such as, "This is not fair, I shouldn't have to take such hard exams," and "How dare they not hire me, it's not fair!" make people feel angry. This anger often prevents the person from learning from the situation and improving the next time. In general, when people turn their preferences into demands, they are thinking irrationally, and they will feel bad. The reality is, "You can't always get what you want" and "People don't behave the way they should or the way you want them to behave."

CRITICAL THINKING / SELF-REFLECTION CORNER

- How often have you thought or said to someone, "It's not my fault. You are to blame"?

- Has anyone ever told you, "it's your fault"?

- How do these statements make you feel?

- Can anything productive come of these statements of blame?

Reality shows us over and over that people are fallible. They make mistakes and so do you! You will be a chronically angry person if you expect that all people will be competent, nice, fair, and respectful at all times.

Work on Your Own Problem Areas

When people experience painful or negative feelings, a few steps can be taken toward eliminating or reducing these unwanted feelings. The first step is to identify the **precipitating event** that has activated a negative feeling or behavior. Next, identify the irrational beliefs about this event. Once the trigger of the emotional distress and the unrealistic beliefs and thoughts about it have been identified, then the next step is to begin disputing the irrational beliefs and substitute more realistic and rational thoughts. Last, an assessment should be made to decide whether changing those thoughts was helpful in changing the negative feelings and behaviors. If not, then there may be other irrational thoughts that are maintaining the negative feelings. The following examples of two common situations illustrate how to implement Ellis's approach.

Example 1: negative feelings of anger and bitterness

Precipitating event: receiving a "C" on an exam

Irrational beliefs: "It's the teacher's fault; he didn't give us a study guide. He didn't tell us the right things to study. The material was too confusing. I should get a 'B' because I always get 'Bs' and 'As'. It's not fair. It's horrible to get a 'C' because now I can't get into graduate school."

Disputation and substitution of realistic beliefs for irrational beliefs: "Where is it written that teachers must provide study guides? They don't all do this. It's really up to me to study and take responsibility for studying. Unfortunately, some teachers don't focus on assisting students in passing exams, and some teachers don't present material clearly. I'd certainly rather earn a 'B' or an 'A' on all exams. Many people get into graduate school even if they get a few 'Cs'. It's always possible to retake a course if need be. Unfortunately, life is not always fair, and things don't always go the way we want."

Evaluation of effect of disputation and substitutions: "I'm feeling less angry and more empowered to take charge of my own studying and grades. Although I'm not exactly happy that life is not fair or that I can't always get what I want, I realize that this is reality and I can't fight reality."

Example 2: negative feelings of depression and thoughts of suicide

Precipitating event: breakup of a romantic relationship

Irrational beliefs: "No one will ever love me again. I can't go on living without him/her. I'm not worthy of love. Something is wrong with me or else why would this happen to me? I'm ugly and fat. I'm stupid and I shouldn't have put so much trust in one person."

Disputations and substitutions: "It is sad and difficult to experience a loss. But where is the proof that no one will ever love me again? As an adult, I can live without another person, although I may feel sad and lonely sometimes while I grieve. But loss is a normal part of life. We all risk the chance of experiencing loss when we become close to someone, because, as sad and disappointing as it is, people change their feelings, they grow in different directions, and it often has nothing to do with anyone but themselves. Just because someone doesn't want me now, it doesn't mean that was always true. People change, and at least I know the truth now. The extent of my grief indicates the attachment and love we both shared. Loss can be a time for both celebrating what I had experienced as well as a time to feel sad at not having that anymore. It is an opportunity to grow and seek new experiences."

Evaluation: "I am still sad but am beginning to believe that I might be able to make it through this breakup. I sure don't like it, but it isn't the end of the world."

REFRAMING CRITICAL AND IRRATIONAL THOUGHTS

Cognitive-restructuring approaches are similar to what strategic therapists call "reframing" and using "positive connotations" (Haley, 1976; Palazzoli, Cecchin, Prata, & Boscolo, 1978). These approaches help people view their problems as possible opportunities for growth and can reshape perceptions of negative events into more positive, more acceptable experiences. Therapists who use reframing techniques first need to understand a client's—and often the entire family's—frame of reference before being able to put the problems in a solvable light. The following examples illustrated how reframing and positive connotations can be used.

Example 1: A 54-year-old woman tells her therapist that she wants to kill herself because she is a burden to her family. Since her back surgery, her children must drive her to doctor appointments and help her clean her house. If she kills herself, she believes, she'll be a good mother by unburdening her children from having to care for her.

Client's frame of reference: She's a good mother, and committing suicide is a sign of being a good mother.

Therapist's reframe: Client would be a bigger burden to her children if she were to kill herself because they will forever feel guilty and sad that she killed herself because she didn't want to be a burden to them. A good self-sacrificing mother would just put up with being taken care of by her children so that they can still feel her love and her presence.

Example 2: A new intern at a battered women's shelter answers a hotline call. The person on the phone is a female who wants to know where the shelter is. The intern figures that since the caller is a woman it would be allright to tell her the address. When the intern tells her supervisor what she did, the supervisor says that it is a felony to give out the address of a battered women's shelter.

Intern's frame of reference: She feels she is horrible and stupid for giving out the address.

Supervisor's reframe: It's a good thing this time that she gave the address to a safe person and that she told me about it right away. Mistakes like these are helpful because they remind all of us about this most important issue. The trainer at the orientation failed to mention this legal issue, and it would have been overlooked if the intern had not brought it to my attention. It would have just been assumed that everyone knew about the policy.

Notice that the reframes and positive-connotation method allow both people to save face and leave the situation with their self-esteem intact.

The main thread that all of these approaches have in common is that individuals can examine their own thoughts that lead to stress and can change them. The change in perception leads to reduction in negative and painful emotions. **Cognitive restructuring** is not only used in American workplaces and private counseling offices, but it is being used effectively in other countries as well. The following two examples explain how it is being used in China.

Example 1: Using cognitive restructuring theory at the Ho-Chunk casino

The management of this casino designed a stress-management program called Rethinking Stress, which teaches employees how to accept responsibility for their own reactions to stress. It does not allow employees to blame their stress on outside forces, but it motivates them to change their own behaviors rather than expecting others to change. Participants in the program reported saving an average of 6.25 hours per week and using an average of 2.92 fewer sick days for stress-related issues (Lee, Dolezalek, & Johnson, 2005).

Example 2: Targeting Work-Related Stress at a Company in China

A company in China has begun a training program in managing emotional intelligence, a twist on conventional stress management. The focus is on helping employees manage their emotions in the face of crisis or change, and even transform negative emotions into positive ones (Caplan, J. 2005).

MAINTAINING A HEALTHY LIFESTYLE

While much stress and burnout come from an individual's thoughts and beliefs, a person's lifestyle and behaviors can also create stress. Eating habits, exercise, and recreational activities play a big part in both controlling and reducing stress. A person's home life and social interests may provide clues to why some people have more difficulties coping with stress and burnout than others do. While feeling productive and fulfilled at work is healthy, using a job as a substitute for living is not. When human services workers' personal lives and needs take a backseat to those of their clients', no one benefits. It does feel good to be needed and respected by clients, but when workers' own needs of being needed and liked are motivations for helping others, the support and help workers provide become confused with the support and help that they need. Such confusion can lead to unwise choices as well as mixed messages (Russo, 1980).

Human services workers must develop and maintain healthy personal lives outside of their jobs. They must eat healthy food and exercise regularly. It is vital to take time to relax and to get involved in activities and interests that are not related to work. When a human services worker (or student) begins feeling stressed or burned out, it may be time to focus on outside interests. If the stress seems unmanageable and overwhelming, seeking the services of a professional counselor is advised. By using these stress-management tactics, workers can make sure that clients receive the most effective and ethical interventions. The mental health of human services workers is probably the most important resource that a worker gives to clients and the agency.

Just as problematic, however, are human services workers who begin to care too little about clients and their jobs. They disengage from their own personal feelings for clients and coworkers and become bureaucratic technicians. They carry out institutional procedures and rely solely on the rules and regulations to make decisions without letting their personal values and feelings get in the way (Russo, 1980). While this may prevent their personal needs from interfering with their work with clients, it may lead to feelings of emptiness and lack of satisfaction at work. Obviously, the trick is to allow oneself to care about clients and the organizational goals while at the same time allowing oneself to be involved in an outside life that fulfills one's needs socially and recreationally.

Improving Interpersonal Communication

While much work-related stress and burnout come from an individual's cognitions and behaviors, at other times conflicts with coworkers, difficulties with work-related responsibilities, and other real job-related problems are to blame. Many of these problems can be eliminated by talking assertively with supervisors. The Health and Safety Executive in the United Kingdom (Goldman & Lewis, 2005, p. 13) recently identified six key areas that may affect work stress and burnout. When workers have problems in any of these areas, they should speak with a manager/supervisor to attempt to resolve the problems.

1. "The demands of the job" Both employee and supervisor must ensure that the employee can cope and handle the job requirements, and if not, training and guidance should be provided.
2. "The degree of employee control over his work." Employees should communicate with supervisors if this is a problem, and supervisors should allow employees to have a say in how they should go about their work.
3. "The level of management and colleague support provided." Supervisors should provide information and support through accessible policies and procedures and give regular and constructive feedback. If employees do not feel this is occurring, they should speak up and ask for more training and positive reinforcement when work activity is productive.
4. "The quality of work relationships." Employees must speak up if they experience intimidation, bullying, or other unacceptable and unprofessional behav-

iors from others. Sometimes this can be done in staff meetings, retreats, or through union representatives. As the study of community workers discovered, talking with coworkers is invaluable in dealing with work stress. Getting along with coworkers is worth fighting for, and to survive at an agency, employees must feel an alliance with at least several other workers. Sometimes open warfare must precede a more cooperative spirit among coworkers. Effective managers must be competent in creating a work environment in which coworkers can get along. At times, an outside mediator may be called upon to manage serious employee conflicts.

5. "Employee role within the organization and how it is managed." An employee's roles and responsibilities should be clearly defined. It can be stressful to not know what is expected. It is very stressful to receive negative evaluations for duties that the employee didn't even know were his or hers. It is the manager or supervisor's job to ensure that each employee knows his or her duties clearly.

6. "The management of change" When an agency makes changes, employees should be involved and allowed opportunities to communicate with management about their feelings and thoughts. Change is scary for employees and management because there is always a risk that new rules and ideas won't work as well as old ones. Employees may worry about being replaced or fired (Goldman & Lewis, 2005).

The key to all of these problems is open communication between employees and management. Of course, that is the ideal solution, not necessarily the way things work out in reality. Some managers and supervisors are incompetent and insecure. They may behave in less than professional ways. If a worker wishes to continue in the agency with this type of management style, then the worker must take responsibility to speak up and attempt assertive resolution. Sometimes it is possible to go above one's immediate supervisor and complain. This is referred to as breaking chain of command and is not usually greeted with open arms. Status quo is threatened when you go around your immediate superiors, and you may pay a price for doing so (Russo, 1980). Some problems must be addressed by upper management, such as in cases of sexual harassment. For the most part, though, most organizations prefer that immediate supervisors and their staff resolve complaints and problems.

Developing mentoring relationships can be helpful in managing job-related stress, especially for beginning human services workers. A mentor is someone that an employee or intern can trust, respect, and communicate with openly. The mentor must be someone that has time to spend answering questions and listening to fears, struggles, and other issues. Usually, a mentor is an experienced human services worker who is available to offer ideas about how to perform job duties and how to get along with coworkers and survive in the system.

AGGRESSIVE, PASSIVE, AND ASSERTIVE BEHAVIORS

Many people confuse being **assertive** with being **aggressive,** and so they behave passively to avoid aggressive behavior. Passive, aggressive, and assertive behaviors are three very different styles of interpersonal communication. When people communicate assertively, stress levels are typically reduced, while aggressive and **passive** styles of communicating often increase stress. Learning how to communicate assertively is helpful to everyone, no matter what they choose to do with their lives. By learning these few assertive tactics, the reader has the opportunity to improve his or her own relationships and reduce stress as well as pass the information on to future recipients of human services. **Assertive** behaviors make it likely that the people get what they want when possible. They allow people to negotiate and express themselves appropriately and respectfully. Before introducing specific assertive techniques, a brief discussion about aggressive and passive communication will be presented.

Aggressive communication usually leaves both parties feeling bad. While someone may get their needs and wants met, the other feels disrespected, unheard, and manipulated. This type of interacting only concerns itself with one person's needs without any regard as to how the interaction affects the other. The person on the receiving end often feels angry, resentful, scared, and bad about him or herself. The aggressive person may temporarily feel powerful and in control, but over time he or she may destroy relationships with others. The aggressive person often appears to have a "chip on his shoulder" and may unwittingly turn others away from him or her. While he or she may get what he or she wants at the moment, he or she is losing the love and respect of others in the long term. Aggressive people intimidate others in order to succeed. How content would you be to have relationships with others based on fear?

Passive people often complement aggressive ones. They keep their feelings and needs inside for fear of creating conflict. They don't speak up but rather let others walk all over them. The price people pay for avoiding conflict is often to be viewed and treated like a doormat. At first, others may think it is positive that someone is so easygoing. Over time though, passive people may lose the respect of others because they don't command respect. Another consequence of being passive is a buildup of resentment. Instead of expressing disagreement and anger directly, passive people often let their angry feelings out indirectly. This is referred to as being passive-aggressive and leads to relationship dissatisfaction. For example, instead of telling her spouse that she is tired of his coming home late for dinner, a wife might simply burn his food and leave it on the table cold.

Simply put, assertive behavior allows people to express their own needs and wants in a way that does not harm others. Assertive people respect themselves and respect anyone else with whom he or she is interacting. While it may not always be possible for everyone to get whatever they want and need all the time, there is frequently room for compromises and negotiations when people relate to one another with respect and empathy. The key to assertive communication is to avoid blaming others or placing responsibility on others for one's own feelings and behaviors. The assertive person expresses needs and wants by making "I" statements instead of "you" and other attacking/blaming statements. In general, when people interact with respect for others as well as for themselves, everyone has a good chance of feeling good about themselves. When people feel good and respected, problems can be solved more readily and conflict can be resolved. The following lists provide examples of aggressive, passive and assertive statements.

Examples of Aggressive, Ineffective Statements

- "You make me so mad!"

- "You shouldn't talk that way to me."

- "You really have issues, don't you?"

- "You made the wrong choice, and now I have to suffer."

- "You never have enough time to spend supervising me."

- "Why does Janice get to leave early? She doesn't even do as much work as everyone else."

Examples of Passive Statements

- "I guess it's allright if you borrow my book, although I do need it to study tonight."

- "Sure, I don't mind skipping lunch today."

- "You need me to work this weekend? I suppose I can always watch the video of my nephew's graduation."

Examples of Assertive Statements

- "I feel angry when you ignore me because your attention and respect is important to me."

- "When we disagree, I would appreciate it if you could lower your voice and not use curse words."

- "I don't understand why you are upset with me right now."

- "I'm upset that what you've done affects me."

- "I feel that I need more supervision time with you. Can that be arranged?"

- "Although it may not be any of my business, I feel confused as to why Janice leaves earlier than the rest of us. Another thing that's bothering me is when she often refuses to pitch in and help the rest of us. Are you aware of this?"

Assertive interacting includes calm, realistic attempts to solve problems without blaming anyone. People think more clearly when they don't feel attacked and are more likely to come up with viable solutions than when they feel blamed. The assertive person must accept that sometimes the best one can achieve is a compromise.

Suppose you loaned your textbook to a classmate who lost it. You need it to study for the final exam. You don't have enough money to buy a new one and neither does the other student. Because you really need the book immediately, you may have to arrange a plan in which you pay for half of the book along with the other student to ensure you get the book soon. Although it isn't exactly fair, you will get what you need. You can always set up a plan for the classmate to reimburse you with small payments over the next few months. The focus should be on how to get the book you need, not on whose fault it is that you don't have it. You are likely to get reimbursed if you handle it assertively instead of passively or aggressively. If you were to yell and scream and blame your classmate, she might just tell you "tough, you're out of luck." If you don't speak up at all, she may just let you pay for a whole new book on your own.

Human services workers may be especially vulnerable to stress, given the nature of their work with clients and their other duties. Of course, handling criticism can be difficult for everyone, but responding assertively may reduce stress. Instead of fighting the criticism, an effective technique to manage the negative feelings associated with being criticized is to simply agree with the criticism or try to more clearly understand it. This gives the person a chance to learn from any mistakes to make improvements. When someone criticizes another person, there is often the tendency to defend or explain oneself. This is not necessary. The best thing to say to a supervisor, coworker, or a client who's being critical of others is, "What you say may be accurate. What exactly is it about my behavior that you find objectionable? What do you think would be a better way to handle things?" Even if they were wrong to make a comment, by saying these things, they are forced into taking responsibility for their criticism. Assertive people don't allow negative remarks to go by easily. They respectfully ask others to communicate without attacking or blaming. The following lists provide some examples of how to handle criticism assertively.

Examples of Handling Criticism from a Supervisor

- Criticism: "You didn't write these case notes very legibly."

- Assertive response: "I guess you're right, they are a bit messy. What would be the best way to fix it?"

- Aggressive response: "So what? Everyone else writes messy too."

- Passive response: "I'm sorry. I was in a hurry and didn't concentrate. I'll do them over."

Examples of Handling Criticism from a Coworker

- Criticism: "You were rude to those clients."

- Assertive response: "Wow, if that is the case, I sure didn't mean to be. What exactly did I do that seemed rude to you?"

- Aggressive response: "They were rude to me first. Whose side are you going to take anyway?"

- Passive response: I'm horrible. I guess I should quit.

Handling Criticism from a Member of a Substance-Abuse Group

- Criticism: "You're too young to be a group counselor. How can you know anything?"

- Assertive response: "Yes, I am young. What is it exactly about my age that bothers you? What would make you feel better?"

- Aggressive response: "Well, at least I went to college. How about you?"

- Passive response: "Yeah, I know. Maybe I'll wait until I get older to run groups."

Maintaining a Sense of Humor

Using humor appropriately to manage stress on the job, even when working with clients, can relieve tension and create a bond between people. True, one should not laugh at client's problems, but humor can be useful in a variety of ways. Psychologists often use humor in promoting healing in their clients (Fry, 1993; McGuire, 1999). If it is a healing process for clients, then it is probably beneficial for anyone experiencing stress. Studies have demonstrated that laughter boosts the immune system and lowers blood pressure (McGuire, 1999). That alone is extremely beneficial for someone who feels stress. Humor also allows people to think about a situation in new ways, and it effectively reduces feelings of anxiety and depression.

Some tips for adding humor into one's life include interacting with funny, playful people; taking time to play everyday, observing children and animals, searching for things to laugh about, and posting cartoons where they can be seen. It's important to avoid sarcasm and abusive humor, as well as to avoid discounting serious emotions by laughing them off. Humor should facilitate, not interrupt, the healing process (McGuire, 1999).

Chapter Summary

Stress occurs daily. It is not abnormal, but must be managed effectively if we are to function at our best. Human services workers may be prone to stress on the job because of ongoing contact with people in crisis and suffering. It is vital that human services workers practice stress management to perform their duties appropriately. Clients deserve to receive services from workers who are not burned out. Cognitive restructuring, assertive communication, talking to coworkers, and recreation are all helpful in managing stress.

Suggested Applied Activities

1. Using the worksheet below, think of a current situation in which you find yourself feeling negative emotions or engaging in destructive behaviors. Fill in the blanks and try to reduce your irrational thoughts and negative feelings.

Worksheet to Help Reduce Irrational Thoughts and Feelings

Negative feelings: _____

Precipitating event: _____

Irrational beliefs: _____

_____

Disputations and substitutions: _____

_____

_____

_____

Evaluation: _____

---

2. The next time someone criticizes you, try to handle the criticism by asking the person what it is about your behavior bothers them so much. Perhaps you might even agree with the criticism and ask for suggestions on how to improve. Don't explain yourself or defend yourself. Evaluate how this type of response makes you feel.

_____

_____

_____

3. Keep track of your daily activities. Make sure you incorporate a fun, playful activity every day. How often do you laugh during a day? Try to engage in activities that make you smile and laugh.

_____

_____

_____

_____

_____

Chapter Review Questions

1. What are five symptoms of burnout?

_____

_____

2. What are five causes of burnout?

_____

_____

3. Name three ways to manage stress on the job?

_____

_____

4. What is the difference between assertiveness and aggressiveness?

_____

_____

5. How might cognitive therapy help reduce stress?

_____

_____

Glossary of Terms

Aggressive is a type of interacting in which a person takes care of his own needs without regard for others.

Assertive is a type of interacting in which a person demonstrates self-respect as well as respect for others.

Burnout refers to job-related anxiety and dissatisfaction that adversely affects job performance and other areas of a person's life.

Cognitive restructuring involves changing the way people think about their experiences.

Disputation is an internal dialogue that helps people think rationally about a situation that was previously thought of as negative and that led to irrational beliefs.

Irrational and self-defeating thoughts are not based on facts but are habitual ways that people think that often make them feel badly.

Morale is the way people feel about the place where they work. When morale is high, workers are happy; when it's low, people are generally dissatisfied and discouraged about their work.

Passive is a type of interacting in which people do not command respect for themselves and their needs but instead take care of others' needs in order to avoid conflict.

Precipitating event is a situation that causes a reaction in an individual.

Self-critical thoughts are negative thoughts that people use to label themselves bad in some way. Rather than thinking through a situation rationally, people simply think of themselves badly and feel terrible.

Stress is a state of being physically, psychologically, emotionally, and intellectually overwhelmed. It can manifest itself in physical symptoms, as well as negative emotions and thoughts about a situation.

Stress management is a group of behaviors used to reduce stress. This includes cognitive restructuring, maintaining a healthy lifestyle, and assertive communication.

Case Presentation and Exit Quiz

General Description and Demographics

Kara is an undergraduate in the human services department of a local university. This is her second semester in the human services program, and she's beginning her first internship, which is at a group home. Kara is an excellent student and her grade-point average has been a 4.0. She has a keen understanding of various theories and counseling techniques, knowledge about case management, and has excelled in her course dealing with cultural issues. Currently, in addition to her internship class, she's taking courses on crisis intervention, child development, self-awareness, and abnormal psychology. Kara's career goal is to be either a social worker or a family counselor. Kara is 20 years old.

The group home where she is interning is an approved agency site for the human services department. It is a nonprofit agency that contracts with the county department of social services for funding. The agency also holds yearly fundraisers to increase its budget. Kara's supervisor, Emma, is a 38-year-old pediatric counselor who has a bachelor's degree in child development. Kara's stated responsibilities include monitoring the children while they do homework, helping children resolve conflicts with one another, supervising children on the playground, and escorting children on field trips. Kara, Emma, and Kara's fieldwork instructor all agreed on these responsibilities.

The children who live at the group home have all been placed there by the courts because they have been physically, sexually, or emotionally abused or severely neglected by their parents. Many of their parents are in jail, mental hospitals, or are substance abusers. The parents have failed to follow through with case plans. Many of the children suffer from behavioral and emotional problems. They often act out their anger and frustration at their situation by lying, stealing, hitting, yelling, and swearing. The group home operates under a behavior-modification model. Children receive rewards when they follow the rules and suffer consequences when they break them. Each child is assigned to a personal therapist, either a licensed clinical social worker or a licensed marriage and family therapist. Some children with extremely severe problems receive treatment from psychologists, and some are on medication prescribed by a psychiatrist. Older children often participate in group counseling. They all go to school at the group home and are only allowed to leave the home when accompanied by a staff member.

Kara's Stress

Kara has always wanted to work with abused children. She was abused physically as a child and wants to help abused children feel better about themselves. When she was first accepted to intern at the group home, she felt excited and couldn't wait to start. After interning there for only three weeks, she finds herself dreading the days she works at the agency. She has begun to oversleep on those days she is supposed to go to the agency, and on weekends, she's been going to a lot of parties and getting drunk. She feels guilty about disliking the agency because she tells herself that she should want to help those poor kids. Kara believes that if she doesn't help them, they will grow up to be losers and she would be partially to blame.

When Kara is at the agency, she handles the children very competently. She usually knows the right things to say and is able to help the children manage their conflicts and aggressive feelings very effectively. In fact, she is so competent that her supervisor has left her alone at the agency while the paid staff all go to lunch. At other times, Kara is left alone because several staff members called in sick. Kara doesn't feel comfortable being there by herself and has told Emma that she feels a little nervous. Emma told Kara not to worry because Kara is more competent than half of the paid staff.

Another of Kara's concerns is that she has been asked to drive some children to dental and medical appointments. She never agreed to do this when she signed her contract. Kara knows she isn't supposed to drive them in her own car because the university doesn't allow it. One day a child became violent when Kara was at the home alone. Kara phoned Emma, but Emma didn't answer her cell phone. Kara called the on-call licensed supervisor, who told her to call the police and she'd be right in.

Kara is afraid to tell her class instructor about what is going on because she thinks that the instructor will be angry or that she will get in trouble for performing duties not on her contract. Kara can't handle another day at the agency. Thank goodness she gets to go to her internship class tomorrow.

Kara finally opens up to her instructor and to the rest of her classmates. She learns that other students have had similar experiences at their internship sites. The students and instructor offer some ideas to Kara about how to manage her stress.

Kara takes their advice, and over the next few weeks she slowly starts to feel better about going to the group home.

Exit Quiz

1. Kara shows which signs of burnout?
   a. physical energy
   b. overly positive self-concept
   c. negative job attitudes
   d. all of the above

2. All but one of the following is probably a cause of Kara's burnout:
   a. conflict between the ideal and the real
   b. dealing with tedious bureaucratic tasks
   c. lack of client motivation and limited capabilities to receive help and help themselves
   d. conflicts between personal values and organizational norms

3. Kara's drinking is
   a. an attempt to manage her stress
   b. evidence that she is an alcoholic
   c. a sign that she shouldn't be a social worker
   d. cause for dismissal

4. Kara's instructor asked her what she was thinking that made her feel guilty about not wanting to go to the group home. Kara replied:
   a. "The children don't really want me there."
   b. "If I don't help them, they may grow up to be losers."
   c. "I really am not qualified to help."
   d. none of the above

5. The instructor tells Kara that working with abused children is difficult for even the most experienced counselor and that most of them go through a period of anxiety and depression when working with this population. This is an example of
   a. assertion training
   b. changing the agency structure
   c. cognitive restructuring
   d. all of the above

6. The instructor has Kara role-play a conversation between Kara and her supervisor Emma. Kara is told to tell Emma what she wants in an assertive manner. Which statement below is not an example of an assertive communication?
   a. "I feel very uncomfortable being alone at the group home and believe it is inappropriate for an intern to be alone with so many abused children."
   b. "You are so unethical leaving me alone. I should report you to the better business bureau."
   c. "I can no longer drive the children in my personal car to doctor appointments. It is against my university's policy for interns."
   d. "I would like to continue working at the group home, but some things need to change for me to be able to continue."

7. What can Kara do to help relieve some of her stress while interning at the group home?
   a. talk to coworkers about her feelings when she's at the agency
   b. engage in recreational activities such as swimming
   c. watch a funny movie
   d. all of the above

Exit Quiz Answers

1. c	4. b	7. d
2. b	5. c	
3. a	6. b	

CHAPTER 11

Ethical Issues in the Human Services

Introduction

The field of human services places a strong emphasis on adhering to specific ethical standards. Recipients of human services are often vulnerable because of the many needs for which they seek help. When people are vulnerable, they may be easy to take advantage of or manipulate. **Ethics** ensure that clients who seek help from human services providers are treated with respect, dignity, and honesty.

What Are Ethics?

Ethics are standards of conduct that human services professionals have agreed are vital to appropriate and effective interventions. Although a variety of professional organizations have determined what they consider ethical behavior to be, there is very little disagreement among these organizations. There seem to be some basic ethical standards that cross over among the various human services disciplines.

In general, "ethical issues usually refer to moral imperatives; the 'shoulds' and 'oughts' directed toward protecting the welfare of those who require services of helping professionals and are regulated by the professions. Legal issues refer to the efforts of governmental administrative agencies, legislatures, and the courts to create rules of law which govern the practice of psychology, psychiatry, social work, and counseling" (Herr & Cramer, 1987, p. 156). Sometimes behaviors that are considered unethical are also illegal.

Why Are Ethics Necessary?

Although following prescribed rules and standards may seem burdensome and diminish autonomy, in fact ethical standards benefit human services workers. By knowing and adhering to ethical standards, human services workers are protected from frivolous lawsuits that some clients might file against workers and agencies. Unless clients can prove in a court of law or with a professional organization that a worker engaged in unethical or illegal behaviors, they aren't likely to win such lawsuits. Conservative ethical practice can be a relief to human services workers because they know they won't be liable for sanctions if they follow approved ethical standards.

Ethical standards also protect the consumer. People who reach out to human services workers deserve to receive competent, objective, and fair services. Ethics ensure that people receive services from qualified workers, workers who understand the personal affect they may have on clients, and from workers who provide confidential services that permit clients to be open and trusting.

A third benefit of ethics is that by having standards written down and standardized, there is less opportunity for bickering among helping professionals. Commonsense would suggest that if the majority agrees that certain behaviors should be practiced, then those who disagree should have to go along with the majority. Of course, there is always room for changing ethics as new technologies arise, new problems arise, and different cultural issues arise. For example, online technology has created an industry where people can access counseling services by logging onto a computer. The ethical standards of the 1980s did not include such services, so various professional organizations have been discussing this issue for the past 10 years until an acceptable ethical standard can be created. Another example has to do with how workers are to handle the **confidentiality** standard when working with people who are HIV-positive. Since it is known to be lethal to others, should a human services worker be forced to breach confidentiality if he finds out an HIV-positive person is having unprotected sex with someone? These are the types of questions that the professional organizations consider and respond to in forming new ethical standards.

Since each major mental health, medical, and social welfare professional organization has its own code of ethics, the reader should obtain a copy of the ethical codes of the profession when he or she is sure about what field he or she wishes to pursue as a career. The written standards are often lengthy and would take up many pages to include in this text. Following is a list of many of the various codes of ethics applicable to the field of human services:

1. Code of Ethics, the American Counseling Association (ACA, 2005)
2. Ethical Principles of Psychologists and Code of Conduct, American Psychological Association (APA, 2002)
3. Code of Ethics, National Association of Social Workers (NASW, 1999)
4. AAMFT Code of Ethics, American Association for Marriage and Family Therapy (AAMFT, 2001)
5. Ethical Standards of the National Organization for Human Services, National Organization for Human Services (NOHS, 2000)
6. Code of Professional Ethics for Rehabilitation Counselors, Commission of Rehabilitation Counselor Certification (CRCC, 2001)
7. CCA Code of Ethics, Canadian Counseling Association, (CCA, 1999)

8. Ethical Standards for School Counselors, American School Counselor Association (ASCA, 2004)
9. Ethical Guidelines for Counseling Supervisors, Association for Counselor Education and Supervision (ACES, 1995)
10. Feminist Therapy Code of Ethics, Feminist Therapy Institute (FTI, 2000)
11. The Principles of Medical Ethics with Annotations Especially Applicable to Psychiatry, (American Psychiatric Association (2001)

There are a multitude of ethical issues reviewed by each of the above professional associations. A discussion of every ethical dilemma and issue is beyond the scope of this chapter. Five ethical issues will be discussed in the sections that follow: 1) **confidentiality,** 2) **dual relationships,** 3) **countertransference,** 4) **values clarification,** and 5) ensuring ethical competence through **continuing education.** These particular issues were selected because most of the professions emphasize these concerns in their stated standards, and they apply to many different types of human services workers and client populations.

Confidentiality

Confidentiality relates to the concept of privacy. Siegel (1979, p. 251) defines it as "the freedom of individuals to choose for themselves the time and the circumstances under which and the extent to which their beliefs, behaviors, and opinions are to be shared or withheld from others." The ethical standard of confidentiality is meant to reassure clients that they can speak freely to a human services worker without the fear that their confidential information will be disclosed. When clients are open and honest, workers can more effectively meet their needs.

The legal counterpart to the ethical concept of confidentiality is referred to as **privilege.** This is the term used in court actions, which "refers to a rule in evidence law that provides a litigant with the right to withhold evidence in a legal proceeding that was originally communicated in confidence" (Swoboda, Elwork, Sales, & Levine, 1978, p. 449). Privileged communication in professional relationships requires mutual trust, such as that between client and attorney, therapist and client, doctor and patient and priest and church member.

When confidentiality is broken, a professional may be considered to have engaged in unprofessional conduct and may be subject to disciplinary action, such as suspended license or mandatory education courses on ethical standards. Many states have statutes that consider violations of confidentiality a misdemeanor and if someone is found guilty they may be imprisoned or required to pay a fine, or both (Benitez, 2004, p. 32).

Privacy for people receiving services in any health care organization is such an important issue that Congress passed legislation in 1996 designed to standardize exactly how information might be disclosed by health care providers nation-wide. The **Health Insurance Portability and Accountability Act (HIPAA)** includes four components that aim to streamline communication among health care providers and afford patients more rights. The first component, privacy requirements, creates rights for patients concerning how their health information is used and disclosed by health care providers. It limits what a health care provider can do with a patient's health information without that patient's knowledge and consent. It also sets up standards that require health care providers to keep patient information confidential and secure. While most human services and health care institutions have been practicing under ethical codes requiring the confidential treatment of patient information, this act ensures that all providers in all states adhere to strict privacy standards. The other three components provide standards regarding security of information, how to secure electronic transactions and set up national identifier require-ments for health care providers.

Exceptions to Confidentiality

While every attempt should be made to ensure a client's privacy, some situations do require that confidentiality be breeched. Situations that have the potential to inflict serious harm or cause destruction need to be revealed.

MANDATORY REPORTING STANDARDS

Since the passage of the Child Abuse Prevention and Treatment Act in 1974, all states in the nation have been required to set up standards for the identifi-cation, treatment, and prevention of child abuse. This created **mandatory reporting standards** for professionals who engage in the care or treatment of minors. Likewise, after the passage of the Elder Abuse and Dependent Adult Civil Protection Act, states set up mandates that required professionals who intervene with the elderly or disabled adult populations to report suspected instances of abuse to appropriate agencies. Where to report abuse varies from state to state. Urban areas usually have agencies specifically designed to man-age abuse reports, whereas rural areas may depend on law enforcement to manage them. Abuse of children, the elderly, and the disabled require breech-ing confidentiality.

DUTY TO WARN

Another area in which workers must breach confidentiality and report disclosures to appropriate agencies is when a client poses a serious threat of physical violence against a reasonably identifiable victim or victims. This exception to confidential-ity is known as the **duty to warn.** The worker must report such danger to law enforcement immediately. Duty to warn is not applicable, when clients pose a danger to themselves but not to others. In cases where clients plan to hurt themselves, workers are not mandated to inform law enforcement. Instead, a worker is permitted to breach confidentiality if it is believed that it is necessary to prevent an act of suicide or self-harm.

OTHER EXCEPTIONS TO CONFIDENTIALITY

Other mandatory exceptions to confidentiality occur when there is a court order, subpoena, or search warrant issued, when a coroner requests records as part of an investigation, and when the client requests that records be shared. The most recent legal mandate that requires exception to confidentiality is contained in the **Patriot Act of 2001.** This federal legislation prohibits disclosing to clients that the FBI sought or obtained personal books, records, papers, documents, and other items of theirs, as well as requires that such items be provided to the FBI (Benitez, 2004, p. 34). Table 11.1 outlines the exceptions to confidentiality.

Table 11.1 Exceptions to Confidentiality

The Exception	The Follow-Through
suspected physical, sexual child abuse and neglect	must report to child protective agency or law enforcement
suspected elderly or disabled adult abuse: neglect, physical, sexual, or financial	must report to adult protective agency or law enforcement
duty to warn: someone poses a serious physical threat to another person	must report to law enforcement
danger to self: someone poses a serious physical threat to himself	not mandatory to report, though may report to prevent harm
court order or subpoena	must disclose to judge
an investigation into a death of a client	must disclose to coroner
when a client signs a release of information	must disclose to the person requested by client
Patriot Act of 2001	must hand over records to FBI, cannot tell client

Dual Relationships

Definition of Dual Relationships

Ethical guidelines suggest that human services workers maintain clear boundaries with their clients about the nature of the relationship. Counselors, social workers, probation officers, teachers, and any other types of human services workers are strongly encouraged to keep their relationship with their clients strictly professional. The sole purpose of the relationship should be for the human services worker to help the client meet his or her needs. The reverse should not be the reason–using clients to meet the needs of the human services worker.

The use of the phrase *dual relationship* means that the connection between a human services worker and a client includes two or more types of relationships and is strongly discouraged, and sometimes illegal, such as in the case of sexual relationships between clients and counselors. This might include any type of social relationship, romantic or sexual relationship, familial relationship, or business relationship. In some areas, especially small, rural towns, this may prove to be difficult because there may be very few human services workers in a community of 500 people, so the chances of relationship crossover would be higher than in heavily populated urban communities. In general, though, human services workers should make every attempt at keeping the relationship with clients professional.

Why Should Dual Relationships Be Avoided?

The primary purpose of the dual relationship ethical standard has to do with the prevention of the exploitation of clients. People who seek the help of human services workers are often vulnerable and therefore may be easy to manipulate. Some human services workers may use their clients to meet their own needs, such as the need to control, need to have someone be dependent, need to have companionships, need for sex and love, or need for money. Although the human services worker may not consciously try to harm or exploit a client through a dual relationship, a client might be emotionally injured if the worker and the client engage in activities outside the helping relationship.

If the relationship were to become personal, the worker might lose objectivity and effectiveness in helping the client. Additionally, if the worker is using the client to meet his or her own needs, then the client's need may become lost and may not be met. Finally, if a personal or business relationship turns sour, the client-worker relationship is also hampered. Several examples of potentially damaging dual relationships are described below.

EXAMPLES OF DUAL RELATIONSHIPS

Example 1: A social worker has been working with a family for six months with three children ages 2, 6, and 14. They live only with their mother because their father was sent to prison for molesting the six-year-old girl. The 14-year old girl is turning 15 and has invited the social worker to her *quincinera,* a coming-out party for adolescent girls that occurs frequently in many Latino families.

Initially, this seems harmless. After all, what needs could the social worker be meeting by attending? How could the family be exploited? Several potential problems might occur. If the social worker attends this affair, how might the 6-year-old girl feel? She may feel that the 14-year-old is getting more attention and feel resentful at the social worker. How will the family explain how they know the social worker to family and friends? They may not have explained the situation to others, and this could prove to be awkward. Also, what if the social worker lets her hair down and has a few drinks and dances with a male guest. How might this affect the professional relationship? If the social worker is a lonely person, she could use this big celebration as an opportunity for her to meet her own needs. What would you do? Would you go to the *quinicera,* or would you politely decline, informing the family that personal involvement outside the office is not permitted?

Example 2: A male mental health counselor at a substance abuse facility has been working with a woman for about three months. During that time, the woman has cleaned up her act and is working full time. The client, who the counselor thinks is very attractive, tells him that she wants to end therapy and would like to start seeing him socially. The counselor would be very interested in dating her. So, because she has terminated therapy with him, is he free and clear to do this?

Could any problems occur if they did begin to date? Would it technically be a dual relationship? In fact, most professional associations recommend at least a six-month cooling off period before a counselor develops a romantic relationship with a former client. The biggest problem with this situation is that she is telling him of her feelings for him while he is still her therapist. These feelings she has for him may be a phenomenon known as **transference,** which occurs frequently between clients and counselors. The client may be feeling attracted to the counselor not because of who he is, but because she has attributed characteristics to him based on unresolved issues with a significant other in her life. She may have had a very distant, rejecting father and had never dealt with the pain of this. Her attraction to the counselor may be an unconscious attempt to have a relationship with a man who will not reject her, to compensate for that which was missing with her father.

If the counselor responds to her request, he may at some point reject her and she would suffer a recurrence of the original wound from her father's rejection. Also, if the client ever needs more counseling, she certainly can't call on him again to help her. Once a relationship turns personal, counselors cannot maintain the objectivity they need. The relationship itself may be the very problem that a client may need further help with, and obviously the previous counselor, who's now part of the problem, could not be impartial. So the correct response if a client tells you they want to date you, is "I feel very complimented that you have feelings for me that way, however, professional ethics are very strict on this matter, and so I must decline your invitation. I am sure you will find someone that can reciprocate these feelings."

Example 3: One of the activities coordinators at a senior center has been interacting with an elderly couple for the past 3 weeks about their family business. They own several restaurants and their daughter has recently quit and moved across the country. They need a nighttime hostess part time. The pay is great! The coordinator has been thinking about getting a part-time job to help pay for her son's college tuition. Should she take the job?

This would definitely be a dual relationship and should be discouraged. You may ask, "Why? Everyone benefits." The couple gets a new hostess, and she gets extra money. What could go wrong? As you can guess, things do go wrong. She may turn out to be an incompetent hostess. How would the couple then fire her? Also, how will the coordinator switch roles from employee at night to in charge program director during the day. Can you picture how awkward this might be?

How to Avoid Dual Relationships

These three examples provide just a small sample of the potential dual relationships that human services workers might face. In general, keep your relationship with clients professional. Do not engage in activities outside work with them. Find your romantic partners, your friends, and business partners elsewhere.

Countertransference

Because human services workers deal with people who share intimate feelings and thoughts, the likelihood of having emotional reactions when working with these people is high. When these emotional reactions are from a worker's unresolved or unacknowledged issues, that worker is experiencing countertransference with the client.

Definition of Countertransference

When clients develop feelings toward human services workers based on unresolved feelings and needs toward significant others, they are experiencing a phenomenon referred to as **transference.** Human services workers may also experience reactions toward clients that are based on their unresolved feelings and needs toward their own significant others. When it is the human services worker having feelings toward clients based on these unresolved feelings, it is referred to as countertransference. If the human services worker were to react to a client based on feelings that in reality were based on a different relationship, the client would certainly be receiving ineffective and inappropriate services.

Countertransference may lead to emotional reactions that may cloud the worker's judgment and lead to **negligence** and incompetence. Countertransference issues can prevent workers from being aware of their own limitations and inappropriate reactions. If inappropriate behavior goes unchecked, workers can be sued for malpractice. The following scenarios are examples of countertransference situations.

EXAMPLES OF COUNTERTRANSFERENCE

Example 1: A social worker begins to feel very angry at a seven-year-old girl whose uncle had been sexually molesting her. The little girl had confided that she wasn't angry with her uncle and in fact missed him. The social worker reacted to this disclosure by telling the girl outright that she should be very angry with her uncle and that he was a bad man. This made the girl cry.

Countertransference Issue: The social worker had been molested by her own uncle when she was 10. She never told anyone and thought that the experience would just fade from her mind. She has always had troubled relationships with men and often feels angry toward them. The social worker is hardly aware of her feelings about the molestation. She has never talked to anyone about her abuse, so she has not had the opportunity to share her own feelings. This case most likely brought to the surface her own angry feelings, and she was in fact responding to her own issues. Nevertheless, reactions like these are inappropriate and are often at the expense of a client.

Example 2: A mental health counselor is running a group for battered women. She becomes very frightened when she hears about the abuse the women had withstood. She stops the conversation from continuing and encourages the women to move on to a new subject.

Countertransference issue: This counselor is currently living in an abusive relationship with her boyfriend. He shoves her, curses at her, and has threatened to physically harm her. She is ashamed and hasn't told anyone. She just hopes he'll be nicer. By blocking the conversation, she helps herself in not dealing with her own situation, but also prevents the members of the group from dealing with theirs.

Example 3: A probation officer visits a parolee who had been released from jail after serving a one-year sentence for burglary. The probation officer arrives and notices that the leftovers to a couple of joints of marijuana are in an ashtray and a mirror is lying across a coffee table with traces of cocaine on it. The parolee quickly hides these things. The probation officer doesn't mention it and instead engages in a very friendly conversation. The parolee hasn't gotten a job yet but is trying. The probation officer doesn't say anything about the evidence of illegal drugs or ask about where the rent money is coming from.

Countertransference issue: The probation officer has a brother who has been a drug addict for many years. The probation officer has spent much time and effort trying to help his brother. This client reminds him of his brother in personality and looks. The probation officer feels sorry for the client and is willing to give him money and take him out to dinner. The client accepts and shows appreciation, something his own brother has never done. The probation officer is using the client to feel appreciated. He may even feel that he can save him, unlike his brother who has been in and out of rehab for years. This is not good for the client because now he is getting away with inappropriate behaviors that may get him into trouble.

How Can Countertransference Be Avoided?

These examples show how issues of countertransference can lead to negligent practice and be harmful to a client. One strong ethical standard for all those in the helping professions is to cause no harm to clients. When workers are unaware of their own needs, feelings, and past experiences, they can do harm.

Of course, not every client triggers countertransference in every human services worker. Ideally human services workers would work on developing the **self-awareness** necessary to identify the issues, problems, and personality types that create issues of countertransference. By doing so, human services workers have a better chance of heading off their own inappropriate reactions. They would be able to take an objective stance if they were aware that their emotional response may be related to their own issues rather than those of the client. Continuous **self-examination** is necessary to prevent countertransference from interfering with ethical practice. This means that human services workers must monitor their reactions during sessions with clients so that they don't act out inappropriately. Human services workers can also consult with colleagues, supervisors, and their own therapists when a client brings out countertransference reactions to ensure the client receives proper intervention.

Values Clarification

Human services workers should also be aware of their own values. Values usually serve as an internal guide for how to behave and feel about life situations. Human services workers must be aware of their own values so they do not force them onto their clients.

Definition of Values Clarification

No one can be completely free of all biases and values. That is certainly true for human services workers. After all, it is their values that influenced them to work in the field of human services. Values clarification is a process during which a human services worker helps clients figure out their own values and decisions. It is not even considered inappropriate for human services workers to share some of their feelings and values about various subjects, as long as they let the client know that these values belong to the worker and that the client does not need to feel obligated to agree with them.

By merely exposing one's values to the client, the human services worker may be helpful in broadening the clients' views, hence giving them more options to assist them in solving problems. Human services workers must be careful to respect the client's values even as they expose their own. The conversation should be more of a values clarification dialogue rather than a "here's how I think, therefore you should . . ." lecture. Remember, clients can be very vulnerable and easy to manipulate. They may momentarily agree with the worker's values, but later may regret accepting these values when they have a chance to think about it more. They may be afraid to disagree with a professional and institute behaviors that go against everything they believe.

Enhancing Values Clarification

Just as self-awareness and self-monitoring are vital to avoiding countertransference, they are just as vital in ensuring that human services workers engage in the process of values clarification appropriately. They should be in tune with their own values and biases. It is essential to monitor oneself so as not to impose one's own values onto clients. The more one knows about what he or she believes to be important, the more one can monitor what is said to clients. All clients deserve to have objective feedback that aims to help clients arrive at solutions that fit their value systems.

When clients' values differ greatly from those their human services workers', workers need to have the self-awareness and integrity to follow ethical standards and either refer the client to someone else who can be objective, or to consult with someone to help them deal appropriately with their clients. Some examples of ethical dilemmas involving values are described below.

EXAMPLES OF VALUES CLARIFICATION

Example 1 (self-awareness practiced): A psychologist did an intake interview with a new client. The client disclosed that he was gay and was having issues with his partner. This psychologist's religious faith believed that homosexuality was a sin and that homosexuals were beyond hope as long as they continued to live a gay lifestyle. Fortunately, this psychologist's self-awareness about his bias made him realize that it would be inappropriate to continue seeing this client. He referred him immediately to another therapist.

Example 2 (self-awareness not practiced): A 17-year-old male is brought to a counselor by his parents. They are appalled that their son is gay and want the counselor to straighten him out. The 17-year-old is fine with being gay but feels anxious and depressed about his parents' reactions. His fear at the thought of his parents' rejection nearly brought him to suicide. The counselor tells the boy that being gay is wrong and that if he becomes heterosexual, all his problems will go away. The counselor advises the boy to go through a type of therapy that would be re-train him to be heterosexual. Despite the counselor's awareness of his own opinionated views about homosexuality, he chose to impose his values on his *client*. He didn't allow for any options. He wasn't self-aware or objective enough to realize that he was overstepping his bounds as a counselor. The damage to his client could be fatal.

Example 3 (self-awareness practiced): A counselor at a free clinic is conducting an intake session with a 15-year-old girl who is pregnant. The girl is not sure what to do. She doesn't know if she should keep the baby, have an abortion, or put the baby up for adoption. The counselor educates the girl on all of these options and helps her examine the pros and cons for each. By the end of the session, the girl has decided to talk with her parents and then come back. The counselor believes that the girl should put the baby up for adoption but never once told her this. She provided all options with equal support. The counselor is aware of her own bias against abortion and against teenage girls keeping and raising babies, but she also knows that it would be unethical to try to persuade the girl in any direction.

Example 4 (self-awareness not practiced): A different counselor at a birth-control clinic sees a 17-year-old girl who is pregnant. The girl is not sure if she wants to keep the baby and is not even sure who the father is. The counselor tells her that abortion is out of the question because it is murder. She also tells her that God will take care of everything and that babies should be with their real moms. The girl should pay for her sin by raising the baby even if it means sacrificing her own adolescence. After all, she committed the sin and now must pay the price. This counselor is obviously way out of line. She has very little awareness about the damage she could be doing to the girl. Her biases are so strong that she doesn't even consider the effect on the client. She is imposing her own values inappropriately. She may think she is giving the best advice, but has not examined why she is doing so except that she believes it is best.

The Benefits of Self-Awareness

What we can learn from these examples is that human services workers do not always know what is best for all clients. Clients have rights. These rights include the right to examine all the facts, be educated, and be heard by an objective worker before having to make decisions. The more self-aware human services workers are, the greater their ability to be objective and ensure client rights are met. Also, the more self-aware human services workers are, the more likely they are to live successfully and serve as appropriate role models for their clients.

Most formal higher education institutions that teach human services oriented courses include topics that focus on the importance of self-awareness and self-examination for those pursuing a career in the helping professions. Some programs may emphasize this aspect more than others, but it would be fair to say that self-monitoring and self-development of human services workers are universally valued by educators and professional workers. Therefore, one way to begin the process of becoming aware of oneself and one's needs as a person is to participate in formal education. Textbooks, such as this one, class exercises, and reaction or reflection papers are common methods for introducing this ethical standard to human services majors. If every course offers just a little bit of opportunity to learn about oneself, then, by the end of one's study, the student should have gained a considerable amount of self-awareness.

Of course human services workers are also encouraged to seek professional counseling or consultation to further the process of self-awareness, especially if problems arise while providing services to clients. This counseling might be in the form of individual, group, marital, or family counseling. It might be for several years or for a couple of sessions depending on the needs of the worker. Many professional workers seek professional counseling periodically throughout their career as the need arises. This is a smart thing to do as it ensures that workers continually monitor themselves as they provide more and more challenging services to a varied client population that may be triggering a multitude of countertransference reactions.

Professional counseling is not required for human services workers. Self-awareness can be gained through personal examination, engaging in meaningful dialogues with co-workers, and reading various books. The vital message is that human services workers should become as aware of their own needs as possible on an ongoing basis so as not to cause any emotional harm to clients.

CRITICAL THINKING / SELF-REFLECTION CORNER

- What are some of your values that might conflict with your objectivity with clients?

- What will you do if these values become an issue for you in your work?

- Do you agree that human services workers shouldn't be friends with their clients?

- Would you accept a gift from a client? Attend a wedding?

Ensuring Ethical Competence with Continuing Education

Learning about oneself and maintaining ongoing self-monitoring is not the only thing that human services workers must do to meet ethical standards. Ethics also require that professional workers participate in training and education beyond that received in a formal education institution where an actual degree is earned. The field of human services is constantly changing, and human services workers must stay current on new ethical guidelines, new treatment and interventions, and current needs of client populations.

One of the benefits of participating in continuing education for the human services worker is often a renewed feeling of motivation and challenge. After participating in conferences and workshops, counselors, teachers, social workers, and other human services workers usually feel less burnt out. These learning opportunities give them a place to discuss a variety of challenging issues with colleagues. They also increase human services workers' knowledge and skill level that leads to increased competency when providing service. New ideas help prevent stagnation of thought and behavior.

An additional benefit of continuing education is that some of the situations that human services workers face at agencies aren't taught at colleges and universities. It would be impossible for any one program to teach every possible skill and piece of information. Clients have such a variety of needs, and those needs constantly change and so many workers must learn about these needs outside of their college experience.

Many professional associations require 30 or more hours of continuing education in order for the counselors, social workers, and doctors to renew their licenses. This indicates the importance of staying current and expanding one's knowledge base beyond the required college curriculum. The reader is encouraged to explore the multitude of continuing education courses available for students and professional workers. They are offered through private organizations, through the various professional associations, and through universities and colleges. Many nonprofit and public human services agencies frequently offer training for their own workers and for those who plan to serve internships at the agency. While much of the material covered in these courses may have been taught as part of college curriculum, these training classes usually provide more detailed, practical, and agency specific knowledge and skills for the participant in an effort to ensure competent practice.

In addition to participating in required continuing education, human services workers are encouraged to consult with colleagues and outside professionals when clients or other activities pose challenges. Many agencies contract with experienced grant writers to ensure that the agency has the best chance at getting funded. When counselors take on clients who have issues in areas in which they have little experience, they often talk with more experienced therapists so they can better serve their clients. Every human services worker from social worker to probation officer, to child-care worker must, from time to time, seek the assistance of others to make sure clients are receiving effective services. Ethical standards encourage professional consultations if it means clients receive competent services. Failure to provide competent service because supervision, consultations, or training was not sought, may be grounds for malpractice law suits under the ethical standard of negligence. When in doubt, seek extra knowledge and consultation. The goal is to provide clients with the best standard of care possible.

Chapter Summary

Ethics are guidelines that various professions follow to ensure that consumers of services are protected and that there is some consistency among various workers in the same profession. In the field of human services, there are several ethical standards that ensure that clients can trust workers enough that they will be honest about their problems, such as the standard of confidentiality. However, there are some exceptions to this ethical standard. Usually, if someone is in danger, human services workers must breach the confidentiality ethic to protect a potential victim. Other ethical codes deal with the worker's need to maintain professional boundaries with clients, engage in ongoing self-examination and training, and avoid imposing the worker's values onto clients.

Suggested Applied Activities

Go to the websites of the following professional organizations and find the page that lists each group's ethical standards. Note the similarities and differences among the organizations' standards of practice.

American Counseling Association (ACA) www.counseling.org

_____

_____

American Psychological Association (APA) www.apa.org

_____

_____

National Association of Social Workers (NASW) www.socialworkers.org

_____

_____

American Association for Marriage and Family Therapy (AAMFT) www.aamft.org

_____

_____

National Organization for Human Services (NOHS)
www.nationalhumanservices.org

_____

_____

Chapter Review Questions

1. What is the definition of ethical standards?

_____

_____

2. What is confidentiality?

_____

_____

3. When must a human services worker breach client confidentiality?

_____

_____

4. Why is a dual relationship with a client considered inappropriate?

_____

_____

5. Give three examples of dual relationships.

_____

_____

6. What is countertransference?

_____

_____

7. What can human services workers do to prevent imposing their values on clients?

_____

_____

8. Why is continuing education important?

_____

_____

Glossary of Terms

Confidentiality is an ethical standard promising that disclosures made by clients to human services workers stay private.

Continuing education is post-graduate training and courses for human services workers once they have begun working in their profession.

Countertransferences are emotions and reactions experienced by human services workers that are brought up during sessions in which clients are dealing with their own problems and issues. In most cases, workers' personal, unresolved issues create these strong, emotional reactions.

Dual relationships are those that come about when a human services worker develops another relationship with a client that is outside their professional one.

Duty to warn is an exception to the promise of confidentiality whereby workers are obligated to take appropriate action when clients appear to be posing serious physical harm to themselves or to others.

Ethics are moral guidelines created by various professional associations that set standards for how human services workers should behave with clients.

Health Insurance Portability and Accountability Act (HIPAA) standardized the way information might be disclosed by health care providers.

Mandatory reporting standards were created after the enactment of the Child Abuse Prevention and Treatment Act and the Elder Abuse and Dependent Adult Civil Protection Act to set a nationwide standard requiring that all instances of suspected physical, sexual, financial abuse, and neglect of children, elderly, and disabled adults be reported to the appropriate authorities.

Negligence is the failure of a human services worker to provide the appropriate standard of care.

Patriot Act of 2001 was enacted after the terrorist attacks of 9/11/01 in order to give the government authorities access to clients' records and disclosures without the knowledge or permission of the client.

Privilege is the legal counterpart to confidentiality that allows a litigant in a court proceeding to withhold evidence if it was communicated in confidence.

Self-awareness is workers' ability to have insight into how their own needs, feelings, and values affect their actions and behaviors, especially regarding their clients.

Self-examination is a process of looking honestly within one's own motives and reactions in an attempt to understand and resolve any emotional or psychological issues.

Values clarification is a human services worker's attempt to help clients sort out their own values rather than to impose outside values on clients.

Case Presentation and Exit Quiz

General Description and Demographics

Mark works at a juvenile diversion program funded by the county probation office, federal grants, and private donations. Mark has his bachelor's degree in human services. His typical duties include running counseling groups for first-time offenders and substance abusers, conducting intake interviews with new clients, and providing crisis-intervention services when necessary. He also conducts educational groups about drug and alcohol abuse. His title is group counselor I, and his supervisor is a licensed marital and family therapist.

Mark recently interviewed a new client. The client, Jason, is a 15-year-old boy who was caught selling marijuana at school. Since this was Jason's first arrest for anything, the judge ordered him to participate in a drug-diversion program for one year instead of sending him to jail. If Jason does not complete the program, he will be subject to jail time.

Jason has always been a popular, above-average student. He has many friends and likes to hang out at the beach. He lives with both of his parents and his 17-year-old sister, Heather. Although he and Heather have been smoking pot for the past three years, their grades have not suffered because of it.

Jason and his parents have their arguments, especially about what time Jason must be home at night. Naturally, Jason wants to stay out as late as Heather, but his parents believe he is too young to be out until 1 a.m. Jason also argues with his parents about doing chores around the house, but what 15-year-old doesn't?

Specific Problems

During Mark's interview with Jason, Jason reveals that he's been cutting himself for that past three months. Jason has razorblade marks all up and down his wrists. Mark asked him if he wanted to kill himself. Jason said that sometimes he does, especially when his parents fight with him and with each other. Jason says that when he's at home he prefers to stay in his room and listen to music because it drowns out his parents' constant bickering. Sometimes, when his mother drinks, she throws things, usually at his dad. But once, she threw a plate at Jason that cut his head open. When they went to the emergency room to get his head stitched up, Jason wanted to protect his mother so he told the doctor that he was fooling around at a party and unintentionally cut his head.

Another time when Jason's mother was drinking, she became enraged because Jason hadn't taken out the trash, so she scratched him on his neck so deeply that Jason started to bleed. Although it was quite painful, he didn't cry. He understands that his mom has a drinking problem.

Jason tells Mark that he gets into fistfights with kids at school when they look at him "the wrong way." He and his friends like to fight; in fact, the next time they're at the beach they're going to beat up this guy who keeps surfing on their territory. They have a plan to surround him and then drag him into the water and hold him under until he almost drowns. Mark asked what the other kid's name was, but Jason didn't know.

As Jason tells Mark about his life, Mark begins to feel inwardly nervous. Mark really likes Jason, and because Mark also loves to surf, he feels he can easily relate to Jason. Also, at one time Mark's mother had a drinking problem, though she's been sober for quite a while. Mark feels that if Jason's mother gets help, she can stop drinking. Mark feels very guilty about reporting the incidents with Jason's mother to child protective services. After all, the emergency room doctor never reported anything. Also, Mark believes that 15-year-old boys can be so obnoxious that their parents can't help but take out their frustrations on them.

Jason invites Mark to his 16th birthday party, which is coming up in a few weeks. Jason says that it will be great. It will be at the beach, with lots of food, drinks, and chicks. It sounds good to Mark because he would probably be at the beach anyway.

Exit Quiz

1. Mark is mandated to
   a. report Jason's suicidal feelings to the police
   b. report Jason's use of pot to the police
   c. report Jason's intention to hurt the intruding surfer to the police
   d. all of the above

2. If Jason's mother agrees to undergo personal counseling for her drinking
   a. Mark must still report the acts of physical violence against Jason to child protective services
   b. Mark may hold off reporting the acts of physical violence against Jason as long as his mother shows improvement and stops drinking
   c. Mark may breach confidentiality and tell the other parents in the group about what Jason's mother did
   d. none of the above

3. If Mark goes to Jason's sixteenth birthday party, he is
   a. helping the trust-building phase of a counseling relationship
   b. engaging in a dual relationship
   c. engaging in acceptable, ethical behavior
   d. all of the above

4. Mark's feelings of guilt about reporting Jason's mother to child protective services may be an indication of
   a. countertransference
   b. his own feelings toward his own mother
   c. Mark's lack of self-awareness
   d. all of the above

5. Because Jason told Mark that he sometimes wants to kill himself
   a. Mark must guard this secret
   b. Mark may talk to Jason's parents about this
   c. Mark must not tell his supervisor about this
   d. none of the above

6. Mark is not familiar with self-mutilation. To engage in good ethical practice, Mark should
   a. read books about the problem
   b. talk to his supervisor about it
   c. attend a conference on the subject
   d. all of the above

7. If Mark were to tell Jason's parents that they should get divorced, he might be
   a. exposing his values
   b. imposing his values
   c. exploring Jason's values
   d. all of the above

8. The fact that Jason felt close enough to Mark on his first visit to invite him to a birthday party might indicate that Jason experienced
   a. delusions of love
   b. clarification of his values
   c. transference toward Mark
   d. none of the above

Exit Quiz Answers

1. c	4. d	7. b
2. a	5. b	8. c
3. b	6. d	

CHAPTER 12

Organizational Structures of Human Services Agencies and Macro-Level Practice

Human Services Agencies

Previous chapters focused on human services workers and people who use human services. This chapter, however, takes a close look at public and nonprofit agencies, which makeup the largest number of human services agencies. Organizational structure and leadership styles are explored as well as other aspects of agency and organizational structure. The advantages and disadvantages of working and receiving services from each type of agency are also discussed.

Additionally, the process of macro-level intervention is examined, including the process of creating new social programs and policy as well as a macro-level community intervention program.

Introduction

While many of the characteristics of human services agencies can be seen in other types of agencies, the focus here is on agencies whose primary function is to meet the emotional, social, family, educational, psychological, and basic welfare needs of individuals, families, and groups. The terms **organization** and **agency** are often used interchangeably but may be used to indicate distinct entities as well.

An organization can be thought of as a purposeful social unit constructed to achieve certain goals or to perform tasks. Organizations are generally "composed of many different individuals who perform specified roles in an effort to provide needed services to certain populations in the community" (Alle-Corliss & Alle-Corliss, 1999, p. 213). Some organizations work directly with people while others are involved with clients indirectly and perform advocacy and **lobbying** functions.

An agency can be defined as an organization that exists to achieve various goals and usually provides services directly or indirectly to the community. The functioning of an **agency** is usually organized through the establishment of positions that work together to provide services. Most people think of an agency as an actual physical establishment where services are provided and consumers visit.

While this same definition is also true for an organization, some organizations don't necessarily provide direct services but are focused instead on fundraising efforts and policy discussions.

Some examples of common agencies would be community centers, counseling clinics, adoption agencies, community service programs, diversion programs, halfway houses, and group homes. Organizations that are not necessarily considered agencies might include the National Organization for Women (N.O.W.), the American Red Cross, and the United Way. While all of the organizations focus on serving people in need, these larger organizations usually farm out the direct services to smaller agencies that are physically located in various communities. The organization may have a national headquarters where decisions and policies are made.

Throughout this chapter, agency and organization may be used synonymously because the distinction between the two terms is small, and in reality, most people use the two terms interchangeably.

General Characteristics of Human Services Agencies

Before beginning a career in the human services, it is wise to understand the general structure of these types of agencies. The characteristics discussed in this section are not necessarily unique to human services agencies, and so this information will be relevant to any type of organization. Human services workers in particular will benefit from knowing about these aspects because they may be a source of work stress some time in the future. Understanding typical issues involved in working at human services agencies allows for more objective reactions when these factors cause problems and conflicts. The structural characteristics presented in this section include agency norms, the **shadow organization**, leadership styles, and **number numbness**.

NORMS

As with any group of people, agencies operate within the scope of both written and unwritten norms. Norms are the rules and guidelines that are understood and followed by members of a group, and a worker can become familiar with an organization by becoming familiar with these norms (Russo, 1980). At times workers may find themselves in conflict with agency norms. Conflicts are not resolved quickly or easily most of the time. When a human services worker's own values are in conflict with an organization's norms, it may be helpful to communicate respectfully and assertively with a supervisor. While this may be scary, it may also be an opportunity to grow. It may also be an opportunity for an organization to modify its norms. An easy-to-understand example has to do with sexual harassment in the workplace. At one time, it was the norm of many agencies to condone or ignore sexual harassment. Eventually, enough workers complained about this behavior to make it illegal at any place of employment. This process took many years but because employees spoke up, change did occur, which was helpful for employees and organizations. In this case, change was a good thing, but as with all change it was risky. Many changes create work for staff members and require that the public be educated about the changes (Russo, 1980). Keeping things the same (status quo) is sometimes preferred because although the status quo may be miserable, the unknown may be worse.

SHADOW ORGANIZATION

In addition to the formal norms of an organization, human services workers should be aware of the informal organizational norms, sometimes referred to as the shadow organization. This is how the agency really operates (Russo, 1980). Although workers should follow the formal guidelines, many times groups of people who work with each other over time develop their own way of doing things. At times, these ways may differ from those written in organizational manuals. Much of the shadow organizational norms are related to social interaction patterns among various staff at the agency. Some agencies do spell out in a manual how to treat others, but often this type of behavior is not written out in formal language and must be learned on-the-job. New employees should take notice of this shadow organization and make decisions about how to interact based on their own values and interpersonal style. For example, a new employee sees the majority of staff gossiping about their boss but feels uncomfortable about this type of behavior. The new employee can decide not to participate in the gossip, rather than report those who are doing it. While it may still feel uncomfortable knowing that others are engaging in the behavior of gossiping, if the new employee were to tell, there could be serious consequences such as getting picked on by others, being given a heavier workload, and even being framed for an illegal activity. **Whistle-blowing** is not always appreciated and should be done when the consequences of the shadow organization are seriously affecting the lives and well-being of others. Another example is the air-traffic controller who recently blew the whistle on fellow workers who were playing chicken with the airplanes (letting the planes almost collide just for the thrill). She reported them and suffered major consequences as a result. But by whistle-blowing, she probably saved the lives of innocent travelers.

LEADERSHIP STYLES

Every agency has administrative positions. These people are in charge of ensuring that the agency runs smoothly and effectively. They must keep track of budgetary concerns, employee performance, and serve as liaison between the agency and the community. Leadership styles vary among administrators. Many have categorized management style into two types: **instrumental** (theory X) and

expressive (theory Y), (Blake & Mouton, 1968; Etzioni, 1965; Guba & Bridwell, 1957; McGregor, 1960; Parsons, Bales, & Shills, 1955). The instrumental leader needs respect from employees, manages hostility among employees with authority, focuses on production, and worries about the budget and how it is distributed. The expressive leader is less able to handle hostility and has a need to maintain close relationships with employees, and shows great concern for people (Etzioni, 1965).

NUMBER NUMBNESS

Regardless of management's leadership style, most agency administrators spend a great deal of time discussing budgets with either board members (if it is a nonprofit agency) or with upper management (if it is a public agency). These human services workers don't deal directly with clients but focus on managing the numbers that keep an agency operating. These numbers include daily averages, daily attendance at programs, rates of pledge payments, credit hours, and of course any donations or payments. They also focus on operating costs, wages, and many others numbers. Maxwell (1973) has labeled this phenomenon number numbness. Human services workers who are motivated by human growth and development and human contact often find these activities boring and stressful. However, an agency can only function at its total capacity after all of the numbers are examined and managed. Of course, program efficiency and client services are important to management, but at times these matters take a backseat to funding activities and operating costs. The bottom line is that an agency cannot provide any human services to clients without an organized financial system. Every agency is accountable to funding sources, and numbers crunching is a large aspect of being accountable.

Human services workers who deal directly with clients (often referred to as **line staff**) must understand their individual role in keeping this financial system operating efficiently. This means that line staff may have to maintain accurate records of their own productivity rates, time spent in various activities, and other data relevant to the operation of the agency. This data can then be used by the data managers to conduct analyses. These analyses are then turned over to management and board members for **evaluation** and recommendations. **Line staff** workers often experience this number numbness as demoralizing because they usually enter the field of human services to provide service and care to clients, not to conduct data analyses. Line staff should guard against developing number numbness themselves. Social workers, counselors, advocates, and other human services workers must leave the numbers crunching to management for the most part, and keep their focus on the clients, while at the same time maintain vital data for those coworkers who must focus on numbers.

Types of Human Services Agencies

The specific structure and operations of both publicly funded and nonprofit agencies, including mental health, social welfare, correctional and educational agencies will be presented.

PUBLIC AGENCIES

Public agencies receive government funding from municipal, state, and federal taxes. The benefit of working in a public setting is its stability, good wages, and benefits, such as health insurance, sick pay, and vacation pay. Some of the disadvantages of working for public agencies might be their focus on accountability, red tape (paperwork), and routine work hours. Sometimes the focus can be shifted away from client needs and put on policy, procedures, and numbers.

Most government-run human services agencies operate under a classic bureaucratic model. Because most federal, state, county, and city agencies employee hundreds and thousands of workers, there is a need for a highly structured approach in organizing these agencies. The classical bureaucratic approach, which can be traced back to the Industrial Revolution during the mid-1800s (Brueggemann, 1996), introduced the idea that when large amount of individuals work together in an orderly fashion, they can accomplish more than the same number of individuals working independently (Netting, Kettner, & McMurtry, 1993). This model allows for efficiency and achievement of organizational goals. This structured approach emphasizes task specialization and matching individual workers to appropriate positions. Management must ensure that workers understand their roles and must maintain worker morale for the good of the organization.

Some people view bureaucracies negatively because of their inflexible rules, mandatory paperwork, accountability, hierarchy, and reluctance to modify programs. Each human services worker must decide if the benefits outweigh some of the annoying aspects of a public agency before beginning a career at one.

Most public agencies operate under a well-organized hierarchy. A **hierarchy** is a way to organize workers by power and authority. Most public agencies develop elaborate and efficient flow charts that visually illustrate the **chain of command**. Typically, more workers are at the bottom of a hierarchy than at the top. The workers at the bottom are generally line staff workers that deal directly with clients and support staff such as administrative assistants. These workers are supervised by the first level of management, who are accountable to middle management, accountable to upper management. Upper management is accountable to funding sources and other government officials (the mayor, the governor, the county board of supervisors). The higher up on the chain of command one is, the more responsibility one has for the operation of the agency.

True Stories From Human Service Workers

Bureaucracy In A Public Mental Health Agency

County facilities have a reputation for being mired in red tape—that is, they require a lot of paperwork. The following example illustrates the type of paperwork a mental health worker might encounter while working for county-operated mental health services.

Example: The author worked for four years at the County of Orange Mental Health Services in southern California, where she first experienced red tape. "I was hired as a mental health worker II while I was working on a master's degree in counseling. While much of my time was spent providing individual counseling (about 50 percent), a good portion of my time was spent in meetings, reviewing cases, and filling out forms. As a mental health worker, I had to complete a psychosocial assessment, a mental-status exam, a multiaxial diagnosis form, a treatment plan, and a progress report for each client I treated. The information on each form had to be linked in content to information on the other forms. This paperwork was burdensome and took several years to learn how to complete effi-

ciently. The worst part for me was that my immediate supervisor's job was to check all of the paperwork to ensure it was completed accurately, and if there were any mistakes, if anything was missing, or if I forgot to sign my name, I would find the chart in my box ordering me to fix my errors. This is an example of red tape. However, I do see the point to it all. The agency was funded primarily by a state program called Medi-Cal, which required paperwork to be completed uniformly so that counselors would be accountable for their services. Once this accountability was satisfactorily provided, the agency would continue to receive funding. Without this funding, clients could not continue to be served."

This example illustrates the link between a line staff worker, management, paperwork, accountability, and funding so typical of bureaucratic organizations. While the author's focus was always on client service, she also realized that completing the paperwork was vital to being able to continue to provide services to clients.

Most organizations frown on jumping chain of command. The preferred mode of communication is from one level of the hierarchy to the next. For example, if a line staff worker complains to upper management without first talking to his or her immediate supervisor, upper management might question why the supervisor wasn't contacted first and may even tell the line staff worker that he or she must talk to the supervisor before upper management will listen to the complaint. Breaking chain of command is often considered a slap in the face to those at the level that was skipped. Most policy documents inform workers of the proper way to communicate in the chain of command.

Public Social Welfare Agencies The Equal Opportunity Act of 1964 provided federal funding for all states to provide financial assistance and basic welfare to those in need. Of course the nature of these welfare programs have changed over the past 40 years, but the states are still responsible for providing medical attention, food, shelter, child care, and utilities to needy children, disabled adults, and the elderly.

Public social welfare agencies also provide child protective services and disabled-adult and elderly protective services. These agencies ensure that these vulnerable populations are safe from physical, sexual, emotional, and financial abuse and from neglect. Thousands of workers are employed in these agencies, and they are typical of bureaucratic organizations.

Public Mental Health Agencies Community mental health centers were first established following the Community Mental Health Act of 1963 and were primarily funded through the Federal Short-Doyle Act. They were created to provide services for people with severe mental disorders such as schizophrenia and for people who were at risk of committing suicide. Each state was required to set up centers where clients could receive medications and crisis management. Many of the larger states funneled the money to the county systems, and "county mental health" facilities became the staple of mental health services for many years. Currently, the name of these centers has changed in many areas to "County Behavioral Health Services." Because in the past mental health facilities had been used by clients who weren't severely impaired, administrators have instituted stricter guidelines for who may receive services. Typically, only those who demonstrate impairment in behavioral functioning are allowed to receive public mental health services, hence the name change to behavioral health. Mental health may have been a bit too general and could have included many types of emotional problems that just weren't severe enough to warrant Short-Doyle funding. Because of these changes, many nonprofit agencies have been created to treat the higher functioning clients who previously used county mental health services.

Public Correctional Agencies Correctional facilities exist at the city, county, state and federal levels. These programs are usually part of a jail or prison system. Because these correctional facilities are often overcrowded, most communities have organized a Department of Probation, funded by state and county government agencies. The Department of Probation allows people convicted of crimes to live in the community while being monitored by probation officers. This system employs thousands of probation and deputy probation officers, juvenile hall counselors, and other human services workers.

Public Educational Agencies All communities fund public schools for children in grades kindergarten through 12. Most communities also fund community college programs and even state-funded universities. Within these schools, special programs exist beyond classroom teaching. The educational system is a clear example of publicly funded human services that operate under a bureaucratic organizational structure.

NONPROFIT AGENCIES

Some nonprofit agencies deal with clients who receive direct services from the agency itself. Other agencies provide an arena for fundraising and community outreach and education. They tend to be more flexible in hiring community college and bachelor level human services workers. The advantage for the worker is a more informal atmosphere where program development and client needs are emphasized and there is autonomy and flexibility in work hours. Workers at nonprofit agencies also have the opportunity to give back to the community, increased job satisfaction for helping people, opportunity for increased responsibilities and training in a new field, opportunity to use professionals skills to make a difference, work with caring and motivated people, and gain rewards beyond a paycheck (McAdam, 1986). The disadvantage is often instability in funding and lower salaries. The focus of these agencies is to provide high quality service to people to meet their needs.

According to Weinstein (1994), more than 983,000 nonprofit organizations operate in the United States. In the 1990s, the average annual salary for people who work in these agencies was about $17,500 compared to $24,000 in the for-profit sector. Nonprofit agencies depend on volunteers but the number of paid employees has increased from 8.8 million in 1977 to 14.4 million from in the 1990s. An estimated 98 million Americans volunteer at nonprofit agencies and the estimated value of this volunteer time is over $170 billion. Weinstein found that nonprofit employers with the largest number of employees were in the following disciplines: health services, educational/research services, religious organizations, social and legal services, civic, social and fraternal organizations, arts and culture, and foundations. Human services are obviously well represented in the nonprofit sector.

Although nonprofits may have some characteristics of the bureaucratic structure found in public agencies, nonprofits tend to follow the **human relations model** of organizational structure. This model can be traced back to the 1929 stock-market crash that preceded the Great Depression. The federal government responded to this economic disaster by implementing New Deal agencies that were established to restore hope in the government as well as assist people in finding employment. These new agencies were structured differently from the organizational bureaucracies that were receiving so much criticism at the time. The New Deal agencies, instead, focused on employee rights and social concerns. The workplace was considered a secondary social system, and concern about employees' needs, interests, and issues had a powerful effect on workplace efficiency and output (Brueggemann, 1996). Organizations with large numbers of workers, such as public and government agencies, found that merging a more structured approach with a focus on employee well-being worked the best. Without structure, chaos might ensue. Although the bureaucratic model wouldn't suggest that worker needs should be ignored, meeting every worker's needs all the time simply isn't practical. Large numbers of employees necessitate some rigidity in policy.

The human relations model became the foundation for many nonprofit agencies. It was a nice fit with the growing sense of humanism and civil rights that was seen in the 1960s and 1970s. Nonprofit agencies became an alternative method of providing service to people who were often resistant to governmental policy and philosophies. This anti-establishment era was ripe for services provided within a human relations organizational structure. Not only were employees more happy under this structure, but many clients were as well. Under this type of management, nonprofit agencies operated in more casual ways than public agencies. The focus was more on client needs and program development rather than on numbers and accountability. This was possible because many of the nonprofit agencies from the 1960s through the 1980s got much of their funding from private donations and fundraising events, and were staffed primarily by volunteers who provided much of the professional services.

During the 1990s and 2000s, nonprofit funding began relying more heavily on special **grants** and funding available through government programs. As a result, these previously autonomous agencies had to become accountable to their government funding sources. The increased availability of funding gave agencies an opportunity to hire paid staff, which may have also increased the need for more structure and policy. Despite the growing complexity of these agencies' infrastructures, they were able to maintain their human relations orientation.

The foundation of most nonprofit agencies is the **board of directors,** which is typically made up of people from the community who have an interest in the agency's purpose and goals. They may be professionals such as lawyers, judges, doctors, teachers, or just average citizens who may have volunteered for similar agencies in the past or have used similar agencies in their own lives. This board usually meets about once a month and receives no pay for their services. Their job is to collaborate with the executive director to oversee all the services provided by the agency. They communicate directly with the executive director of the agency and may speak on behalf of the agency at fundraising events. They may advise the executive director of the agency about how to seek funding, how to evaluate the agency programs, and when an employee may need to be terminated. They play a large role in the hiring and firing of the agency executive director.

Executive directors usually work directly with agency boards as well as its employees. Directors often have advanced degrees and oversee all services at an agency. They also work directly with the agency's various program coordinators at the agency, an assistant director, and spend a great deal of time on fundraising activities and grant writing. They represent their agencies at fundraisers and often participate in public meetings and social activities that might benefit the agency.

True Stories From Human Service Workers

Working at a Nonprofit Agency

Working at nonprofit agencies has its advantages and disadvantages. The climate is probably best for people who enjoy autonomy at work and can cope with occasional uncertainties and minimal pay.

Example 1: Jan Tyler, program director at Heritage House, a drug and alcohol rehab program in Costa Mesa, CA, says, "I manage the agency by consensus as much as possible. Some of the benefits in working at the agency is seeing lives change and improve dramatically and having a part in it. Some disadvantages in working for this nonprofit agency is that finding and hiring qualified personnel is very difficult. Also, low pay, burnout, and intense emotional involvement of the staff with each other and with clients are disadvantages."

Example 2: According to Brenda Titus, of Sexual Assault Victim Services, "A major advantage in working for a nonprofit agency is that the type of work performed by each individual is necessary and results in observable positive outcomes. A major disadvantage is that funding for the agency is often unreliable."

Nonprofit agencies focus on service to clients and a truly caring environment is evident. Along with these positive aspects, unfortunately is the reality that funding is precarious.

Directors are often in charge of hiring, training, monitoring, and terminating staff and also monitor client activities and ensure regulations are followed.

Most nonprofit agencies also employ an assistant to the director and program coordinators. These employees meet with the director and together, the day-to-day operation of the agency is organized and planned or modified. This includes the management of volunteers, budget, fundraising activities, and direct services.

Some agencies are fortunate to have enough in their budget to employ line staff workers who provide direct services to the clients. Other agencies depend on volunteers to provide all direct services. Most agencies have paid employees, as well as volunteers and interns. Nonprofit agencies simply could not operate without volunteers. They truly are the foundation of the nonprofit agency.

Some nonprofit agencies have grown in size (i.e., the American Red Cross and the United Way) and must operate under a more classical bureaucratic structure to efficiently organize the thousands of people working at the agency. Other nonprofit agencies are relatively small in terms of numbers of workers and can efficiently operate with more flexibility, and workers often experience a sense of autonomy and personal support in these smaller agencies.

Nonprofit Social Welfare Agencies Some communities have created nonprofit agencies that provide services for homeless people and others who may need food, child care, and clothing. These services may be provided through homeless shelters, church programs, or other agencies such as day care centers. The focus is providing for basic needs until people can get back on their own feet and provide for themselves. These agencies have become vital in recent decades as governmental funding for financial assistance has been reduced.

Other nonprofit agencies have been developed to assist the child protective welfare system. Various group homes have been created that work collaboratively with county social workers to provide housing for abused children. Also, various nonprofit agencies have been created to provide parenting education for abusive parents who may have lost their children to county child protective services.

Nonprofit Mental Health Agencies Many U.S. agencies provide mental health counseling for a low fee to its clients. They can offer lower fee services because the programs are funded by grants, donations, and fundraisers. These agencies use more paraprofessionals, volunteers, and interns than public agencies. They are the ideal setting for interns to learn and gain experience and for people to receive the help they need at a low cost.

Nonprofit Agencies that Deal with Correctional Issues Some facilities contract with governmental agencies to provide monitoring, education, and counseling for people who have violated the law. Some are residential, such as halfway houses (places where convicts may live for up to one year after release from prison), while others are diversion programs at community centers for first-time offenders, such as a teenager caught with drugs. Other facilities offer drug testing and adjunct services, such as counseling, drug education, or anger management groups, for those on probation. These nonprofit programs usually work closely with government officials to ensure proper services are provided and used by the client, who is often mandated by a judge to use the services.

Nonprofit Educational Programs There may be some agencies that provide tutoring services for children and adults. One example might be a local library that provides remedial reading courses for adults. These services are usually provided by volunteers. There may not be many opportunities for paid employment in tutoring programs. However, one may tutor privately at any level for pay.

CRITICAL THINKING / SELF-REFLECTION CORNER

- What motivates you in a job? Pay? Autonomy? Helping others? Power?

- Would you see yourself fitting in better at a nonprofit agency or a public agency? Why?

- Can you see yourself serving in an administrative position? In what way? If not, why not?

Macro-Level Practice

Introduction

Macro-level practice focuses on working with organizations, such as nonprofit agencies and public agencies, and communities. It may entail examining major social issues, examining current social policies, and current organizational programs. According to Brueggemann (1966), macro-level practitioners "try to correct social conditions that cause human suffering and misery. . . . They work to develop new programs and changes in policies" (p. 3). Kirst-Ashman & Hull (1993) describe macro-level practice as a process that focuses on changing or improving policies or procedures that regulate distribution of resources to clients, developing new resources when clients' needs cannot be met with available ones, and helping clients obtain their due rights.

Brueggeman (1996, pp. 4–5) classifies macro-level practice as involving organizational, community, and societal/policy-related activities. Some of the tasks at the organizational level include supervising professional staff, working with communities, participating in budgeting, writing **proposals** and grants, and developing programs.

Community activities include negotiating and bargaining with diverse groups, encouraging consumer participation in decision making, establishing and carrying out interagency agreements, and advocating for client needs.

Societal policy-related activities include **coalition** building, lobbying, testifying, tracking legislative developments that directly affect clients, and carrying out efforts designed to affect legal and regulatory frameworks.

All of these activities are the foundation for the creation and development of new social programs, modification of existing programs, and elimination of obsolete or ineffective programs. In the field of human services, there is a never ending need to meet the changing needs of client populations. For example, in 1975, there was no need to create agencies that serviced clients suffering from AIDS-related problems because HIV/AIDS had not yet become a social problem. However, by the mid-1990s, many programs and legislation had been created to deal with this issue.

The following sections describe two macro-level interventions: creating new programs and policies and providing direct macro-level community intervention through community disaster trauma response.

Creating New Programs

For the macro-level practitioner, the community is the client just as an individual is a client to the micro-level practitioner. A community has its own resources and limitations and coping mechanisms to deal with problems, and it must take responsibility for its actions just as an individual or family does (Homan, 1994). Macro-level practitioners engage in the process of examining these aspects of the community to assess its needs just as the micro level practitioner examines an individual or family regarding these aspects when assessing their needs. The first step then, in macro-level practice is community/organizational **needs assessment.** This assessment is then followed by several other activities and decisions.

FIVE STEPS INVOLVED IN CREATING NEW PROGRAMS

New programs or agencies are often created by macro-level human services workers. Likewise, the impetus for legislative social changes often comes from macro-level practitioners. Following are the steps generally taken when new programs and policies are being developed.

Conducting a Needs Assessment As with any research project, a community needs assessment begins with a problem statement. Interested macro-level practitioners who have observed a need or problem in a community may decide that change is necessary to improve the problem. Much of the focus of any needs assessment is based on the values of the macro-level workers and what they think is important for the target population of interest. Once they choose the problem for a target population, the macro-level practitioner conducts surveys, collects statistics from prior research and data analysis, and researches the background and history of the problem. This data is compiled and used in gaining support from community leaders, community professionals, and the target population for their project.

Gaining Community Support As mentioned previously, nonprofit agencies operate under the direction of a Board, primarily made up of community leaders and professionals. If the project is going to be a nonprofit agency, the macro-level practitioners must gain the commitment of people like this for their project. The data collected in the needs assessment is presented to these potential board members and then a proposal is developed. If the project is going to be legislative change, coalition building is necessary. A coalition may be described as a "loosely developed association of constituent groups and organizations, each of whose primary identification is outside the coalition" (Netting et al., 1993, p. 113). Coalitions are vital when there is a need for action and cooperation. The coalition is able to present a strong voice in the pursuit of funding and legislative change. An example of a coalition to help pass an **initiative** for increased funding for schools might be made up of a national teacher's association, the national PTA association, and the police association. One often sees these groups listed on literature about an upcoming initiative. With the support of the community, the project can move on to the next step.

Deciding Whether to Focus on a New Policy or a New Program Based on the research conducted and the feedback of the community, the macro-level workers decide whether their project will part of an existing program, be a modification of an existing program, be a new agency, or whether it will be a new legislative policy. It must also be decided whether the project will be funded at the city, county, state, or federal level, or whether it will be a nonprofit agency.

Engaging in Political Action or Fundraising Activities If the project is focused on the creation of legislative changes, lobbying is necessary. Lobbying is a specialized form of persuasion that is central to most levels of government. Lobbyists seek access to lawmakers to influence policy making and decision making (Alle-Corliss & Alle-Corliss, 1999). For some social policy change, lawmakers assume full responsibility in enacting legislative change. Other social policy changes are put in the hands of voters. Certain social policy changes may be enacted if enough voters sign a petition to have the policy placed on an official ballot where voters have an opportunity to decide whether the policy should be passed. Election time is usually preceded by a media blitz in which backers (coalitions) of the initiative try to persuade voters to pass the proposal.

If the project is the creation of a new nonprofit agency or a new program at an existing agency, acquiring funding for the new program is the next process. This usually entails writing proposals to receive grants from various organizations who offer money for such programs. These grant funding organizations may be government operated, private organizations, or nonprofit agencies such as the United Way. The program proposal must describe the nature of the program, the target population, the social problem to be addressed by the agency, budget, and staffing plans, fundraising plans, and how the program will be implemented and evaluated.

Implementing and Evaluating the Policy or Program Once the agency is open and operating for about one year, program evaluators usually collect data about the numbers served at the agency, conduct surveys about the effectiveness of the agency, and discuss agency operations with the board of directors. This evaluation is performed by outside contractors who specialize in program evaluation and indicates that an agency is successfully performing the function for which it was designed. The evaluation is also useful in providing feedback to the agency director and the board of directors regarding any modifications that should be made at the agency. Sometimes, the evaluation indicates that the agency was ineffective and should not receive further funding.

Implementation of a change in social policy through the legislative and initiative process may take many years to occur. One hopes that there would be immediate results and that does happen such as when taxes on tobacco purchases were increased in California and the money was given to public schools.

Other legislation might not be implemented as quickly because some groups may appeal it in court as unconstitutional or otherwise inappropriate such as when Californians voted to disallow illegal immigrants access to public services. Although voters passed the initiative, in the 1990s, it still has not been enforced by public agencies as it should be according to the policy set forth on the initiative.

Figure 12.1 describes the qualifications and guidelines needed to apply for a **grant** from the Office on Violence Against Women. Groups and agencies meeting the qualifications must write a grant proposal to apply for funding that would start or maintain a community program.

As evidenced in Figure 12.1, grant writing is detailed and technical. Therefore, any agency lucky enough to employ a competent grant writer would be willing to pay that person fairly well. They are the ones who bring funding to an agency after all. Grant writing and program evaluation are viable human services occupations, and many people work as independent contractors writing grants for various agencies that are in search of funding.

Another technical skill related to grant writing is conducting program evaluations. Most funding sources require that the programs they fund be evaluated within a year of funding to sustain funding in the future. To complete a thorough evaluation, programs need to maintain detailed data bases and records of their services. Evaluators then report on the success of the services, the benefits the program provides to the community, as well as the program's deficiencies. As with grant writing, outside, independent contractors often conduct program evaluations. For people who enjoy research, writing, and compiling data, this is an excellent occupation. The pay is great, the hours are flexible, and the work is meaningful.

Providing Direct Macro-level Intervention

At some point, grants receive funding and programs are implemented. While it may be true that most programs are implemented at agencies and services provided are given to individuals and families at micro and mezzo levels, some programs are definitely macro in scope because they focus on an entire community surviving a trauma. Probably the most familiar type of macro-level intervention that deals with an entire community has been sponsored and organized by the **American Red Cross.** Because of the many community disasters of the past decade, these macro-level interventions have become universally recognized and many people have volunteered their time and donated their money to these programs.

RESPONSE TO TRAUMATIC COMMUNITY DISASTERS

During the past decade, the United States has been hit with a variety of natural and **man-made disasters.** The most recent example of a **natural disaster** was Hurricane Katrina in 2005, which devastated most of New Orleans as well as

INTRODUCTION

The Grants to Encourage Arrest Policies and Enforcement of Protection Orders Program (Arrest Program) encourages jurisdictions to treat domestic violence as a serious violation of criminal law. The Arrest Program also promotes mandatory or pro-arrest policies as an effective domestic violence intervention that is part of a coordinated community response. Arrest should be one element in a comprehensive criminal justice system response to hold offenders accountable and enhance victim safety.

Arrest, accompanied by a thorough investigation and meaningful sanctions, demonstrates to offenders that they have committed a serious crime and communicates to victims of domestic violence that they do not have to endure an offender's abuse. Arrest should be followed by immediate arraignment and a thorough investigation. Orders of protection should be enforced, and cases should be vigorously prosecuted. Designated dockets can enhance the management of domestic violence cases and expedite the scheduling of trials. Frequent judicial oversight and the use of graduated sanctions can help courts monitor the behavior of domestic violence offenders. Probation and parole agencies should closely monitor offenders and strictly enforce the terms and conditions of probation or parole.

At each juncture in the criminal justice process, actions should be guided by concerns for victim safety. Mechanisms should be put in place to allow the voices and experiences of victims of domestic violence, particularly those who have sought assistance from the criminal justice system, to inform the development of policies. These mechanisms should ensure that the diverse experiences of victims are considered—particularly the experiences of women of color, immigrant victims, the elderly, victims with disabilities, and victims from other traditionally underserved segments of the community.

Criminal justice agencies must collaborate among themselves and in respectful partnership with victim advocates from nonprofit, nongovernmental victim service agencies, including local shelters, victim advocacy organizations, and domestic violence coalitions, to ensure that victim safety is a paramount consideration in the development of any strategy to address domestic violence. Nonprofit, nongovernmental agencies may include faith-based or community-based organizations.

The Arrest Program challenges victim advocates, police officers, pretrial services personnel, prosecutors, judges and other court personnel, probation and parole officers, and community leaders to work together to craft solutions to respond to domestic violence.

SCOPE OF PROGRAM

Ensuring victim safety and offender accountability are the guiding principles underlying the Arrest Program. The scope of this program includes the statutory program purposes and the special interest categories outlined below. Proposed projects need not address multiple program purposes or special interest categories to receive support.

(continued)

Figure 12.1 Program Brief for Grants to Encourage Arrest Policies and Enforcement of Protection Orders Program from the Office on Violence Against Women

PROGRAM PURPOSE AREAS

The Violence Against Women Act of 2000 directs that Program funds be used to:

Implement mandatory arrest or pro-arrest programs and policies in police departments, including mandatory or pro-arrest programs and policies for protection order violations.

Develop policies, educational programs, and training in police departments to improve tracking of cases involving domestic violence and dating violence.

Centralize and coordinate police enforcement, prosecution, or judicial responsibility for domestic violence cases in groups or units of police officers, prosecutors, probation and parole officers, or judges.

Coordinate computer tracking systems to ensure communication between police, prosecutors, parole and probation officers, and both criminal and family courts.

Strengthen legal advocacy service programs for victims of domestic violence and dating violence, including strengthening assistance to such victims in immigration matters.

Educate judges in criminal and other courts about domestic violence and improve judicial handling of such cases.

Provide technical assistance and computer and other equipment to police departments, prosecutors, courts, and tribal jurisdictions to facilitate the widespread enforcement of protection orders, including interstate enforcement, enforcement between States and tribal jurisdictions, and enforcement between tribal jurisdictions.

Develop or strengthen policies and training for police, prosecutors, and the judiciary in recognizing, investigating, and prosecuting instances of domestic violence and sexual assault against older individuals (as defined in section 102 of the Older American Act of 1965) and individuals with disabilities (as defined in section 3(2) of the Americans with Disabilities Act of 1990).

PROGRAM PRIORITY AREAS

By statute, 42 U.S.C. Section § 3796(hh-1)(b) priority will be given to applicants that:

Illustrate that the jurisdiction does not currently provide for centralized handling of cases involving domestic violence by police, prosecutors, and courts;

Demonstrate a commitment to strong enforcement of laws, and prosecution of cases involving domestic violence, including the enforcement of protection orders from other States and jurisdictions (including tribal jurisdictions);

(continued)

Figure 12.1 *Continued*

Have established cooperative agreements or can demonstrate effective ongoing collaborative arrangements with neighboring jurisdictions to facilitate the enforcement of protection orders from other States and jurisdictions; and

Intend to utilize grant funds to develop and install data collection and communication systems, including computerized systems, and training on how to use these systems effectively to link police, prosecutors, courts, and tribal jurisdictions for the purpose of identifying and tracking protection orders and violations of protection orders in those jurisdictions where such systems do not exist or are not fully effective.

SPECIAL INTEREST CATEGORIES

The Office on Violence Against Women (OVW) is interested in funding States, Indian tribal governments, State and local courts, or units of local government that have implemented—or plan to implement—promising approaches that respond to domestic violence as a serious violation of criminal law. Although applications that address any of the statutory program purposes outlined above are eligible for funding, OVW is especially interested in supporting projects that address the following special interest categories. All applicants are required to collaborate with nonprofit, nongovernmental victim service agencies.

The following list does not imply any order of priority.

Involve faith-based and/or community-driven initiatives to address violence against women among diverse and traditionally underserved populations.

Include dedicated parole and probation officers within existing or newly created domestic violence units to actively participate in holding perpetrators accountable.

Develop innovative programs to improve judicial handling of domestic violence cases. For example, specialized courts or dockets for domestic violence cases, enhanced judicial monitoring of domestic violence offenders, or the creation or enhancement of technology to provide prosecutors and judges access to case information on prior arrests.

Develop and implement coordinated initiatives to address incidents of sexual assault and/or stalking occurring in the context of domestic violence.

Address system accountability by conducting a safety audit of the jurisdiction's criminal justice system.

PROGRAM ELIGIBILITY

Eligible grantees for this program are States, Indian tribal governments, State and local courts, and units of local government. For purposes of this program, a unit of local government is any

(continued)

Figure 12.1 *Continued*

city, county, township, town, borough, parish, village, or other general-purpose political subdivision of a State; an Indian tribe that performs law enforcement functions as determined by the Secretary of Interior; or, for the purpose of assistance eligibility, any agency of the District of Columbia government or the U.S. Government performing law enforcement functions in and for the District of Columbia and the Trust Territory of the Pacific Islands. Police departments, pretrial service agencies, district or city attorneys' offices, sheriffs' departments, probation and parole departments, shelters, nonprofit, nongovernmental victim service agencies, and universities are not units of local government for the purposes of this grant program. These agencies or organizations may assume responsibility for the development and implementation of the project, but they must apply through a State, State or local court, Indian tribal government, or unit of local government.

By statute, to be eligible to receive funding through this program, applicants must:

Certify that their laws or official policies encourage or mandate arrests of domestic violence offenders based on probable cause that an offense has been committed and encourage or mandate arrest of domestic violence offenders who violate the terms of a valid and outstanding protection order.

Demonstrate that their laws, policies, or practices and their training programs discourage dual arrests of offender and victim.

Certify that their laws, policies, or practices prohibit issuance of mutual restraining orders of protection except in cases where both spouses file a claim and the court makes detailed findings of fact indicating that both spouses acted primarily as aggressors and that neither spouse acted primarily in self-defense.

Certify that their laws, policies, and practices do not require, in connection with the prosecution of any misdemeanor or felony domestic violence offense, or in connection with the filing, issuance, registration, or service of a protection order, or a petition for a protection order, to protect a victim of domestic violence, stalking, or sexual assault, that the victim bear the costs associated with the filing of criminal charges against the offender, or the costs associated with the filing, issuance, registration, or service of a warrant, protection order, petition for a protection order, or witness subpoena, whether issued inside or outside the State, tribal, or local jurisdiction.

"Grants to Encourage Arrest Policies and Enforcement of Protection Orders Program," from the Office on Violence Against Women, within the U.S. Department of Justice, found at www.usdoj.gov/ovw.

Figure 12.1 *Continued*

many regions of Mississippi and Alabama. The victims of disasters such as these received services designed to help them get back on their feet. Other natural disasters, such as earthquakes, fires, and tornados, have devastating economic and emotional effects on millions of people.

Most readers will remember the terrorist attacks on the World Trade Center on September 11, 2001, referred to as 9-11. This **man-made disaster** affected millions of people worldwide and began a war on terrorism. The bombing of the Oklahoma City federal building in 1995 and the 1942 Coconut Grove nightclub fire in Boston are examples of other man-made disasters that affected thousands of lives (Kanel, 2007). Many community volunteers and professionals worked together to assist the many people suffering after these disasters.

Macro-level analyses of community response to both natural and man-made disasters of the past decades have shown four phases of community disaster that are the reactions a community has to the psychological and physical consequences of disasters:

- heroic, or impact, phase

- honeymoon, or immediate post-disaster, phase

- disillusionment, or recoil and rescue, phase

- reconstruction, or recovery, phase
  (Mental Health Center of North Iowa website, June 2005; National Center for Posttraumatic Stress Disorder website, June 2005).

Heroic, or Impact, Phase During the heroic/impact phase, the goal is to get the victims to a safe place where basic needs such as food and water can be met. Once food and water arrived, the victims need to be housed in a safe and sanitary environment. The general goal is to save lives and property. Altruism is prominent while people expend much energy in helping others to survive. Everyone pitches in and is motivated to help.

Honeymoon, or Immediate Post-Disaster, Phase The honeymoon, or immediate post-disaster, phase may last from one week to six months. During this time period, there is a sense by the survivors that the community is available to offer support and resources. They have survived the disaster physically, and realize that they are not alone to recover. They feel a profound sense of having shared something very intense with others.

Disillusionment, or Recoil and Rescue, Phase Unfortunately, survivors soon realize that the help and utopia they had envisioned doesn't usually occur. In this disillusionment, or recoil and rescue, phase, survivors start to lose that sense of shared community and must concentrate on resolving their own problems. Often, outside agencies leave the affected area, and community groups may not respond to the ongoing needs of survivors. Some people believe that many Katrina survivors are in this phase as they have yet to completely rebuild their lives, and it seems that the strong community and national support offered during the first six months post disaster have weakened.

Reconstruction and Recovery Phase   In this final stage, survivors assume responsibility for re-building their own lives. The reconstruction and recovery phase may last years, depending on the damage and community support available.

Throughout the years, many human services workers have serviced the victims of these disasters to aid them in overcoming their feelings of powerlessness, grief, and fear. Trauma response models are very similar to crisis intervention in that the trauma workers must actively listen to the victims, provide them with information, connect them with resources, and ensure they remain safe. The majority of workers that assist victims of traumas like these are volunteers working at the micro and mezzo levels of intervention. Of course certain institutions such as the American Red Cross and the United Way provide services related to community disasters at the macro-level in that they employ permanent administrative employees to ensure continuity of service from the multitude of community agencies providing trauma response. Holding fundraisers, coordinating volunteers, and collaborating with many agencies throughout the nation is a full-time job. Workers who perform these jobs often work long hours for average pay, but the intrinsic satisfaction in knowing that meaningful services are being provided to millions seems to motivate people to continue working and volunteering for these agencies. While micro- and mezzo-levels of intervention are vital for individuals and families, macro-level intervention ensures that current needs of communities are provided for through careful research and evaluation of evolving issues and new problems when they arise.

Chapter Summary

Both public and nonprofit human services agencies serve similar functions in the community. They both provide services to similar populations with the aim of preventing and eliminating a variety of social problems, deviant behaviors, and other emotional disorders. While both types of agencies may use the bureaucratic or the human relations approach to management, human services workers will probably see a combination of both types of structure. Traditionally, public agencies have operated within a bureaucratic structure because of the large numbers of employees working for city, county, state, and federal agencies. Bureaucracy may be useful for these agencies to aid in maintaining accountability and preventing chaos.

Nonprofit agencies have traditionally been able to function under the human relations model because of the smaller number of staff usually employed at the agency. Because nonprofits use volunteers to keep the agency operating, they often encourage a more supportive, family-like organization to ensure that volunteers feel welcome and appreciated. Also, because nonprofit agencies tend to pay lower than public agencies, workers may benefit from the human relations model because workers are rewarded by the support and caring attitude of supervisors and increased job challenges.

Funding for public agencies is typically through taxes paid to various levels of government while funding for nonprofit agencies is through grants, fundraisers, and charitable donations. Volunteers make up the largest number of workers at nonprofit agencies while most workers at public agencies are paid employees.

Human services agencies are designed to meet the needs of the community in which it exists. They may be structured in classical bureaucratic style if the numbers of workers is high such as in government operated agencies. Nonprofit agencies usually employee smaller numbers of workers and may be managed under a human relations style of administration. Government operated agencies tend to be more rigid and operate under chain of command. There is much focus on accountability and standardized paperwork. Nonprofit agencies focus on providing support to employees and volunteers and emphasize program effectiveness. Funding for nonprofit agencies is more tenuous than for public agencies.

Macro-level practice focuses on ensuring that the social problems and needs of the community are met by the development of community resources. Macro-level practitioners work to create social changes by changing laws and by developing programs in the community. Macro-level intervention also includes programs such as trauma response to community disasters.

Now that most of the practices and theories related to the field of human services have been presented, the reader is encouraged to review the Appendix. By answering some of the questions, the reader may begin to have an idea about the specific human services career path for which she or he may be best suited. Of course, this path may change throughout one's life, but it may serve as a beginning guide.

Suggested Applied Activities

1. Think of an agency that you would like to create in your community. Outline a proposal using the following questions to guide you: What populations will your agency serve? Why is there a need for this agency? What services currently exist for this population, and why are they not enough to meet the needs of the population? Which community leaders support your program? How will it be staffed? Who will be on your board of directors? Describe the services that will be delivered? How will you evaluate the agency and its effectiveness?

   _____

   _____

   _____

   _____

2. Think of three propositions that you would like to see pass on a ballot. Do you think they would have a chance? How could you lobby for them to pass?

   _____

   _____

   _____

Chapter Review Questions

1. How is a public agency funded usually?

   _____

   _____

2. How are nonprofit agencies funded?

   _____

   _____

3. What are two aspects of a bureaucratic-run agency?

_____

_____

4. What is the difference between theory X and theory Y in terms of organizational practice?

_____

_____

5. What is a board of directors?

_____

_____

6. How might you conduct a needs assessment?

_____

_____

7. What is red tape?

_____

_____

8. What is chain of command?

_____

_____

9. What are the phases of community disasters?

_____

_____

Glossary of Terms

Agency is an organization that works to achieve various goals and usually provides services directly or indirectly to a community.

American Red Cross is an organization established to assist people who have been devastated by disaster.

Board of directors is a group of people who serve as an advisory council for a nonprofit agency.

Chain of command is the hierarchal structure found in bureaucracies in which lower-level employees must communicate only with the person directly above them in the hierarchy.

Coalition is a group of associations and organizations that work together to create social change or develop programs.

Disillusionment, or recoil and rescue, phase is the third stage of response after a disaster during which survivors begin to feel that the focus of attention is turning away from their problems and start to realize that they must take care of themselves.

Evaluation is conducted by a funding source in which an evaluator examines the effectiveness and problems of a program that is receiving the funding.

Expressive leadership style is a management style that focuses on minimizing interpersonal hostility and on fostering close, supportive relationships among employees.

Grants are funding offers from either government agencies or private foundations to agencies that have submitted an application for funding.

Heroic, or impact, phase is the first phase in a series of responses in the aftermath of a disaster when the focus is on helping people survive and get their basic needs met.

Honeymoon, or immediate post-disaster, phase is the second stage in the aftermath of a disaster when people experience intense altruism and survivors feel hopeful that resources will be available.

Human relations model is an approach to management that focuses on the needs of its employees and social forces in the workplace.

Initiative is a balloted proposal for legislative change that citizens vote on during general elections.

Instrumental leadership style is a rigid style of management whose main concern is with production and profit margins and respect for the organization's hierarchical structure.

Line staff are human services workers who deal directly with clients.

Lobbying is a form of political persuasion in which interested parties attempt to influence policymaking.

Macro-level practices are interventions at the community, county, or state level that focus on working with and creating organizational and social policy.

Man-made disasters are devastating events caused by humans, rather than by the forces of nature, that damage and threaten the lives of the people in a community, such as acts of war and terror or plane crashes and train wrecks.

Natural disasters are natural events, such as fire, flood, earthquakes, and hurricanes, that damage and destroy community and personal property and threatens the lives of its residents.

Needs assessments use neighborhood interviews and surveys to determine what a community believes are its problems.

Number numbness occurs when human services workers focus on budget, accountability, policy, and procedures rather than on program development and human needs.

Organization is a purposeful social unit constructed to achieve certain goals or to carry out a task.

Phases of community disaster is the concept that communities experience the aftermath of disasters in specific stages

Proposal is a document in which the details of a new program are described.

Reconstruction, or recovery, phase is the fourth stage following a disaster during which survivors take responsibility for rebuilding their lives.

Shadow organization refers to the informal norms and behaviors found at most agencies that often dictate acceptable ways to interact and communicate with colleagues, staff, and supervisors.

Whistle-blowing occurs when a worker speaks up about questionable practices that may be detrimental to the operation of an organization.

Case Presentation and Exit Quiz

Janice Nash just accepted a position as an elementary-school teacher at a public school. For the past five years, Janice had been working for a government-funded program for low-income preschoolers called Head Start while she was working on her teaching credentials. That had been her only work experience. She started volunteering during high school at the Head Start preschool, and, after two years, she was hired as a teacher/outreach coordinator. She earned some of her internship credit at Head Start when they increased her responsibilities to include training and supervising new volunteers.

Janice will be teaching second grade at her new job. When Janice arrives for orientation, she is overwhelmed. Her classroom is huge compared to the classrooms at Head Start. More than 50 other teachers from the school are at the first staff meeting. The principal is a 58-year old woman with a doctoral degree in education. She is dressed in a pantsuit and speaks in a very formal manner. At Head Start, the head teacher had been a 35-year-old woman with a bachelor's degree in child development, and staff members were all on a first-name basis with each other and interactions were informal. At this new school, the principal addressed teachers more formally, using their last names, and even referred to herself as Dr. Blain.

At the meeting, Janice receives many forms, schedules, attendance rosters, and other paperwork that she must complete daily. Janice is told that by next week, she must turn in daily lesson plans for the next six months. Each lesson plan must meet state standards and use the required texts and contain material that prepares students for the state-mandated testing in April.

Teachers did not mingle or speak with each other or with the principal. Janice had been accustomed to being involved in the planning of the programs at Head Start. When she was supervising volunteers, she'd take time to introduce each new volunteer to the other volunteers and staff members at each meeting. All the other teachers seemed to know what they were doing. They had all been teaching at the school for at least three years. Janice is the only new teacher.

One teacher, Mrs. Baker, introduces herself to Janice after the meeting . They are both teaching second grade. Mrs. Baker had been teaching 14 years and last year was named teacher of the year. She tells Janice that things will all work out, but that it takes time to get used to Dr. Blain. Mrs. Baker informs Janice that principals stay at the school for about five years, so they might have better luck next time. Mrs. Baker tells Janice that as long as she does the required paperwork and has her lesson plans documented appropriately, Dr. Blain will stay off her back. Mrs. Baker told Janice that some of the teachers are sometimes uncooperative and may even try to sabotage the work of a new teacher. Mrs. Baker suggests that Janice lay low and discover who she feels comfortable with before she gets too close to anyone.

After her talk with Mrs. Baker, Janice was approached by Dr. Blain. Dr. Blain explains that when Janice has any questions or problems, she should first go to one of the vice principals for help. If they couldn't help her, then she'll be referred to Dr. Blain directly.

Exit Quiz

1. Dr. Blain operates under which management style?
   a. expressive
   b. theory Y
   c. instrumental
   d. theory Z

2. The head teacher at Head Start operates under which management style?
   a. expressive
   b. theory X
   c. instrumental
   d. theory Z

3. The focus on attendance, policy, and daily reports may lead some teachers to experience
   a. a heightened sense of job enrichment
   b. a feeling of meaning in their lives
   c. number numbness
   d. all of the above

4. Mrs. Baker was telling Janice about:
   a. the shadow organization
   b. how to win teacher of the year
   c. how to make Dr. Blain like her
   d. all of the above

5. If some of the teachers behave in negative ways with Janice, she should
   a. go straight to Dr. Blain
   b. try to get back at them
   c. talk about them to other teachers behind their backs
   d. none of the above

6. Janice should go to the vice principal with problems to
   a. avoid Dr. Blain
   b. adhere to chain of command
   c. learn about the shadow organization
   d. none of the above

7. Head Start most likely follows the
   a. bureaucratic model
   b. theory X model
   c. human relations model
   d. none of the above

Exit Quiz Answers

1. c	4. a	7. c
2. a	5. d	
3. c	6. b	

References

CHAPTER 1   What Are Human Services?

Alle-Corliss, L., & Alle-Corliss, R. (1998). *Human service agencies: An orientation to fieldwork.* Pacific Grove, CA: Brooks/Cole.

Corey, G., & Corey, M. S. (1993). *Becoming a helper* (2nd ed.). Pacific Grove, CA: Brooks/Cole.

DeMuro, P., & Rideout, P. (2002). *Team decision-making: Involving family and community in child welfare decisions.* Baltimore: Annie E. Casey Foundation. Available at: www.aecf.org/initiatives/familytofamily/tools.htm

Kramer, R. M. (1981). *Voluntary agencies in the welfare state.* Berkeley, CA: University of California Press.

Maslow, A. (1968). *Toward a psychology of being* (2nd ed.). New York: Harper & Row.

Neukrug, E. (1994). *Theory, practice and trends in human services.* Pacific Grove, CA: Brooks/Cole.

Rosenthal, H. (2003). *Human services dictionary.* London: Psychology Press.

Zastrow, C. (1995). *The practice of social work* (3rd ed.). Pacific Grove, CA: Brooks/Cole.

CHAPTER 2   A Brief History of Human Services

Addams, J. (1912). *Twenty years at Hull House.* New York: MacMillan.

Clodd, E. (1997). *Animism: The seed of religion.* Whitefish, MT: Kessinger Publishing.

Columbia electronic encyclopedia (6th ed.). (2006). New York: Columbia University Press.

Compayri, G. (2002). *Horace Mann and the public school in the United States* (M. D. Frost, Trans.). Portland, OR: University Press of the Pacific.

Davis, K. G. (1990). *Don't know much about history.* New York: Perennial.

Dean, D. (1996). *Law-making and society in late Elizabethan England: The parliament of England, 1584–1601* In Fletcher, A., Guy, J., & Morrill, J. (Series Eds.). *Cambridge studies in early modern British history.* Cambridge, England: Cambridge University Press.

El-Hai, J. (2004). *The lobotomist: A maverick medical genius and his tragic quest to rid the world of mental illness.* New York: Wiley.

Grob, G. (1994). *The mad among us: A history of the care of America's mentally ill.* New York: Free Press.

Harper, R. F. (2002). *The code of Hammurabi, king of Babylon.* Portland, OR: University Press of the Pacific.

Hollingshead, G. (2004). *Bedlam.* New York: HarperCollins.

The Holy Bible (Revised Standard Version, W. Tyndale, Trans.). New York: Thomas Nelson & Sons.

Howard, A. (1972). *Legislative history of S 1305 and S 1769: Bills to amend the economic opportunity act of 1964 to authorize a legal services program by establishing a national legal services corporation.* Chicago: University of Chicago Law School.

Lindemann, E. (1944). Symptomatology and management of acute grief. *American Journal of Psychiatry, 101*, 141–148.

Lombroso, C., & Ferrero, G. (2004). *Criminal woman, the prostitute and the normal woman* (N. H. Rafter & M. Gibson, Eds. and Trans.). Durham, NC: Duke University Press. (Original work published in Italian in 1893).

Miles, S. H. (2003). *The Hippocratic Oath and the ethics of medicine.* New York: Oxford University Press.

Mommsen, T. E. (1942). Petrarch's conception of the Dark Ages. *Speculum, 17* (2), 226–242.

Roe v. Wade [Online]. (2006, October). Available at http://en.wikipedia.org/wiki/Roe_v._Wade

Slaikeu, K. A. (1990). *Crisis intervention: A handbook for practice and research* (2nd ed.). Boston: Allyn & Bacon.

Summers, M. (1969). *Malleus maleficarum.* New York: Beaufort Books.

Weiner, D. B. (1979). The apprenticeship of Philippe Pinel: A new document, observations of citizen Pussin on the insane. *American Journal of Psychiatry, 136*, 1128–1134.

Wikipedia. *Roe v. Wade.* retrieved 8/30/2006 from http://en.wikipedia.org/wiki/Roe_v._Wade

CHAPTER 3   Human Service Workers

Kazdin, A. E. (2001). *Behavior modification in applied settings* (6th ed.). Pacific Grove, CA: Brooks/Cole.

Mental Health Assoc. of Los Angeles. (1997). *Human resource needs assessment: Human services industry.* Los Angeles: Author.

Natl. Assoc. of Social Workers. (2006) *Certified Social Work Case Manager* [Online]. Available at www.socialworkers.org/credentials/credentials/casemgmt.asp

Southern Regional Education Board (1969). *Roles and functions for different levels of mental health workers* (pp. 29–30). Atlanta, GA: Author.

CHAPTER 4   Communication Skills and Personal Characteristics of Human Service Workers

Caplan, G. (1964). *Principles of preventive psychiatry.* New York: Basic Books.

Carkhuff, R., & Berenson, B. (1967). *Beyond counseling and therapy.* New York: Holt, Rinehart & Winston.

Corey, G. (2005). *Theory and practice of counseling and psychotherapy* (7th ed.). Pacific Grove, CA: Brooks/Cole.

Hutchins, D. E., & Cole, C. (1992). *Helping relationships and strategies* (2nd ed.). Pacific Grove, CA: Brooks/Cole.

Ivey, A. E., Gluckstern, N. B., & Ivey, M. G. (1997). *Basic attending skills* (3rd ed.). North Amherst, MA: Microtraining Associates.

Kanel, K. (2002). Mental health needs of Spanish-speaking Latinos in southern California. *Hispanic Journal of Behavioral Sciences, 24* (1), 74–91.

Kanel, K. (2007). *A guide to crisis intervention* (3rd ed.). Pacific Grove, CA: Brooks/Cole.

Okun, B. (1992). *Effective helping* (4th ed.). Pacific Grove, CA: Brooks/Cole.

Rogers, C. (1958). The characteristics of a helping relationship. *Personnel and Guidance Journal, 37*, 6–16.

Rogers, C. (1970). *On encounter groups.* New York: Harper & Row.

CHAPTER 5   Biological and Psychological Theories of Causality

Adler, A. (1959). *Understanding human nature.* New York: Premier Books.

American Psychiatric Assoc. (1994). *Diagnostic and statistical manual of mental disorders* (4th ed.). Washington, DC: Author.

Bateson, G., Jackson, D. D., Haley, J., & Weakland, J. (1956). Toward a theory of schizophrenia. *Behavioral Science, 1,* 251–264.

Beck, A. T., Rush, A., Shaw, B., & Emery, G. (1979). *Cognitive therapy of depression.* New York: Guilford Press.

Bowen, M. (1992). *Family therapy in clinical practice.* New York: Jason Aronson.

Brenner, C. (1974). *An elementary textbook of psychoanalysis.* Garden City, NY: Anchor Books.

Canda, E. R. (2005, fall semester). *Spiritual aspects of social work practice: Course description and syllabus* [Online]. Lawrence, KS: University of Kansas. Available at www.socwel.ku.edu/canda/SW_SYLB/SW870syllabus.htm

Chudler, E. H. (2006). Neurotransmitters and neuroactive peptides. *Neuroscience for kids* [Online]. Available at http://faculty.washington.edu/chudler/chnt.html

Corey, G. (2005). *Theory and practice of counseling and psychotherapy.* Pacific Grove, CA: Brooks/Cole.

Ellis, A. (1962). *Reason and emotion in psychotherapy.* Secaucus, NJ: Citadel Press.

Freud, S. (1966). *The complete introductory lectures on psychoanalysis.* (J. Strachey, Trans.). New York: W.W. Norton. (Original work published 1933)

Gabbard, G. O. *Psychodynamic psychiatry in clinical practice* (3rd ed.). Washington, DC: Psychiatric Press.

Genetic disorder [Online]. (2006, October). Available at http://en.wikipedia.org/wiki/Genetic_disorder

Glasser, W. (1975). *Reality therapy: A new approach to psychiatry.* New York: Harper & Row.

Guntrip, H. (1973). *Psychoanalytic theory, therapy, and the self.* New York: Basic Books.

Haley, J. (1976). *Problem-solving therapy: New strategies for effective family therapy.* San Francisco: Jossey-Bass.

Laing, R. D., & Esterson, A. (1977). *Sanity, madness, and the family.* New York: Penguin Books.

Madanes, C. (1981). *Strategic family therapy.* San Francisco: Jossey-Bass.

Mahler, M. S., Pine, F., & Bergman, A. (1975). *The psychological birth of the human infant: Symbiosis and individuation.* New York: Basic Books.

Meichenbaum, D. (1985). *Stress inoculation training.* New York: Pergamon.

Meichenbaum, D. (1986). Cognitive behavior modification. In F. H. Kanfer & A. P. Goldstein (Eds.), *Helping people change: A textbook of methods* (pp. 346–380). New York: Pergamon.

Minuchin, S. (1974). *Families and family therapy.* Cambridge, MA: Harvard University Press.

Pavlov, I. P. (1927). *Conditioned reflexes* (G. V. Anrep, Trans.). New York: Liveright.

Perls, F. (1969). *Gestalt therapy verbatim.* Moab, UT: Real People Press.

Rogers, C. (1961). *On becoming a person.* Boston: Houghton Mifflin.

Rogers, C. (1970). *Carl Rogers on encounter groups.* New York: Harper & Row.

Rogers, C. (1987). Steps toward world peace, 1948–1986: Tension reduction in theory and practice. *Counseling and Values, 32*(1), 12–16.

Satir, V. (1983). *Conjoint family therapy* (3rd ed.). Palo Alto, CA: Science and Behavior Books.

Skinner, B. F. (1948). *Walden II.* New York: Macmillan.

Skinner, B. F. (1953). *Science and human behavior.* New York: Macmillan.

Whitaker, C. A. (1976). The hindrance of theory in clinical work. In P. J. Guerin, Jr. (Ed.), *Family therapy: Theory and practice.* New York: Gardner Press.

Wolpe, J. (1990). *The practice of behavior therapy* (4th ed.). Elmsford, NY: Pergamon.

Wynne, L., Tyckoff, I., Day, J., & Hirsch, S. H. (1958). Pseudo-mutuality in schizophrenia. *Psychiatry, 21,* 205–220.

Yalom, I. D. (1980). *Existential psychotherapy.* New York: Basic Books.

Yalom, I. D. (1985). *The theory and practice of group psychotherapy.* New York: Basic Books.

Zylstra, S. (2006). Untitled [Letter to the editor]. *The Therapist, 18* (1), 6.

CHAPTER 6   Sociological Theories of Causality

Abudabbeh, N., & Aseel, H. A. (1999). Transcultural counseling and Arab Americans (2nd ed.). In J. McFadden (Ed.) *Transcultural counseling* (pp. 283–296). Alexandria, VA: American Counseling Assoc.

Al-Abdul-Jabbar, J., & Al-Issa, I. (2000). Psychotherapy in Islamic society. In I. Al-Issa (Ed.), *Al-Junun: Mental illness in the Islamic world,* (pp. 277–293). Madison, CT: International Universities Press.

Al-Krenawai, A., & Graham, J. R. (2000). Culturally sensitive social work practice with Arab clients in mental health settings. *Health & Social Work, 25* (1), 9–22.

Allison, S. R., & Vining, C. B. (1999). *Native American Culture and Language, 24* (1/2), pp. 193–207.

American Psychiatric Assoc. (1980). *The diagnostic and statistical manual of mental disorders* (3rd ed.). Washington DC: Author.

Canda, E. R. (2005, fall semester). *Spiritual aspects of social work practice: Course description and syllabus* [Online]. Lawrence, KS: University of Kansas. Available at www.socwel.ku.edu/canda/SW_SYLB/SW870syllabus.htm

Delgado, M. (1998). *Social service in Latino communities: Research and strategies.* New York: Haworth.

Doyle, J. (2007). In K. Kanel *A Guide to Crisis Intervention* (3rd ed., pp. tk–tk). Pacific Grove, CA: Brooks/Cole.

Dufort, M., & Reed, L. (Eds.). (1995). *Learning the way: A guide for the home visitor working with families on the Navajo reservation.* Watertown, MA: Hilton/Perkins Project of Perkins School for the Blind and Arizona Schools for the Deaf and Blind.

Gilbert, L. A., & Scher, M. (1999). *Gender and sex in counseling and psychotherapy.* Boston: Allyn & Bacon.

Hare-Mustin, R. T. (1983). An appraisal of the relationship between women and psychotherapy: 80 years after the case of Dora. *American Psychologist, 32,* 889–890.

HinduNet (2003) *Hindu Universe* [Online]. Available at www.hindunet.org/god/summary/index.htm

Hogan-Garcia, M. (1999). *The four skills of cultural diversity competence.* Pacific Grove, CA: Brooks/Cole.

Hsu, J., Tseng, W., Ashton, G., McDermott, J., & Char, W., (1985). Family interaction patterns among Japanese American and Caucasian families in Hawaii. *American Journal of Psychiatry, 142,* 577–581.

Kanel, K. (2005). *Ataque de nervios: Is it time to designate it as a clinical syndrome on its own?* Unpublished manuscript.

Kim, B. S. K., Atkinson, D. R., & Umemoto, D. (2001). Asian cultural values and counseling process: Current knowledge and directions for future research. *The Counseling Psychologist, 29,* 570–603.

Kim, B. S. K., Liang, C. T. H., & Li, L. C. (2003). Counselor ethnicity, counselor nonverbal behavior, and session outcome with Asian American Clients: Initial findings, *Journal of Counseling & Development, 81* (2), 202–207.

Koss-Chioino, J. D. (1999). Depression among Puerto Rican women: Culture, etiology and diagnosis. *Hispanic Journal of Behavioral Sciences, 21* (3), 330–350.

Liebowitz, M. R., Salman, E., Jusion, C. M., Garfinkel, R., Street, L., Cardenas, D. L., Silvestre, J., Fyer, A. J., Carrasco, J. L., Davies, S., Guarnaccia, J. P., & Klein, D. (1994). Ataque de nervios and panic disorder. *American Journal of Psychiatry 151* (6), 871–875.

Loza, N. (2001, May). *Insanity on the Nile: The history of psychiatry in pharaonic Egypt.* Paper presented at the Second Biannual National Conference on Arab American Health Issues, Dearborn, MI.

Marieskind, H. I. (1980). *Women in the health system.* St. Louis, MO: Mosby.

Mattes, L. J., & Omark, D. R. (1994). *Speech and language assessment for the bilingual handicapped.* San Diego, CA: College-Hill Press.

Nassar-McMillan, S. C. & Hakim-Larson, J. (2003). Counseling considerations among Arab Americans. *Journal of Counseling & Development, 81* (2), 150–159.

Nassar-McMillan, S. C. (1999, May). *Mental health considerations in the Arab community.* Paper presented at the Conference on Arab American Health Issues, Dearborn, MI.

Native American Research and Training Center. (1995). *Some alarming facts.* Tucson, AZ: University of Arizona.

Nydell, M. (1987). *Understanding Arabs: A guide for westerners.* Yarmouth, ME: Intercultural Press.

O'Brien, E. M. (1992). American Indians in higher education. *Research Briefs, 5* (5). Washington, DC: American Council on Education, Policy Analysis and Research.

Oquendo, M. A., (1995). Differential diagnosis of ataque de nervios. *American Journal Orthopsychiatry, 65* (1), 60–64.

Peel District School Board. (2002). *Ableism* (Issue Paper No. 2) [Online]. Toronto, ON: Author. Available at www.gobeyondwords.org/ableism.html

Rubio, M., Urdaneta, M., & Doyle, J. L. Psychopathological reaction patterns in the Antilles command. *US Armed Forces Medical Journal, 6,* 1767–1772.

Schaefer, R. T. (1988). *Racial and ethnic groups.* Glenview, IL: Scott, Foresman.

Schechter, D. S., Marshall, R., Salman, E., Goetz, D., Davies, S., & Liebowitz, M. R. (2000). Ataque de nervios and history of childhood trauma. *Journal of Traumatic Stress, 13* (3), 529–534.

Sears, D. O., Peplau, L. A., & Taylor, S. E. (1991). *Social psychology.* Englewood Cliffs, NJ: Prentice Hall.

Seekins, T. (1997). Native Americans and the ADA. *The Rural Exchange, 10*(1).

Shields, S. A. (1995). The role of emotion, beliefs, and values on gender development. In N. Eisenberg (Ed.), *Review of personality and social psychology,* Vol. 15 (pp. 212–232). Thousand Oaks, CA: Sage.

Smith, G. H. (1989). *Atheism: The case against god.* Buffalo, NY: Prometheus Books.

Uba, L. (1994). *Asian Americans: Personality patterns, identity, and mental health.* New York: Guilford Press.

U.S. Census Bureau. (2001). *Statistical abstracts of the United States.* Washington DC: Author.

U.S. Census Bureau. (2004). *Statistical abstracts of the United States.* Washington DC: Author.

Vogel, D. L., Epting, F., & Wester, S. R. (2003). Counselors' perceptions of female and male clients. *Journal of Counseling & Development, 81* (2), 131–141.

Zogby, J. (2001). *What ethnic Americans really think: The Zogby culture polls.* Washington, DC: Zogby International.

Zylstra, S. (2006). Untitled [Letter to the editor]. *The Therapist, 18*(1), 6.

CHAPTER 7 Populations That Utilize Human Services

Alzheimer's Assoc. (2004). *Alzheimer's disease statistics* (Fact Sheet). Chicago: Author.

American Psychiatric Assoc. (1994). *Diagnostic and statistical manual of mental disorders* (4th ed.). Washington, DC: Author.

Bendau, M. C. (Producer and Director). (1992). *Gangs: Dreams under fire* [videotape]. Los Angeles: Franciscan Communications.

Berkeley Planning Associates. (1997). *Disabled women rate caregiver abuse and domestic violence number one issue.* Berkeley, CA: Dept. of Education.

Briere, J., & Gil, E. (1998). Self-mutilation in clinical and general population samples: Prevalence, correlates, and function. *American Journal of Orthopsychiatry, 68,* 609–620.

Centers for Disease Control and Prevention. (2002). Guidelines for preventing opportunistic infections among HIV-infected persons: Recommendations of the U.S. Public Health Service and the Infectious Diseases Society of American. M M W R 51: (R R-8).

Centers for Disease Control. (2004). *Basic statistics* [Online]. Atlanta, GA: Author. Available at www.cdc.gov/hiv/topics/surveillance/basic.htm

Colliver, J., & Epstein J. (2006). Substance dependence, abuse, and treatment. In *Results from the 2005 National Survey on Drug Use and Health: National Findings* (Office of Applied Studies, NSDUH Series H-30, DHHS Publication No. SMA 06-4194, Chapter 7). Rockville, MD: Substance Abuse and Mental Health Services Administration. Available at www.drugabusestatistics.samhsa.gov/nsduh/2k5nsduh/2k5results.htm#Ch7

Comer, R. J. (1995). *Abnormal psychology* (2nd ed.). New York: Freeman Publishing.

Corey, G. (2005). *Theory and practice of counseling and psychotherapy* (7th ed.) Pacific Grove, CA: Brooks/Cole.

Corsini, R. J., & Wedding, D. (2005). *Current psychotherapies* (7th ed.). Pacific Grove, CA: Brooks/Cole.

Darche, M. A. (1990). Psychological factors differentiating self-mutilating and non-self-mutilating adolescent inpatient females. *The Psychiatric Hospital, 21,* 31–35.

Department of Health and Human Services. (2003, February, 7). Annual update of the HHS poverty guidelines. *Federal Register, 68*(26), 6456–6458.

Department of Health and Human Services. (2004, February, 13). HHS poverty guidelines. *Federal Register, 69*(30), 7336–7338.

DiClemente, R. J., Ponton, L. E., & Hartley, D. (1991). Prevalence and correlates of cutting behavior: Risk for HIV transmission. *Journal of the American Academy of Child and Adolescent Psychiatry, 30,* 735–739

Federal Interagency Forum on Aging-Related Statistics. (2005). *Older Americans 2004: Key indicators of well-being* [Online]. Washington, DC: Author. Available at www.agingstats.gov/chartbook2004/population.html#indicator%207

Fleming P. L., Byers, R. H., Sweeney, P.A., Daniels, D., Karon, J. M., & Janssen. *HIV prevalence in the United States, 2000* [Abstract 11]. Presented at the Ninth Conference on Retroviruses and Opportunistic Infections. Seattle, WA: February 24–28, 2002.

Hammer, H., Finkelhor, D., & Sedlak, A. J. (2002) *Runaway/thrownaway children: National estimates and characteristics* (NISMART Bulletin Series [2002, October], NCJ No. 196469). Washington, DC: Office of Juvenile Justice and Delinquency Prevention.

Heise, L., Ellsberg, M., & Gottemoeller, M. (1999). Ending violence against women. *Population Reports* (Series L, No. 11). Baltimore: Population Information Program of the Johns Hopkins University School of Public Health. Volume XXVII, Number 4 December, 1999

Kanel, K. (2007). *A guide to crisis intervention* (3rd ed.). Pacific Grove, CA: Brooks/Cole.

Kaplan , J. E., Masur H., & Holmes, K. K. (2002) *Guidelines for preventing opportunistic infections among HIV-infected persons: Recommendations of the U.S. Public Health Service and the Infectious Diseases Society of America* (PMID: 12081007, MMWR Recomm Rep. 2002

June 14; 51(RR-8): 1–52) Bethesda, MD: Natl. Institutes of Health. Available atwww.ncbi.nlm.nih.gov/entrez/queryd.fcgi?itool=abstractplus&db=pubmed&cmd=Retrieve&dopt=abstractplus&list_uids=12617574

Kenner, K. L. (1996). *Gangs.* Santa Barbara, CA: ABC-Clio.

Kilpatrick, D. G., Edwards, C. N., & Seymour, A. E. (1992). *Rape in America: A report to the nation.* Arlington, VA: Natl. Crime Victims Center.

Lloyd, E. E. (1998). Self-mutilation in a community sample of adolescents. (Doctoral dissertation, Louisiana State University, 1998). *Dissertation Abstracts International 58,* 5127.

Natl. Institute of Justice, U.S. Department of Health and Human Services, & Centers for Disease Control and Prevention. (1998). *Prevalence, incidence, and consequences of violence against women: Findings from the national violence against women survey.* Washington, DC: U.S. Department of Justice.

Nelson, B. (1984). *Making an issue of child abuse.* Chicago: University of Chicago Press.

Orange Caregiver Resource Center, Orange County Office on Aging and South County Senior Services. (no date). *Orange County Caregiver's Resource Guide.* Fullerton, CA: Author.

Oswald, W. T. (2005). *Broadening our approach: Attacking poverty at its roots.* Paper presented at the Western Regional Conference of the National Organization of Human Services, Fullerton, CA.

Rogers, J. R., Gueulette, C. M., Abbey-Hines, J., Carney, J. V., & Werth, J. L., Jr. (2001). Rational suicide: An empirical investigation of counselor attitudes. *Journal of Counseling and Development, 79,* 365–372.

Ross, S., & Heath, N. (2002). A study of the frequency of self-mutilation in a community sample of adolescents. *Journal of Youth and Adolescence, 31,* 67–77.

Sedlak, A. & Broadhurst, D. (1996). Executive summary. *The Third National Incidence Study of Child Abuse and Neglect* (NIS 3). Washington, DC: U.S. Department of Health and Human Services.

Silverman, J. G., Raj, A., Mucci, L. A., & Hathaway, J. E. (2001). Dating violence against adolescent girls and associated substance abuse, unhealthy weight control, sexual control, sexual risk behavior, pregnancy, and suicidality. *Journal of the American Medical Assoc., 286* (5).

Simpson, C., Pruitt, R., Blackwell, D., & Sweringen, G. S. (1997, April). Preventing teen pregnancy: Early adolescence. *ADVANCE for Nurse Practitioners,* 24–29.

Tower, C. C. (1999). *Understanding child abuse and neglect* (4th ed.). Boston: Allyn & Bacon.

Tyiska, C. G. (1998). *Working with victims of crime with disabilities* (Bulletin No. NCJ 172838 [Online]). Washington DC: Office for Victims of Crime, U.S. Department of Justice. Available at www.ojp.usdoj.gov/ovc/publications/factshts/disable.htm

U.S. Census Bureau. (1990). *Statistical abstracts of the United States.* Washington DC: Author.

U.S. Census Bureau. (2000). U.S. *census of population and housing profiles of general demographic characteristics.* Washington DC: Author.

U.S. Census Bureau. (2004). *How the Census Bureau measures poverty* [Online]. Washington, DC: Author. Available at www.census.gov/hhes/poverty/povdef.html

U.S. Census Bureau. (2006). Vital statistics. In *Statistical abstract of the United States.* Washington, DC: Author.

Walker, L. E. A. (1984). *Battered Woman Syndrome.* New York: Springer Publishing.

Wallace, R. C., & Wallace, W. D. (1985). *Sociology.* Boston: Allyn & Bacon.

Wyman, S. (1982). *Suicide evaluation and treatment.* Paper presented at a seminar of the California Assoc. of Marriage and Family Therapists, Orange County Chapter.

Young, M. E., Nosek, M. A., Howland, C. A., Chanpong, G., & Rintala, D. H. (1997). Prevalence of abuse of women with physical disabilities. *Archives of Physical Medicine and Rehabilitation. 78,* 534–538.

CHAPTER 8   Micro- and Mezzo-Level Assessments and Interventions

Alle-Corliss, L., & Alle-Corliss, R. (1999). *Advanced practice in human services agencies.* Pacific Grove, CA: Brooks/Cole.

DeLeon, P. H., Uyeda, M. K., & Welch, B. L. (1985). Psychology and HMDS: New partnerships or new adversary? *American Psychologist, 40* (10), 1122–1124.

Herr, E. L., & Cramer, S. H. (1987). *Controversies in the mental health professions.* Muncie, IN: Accelerated Development.

Hollis, J. W., & Donn, P. A. (1980). *Psychological report writing theory and practice.* Muncie, IN: Accelerated Development.

Kanel, K. (2007). *A guide to crisis intervention* (3rd. ed.). Pacific Grove, CA: Brooks/Cole.

Lancer, D. (2004). Recovery in the twelve steps. *The Therapist, 16* (6), 68–71.

Newton, J. (1988). *Preventing mental illness.* London: Routledge & Kegan Paul.

Price, R. H., Cowen, E. L., Lorion, R. P., & Ramos-McKay, J. (1988). *Fourteen ounces of prevention: A casebook for practitioners.* Washington, DC: American Psychological Assoc.

Tulkin, S. R., & Frank, G. W. (1985). The changing role of psychologists in health maintenance organizations. *American Psychologist, 40* (10), 1125–1136.

Wyman, S. (1982). *Suicide evaluation and treatment.* Paper presented at a seminar of the California Assoc. of Marriage and Family Therapists, Orange County Chapter.

CHAPTER 9   Human Services Delivery to Client Populations

Bancroft, L., & Silverman, J. (2003). *The batterer as parent.* Thousand Oaks, CA: Sage Publications.

Bowker, L., Arbitell, M., & McFerron, R. (1988). On the relationship between wife beating and child abuse. In K. Yllo & M. Bograd (Eds.), *Feminist perspectives on wife abuse.* Thousand Oaks, CA: Sage Publications.

Committee on the Judiciary, U.S. Senate, 102nd Congress. (1992). *Violence against women: A majority staff report* (p. 3). Washington, DC: Author.

Kanel, K. (2007). *A guide to crisis intervention* (3rd ed.). Pacific Grove, CA: Brooks/Cole.

Langford, L., Isaac, N. E., & Kabat, S. (1999). *Homicides related to intimate partner violence in Massachusetts, 1991–1995.* Boston: Peace at Home.

Magallon, T. (1987, June). Counseling patients with HIV infections. *Medical Aspects of Human Sexuality,* 129–147.

Natl. Institute on Alcohol Abuse and Alcoholism. (1999). *Brief intervention for alcohol problems.* (Alcohol Alert No. 43). Bethesda, MD: Author.

Natl. Institute on Drug Abuse. (1999) *Principles of drug addiction treatment: A research based guide* (NIH Publication No. 99-4180). Bethesda, MD: Author. Available at www.drugabuse.gov/PDF/PODAT/PODAT.pdf

Nowinski, J. (2000). *Twelve-step facilitation.* (NIH Publication No. 00-4151 [Online]). Bethesda, MD: Natl. Institute on Drug Abuse, Natl. Institutes of Health. Available at www.drugabuse.gov/ADAC/ADAC10.html

Price, R. E., Omizo, M. M., & Hammitt, V. L. (October 1986). Counseling clients with AIDS. *Journal of Counseling and Development, 65,* 96–97.

Rennison, C. M. (2003, February). Intimate partner violence, 1993–2001(NCJ 197838). *Bureau of Justice Statistics crime data brief.* Washington, DC: U.S. Department of Justice.

Slader, S. (1992). *HIV/IV drug users*. Paper presented at a meeting held at California State University, Fullerton.

Wyman, S. (1982). *Suicide evaluation and treatment*. Paper presented at a seminar of the California Assoc. of Marriage and Family Therapists, Orange County Chapter.

CHAPTER 10   Stress Management

Anonymous (2005). The change agenda. *Management Today, 45*.

Caplan, J. (2005). Training: What's hot in 2005. *China Staff, 11*(2), 20–24.

Chang, J. (2005). Pressure points. *Sales and Marketing Management, 157*(4), 18.

Ellis, A. (1962). *Reason and emotion in psychotherapy*. Secaucus, NJ: Citadel Press.

Ellis, A. (2001). *How to control your anxiety before it controls you*. New York: Citadel Press.

Freudenberger, H. J. (1975). The staff burnout syndrome in alternative institutions. *Psychotherapy: Theory, Research and Practice, 12*, 73–82.

Fry, W. F., & Salameh, W. A. (Eds.). (1993). *Advances in humor and psychotherapy*. Sarasota, FL: Professional Resources Press.

Goldman, L., & Lewis, J. (2005). The emphasis on stress. *Occupational Health, 57* (3), 12–14.

Gomez, J. S., & Michaelis, R. C. (1995). An assessment of burnout in human service providers. *Journal of Rehabilitation, 61*, 23.

Haley, J. (1976). *Problem solving therapy*. San Francisco: Jossey-Bass.

Kanel, K. (2007). *A guide to crisis intervention* (3rd ed.). Pacific Grove, CA: Brooks/Cole.

Lee, C., Dolezalek, H., & Johnson, G. (2005). Top 10. *Training, 42* (3), 26–41.

Maslach, E., & Jackson, S. E. (1986). *Maslach burnout inventory: Manual* (2nd ed.). Palo Alto, CA: Consulting Psychologists Press.

McGuire, P. A. (1999). More psychologists are finding that discrete uses of humor promote healing in their patients [Online]. *APA Monitor Online, 30* (3). Available at www.apa.org/monitor/mar99/humor.html

Mendoza, M. (2005, April). Breaking point. *Human Resources*, 24–27.

Palazzoli, M. S., Cecchin, G., Prata, G., & Boscolo, L. (1978). *Paradox and counterparadox*. New York: Aronson.

Pines, A., & Maslach, C. (1978). Characteristics of staff burnout in mental health settings. *Hospital and Community Psychiatry, 29*, 223–233.

Russo, J. R. (1980). *Serving and surviving as a human-service worker*. Prospect Heights, IL: Waveland Press.

Sparks, P. J., Simon, G. E., Katon, W. J., Altman, L., C., Ayars, G. H., & Johnson, R. L. (1990). An outbreak of illness among aerospace workers. *Western Journal of Medicine, 153*, 28.

Vettor, S. M., & Kosinski, F. A., Jr. (2000). Work-stress burnout in emergency medical technicians and the use of early recollections. *Journal of Employment Counseling, 37*, 216.

CHAPTER 11   Ethical Issues in the Human Services

American Assoc. for Marriage and Family Therapy. (2001). *AAMFT code of ethics*. Washington, DC: Author.

American Counseling Assoc. (2005). *Code of ethics*. Alexandria, VA: Author.

American Psychiatric Assoc. (2001). *Principles of medical ethics with annotations especially applicable to psychiatry*. Washington, DC: Author.

American Psychological Assoc. (2002). Ethical principles of psychologists and code of conduct. *American Psychologist, 57*(12), 1060–1073.

American School Counselor Assoc. (2004). *Ethical standards for school counselors*. Alexandria, VA: Author.

Assoc. for Counselor Education and Supervision. (1995). Ethical guidelines for counseling supervisors. *Counselor Education and Supervision, 34*(3), 270–276.

Benitez, B. R. (2004). Confidentiality and its exceptions (including the U.S. Patriot Act). *The Therapist, 16*(4), 32–36.

Canadian Counselling Assoc. (1999). *CCA code of ethics.* Ottawa: Author.

Commission of Rehabilitation Counselor Certification. (2001). *Code of professional ethics for rehabilitation counselors.* Rolling Meadows, IL: Author.

Feminist Therapy Institute. (2000). *Feminist therapy code of ethics* (rev. 1999). San Francisco: Author.

Herr, E. L., & Cramer, S. H. (1987). *Controversies in the mental health professions.* Muncie, IN: Accelerated Development.

Jensen, D. G., (2003). HIPAA overview. *The Therapist, 15*(3), 26–27.

Natl. Assoc. of Social Workers. (1999). *Code of ethics.* Washington, DC: Author.

Natl. Organization for Human Services. (2000). Ethical standards of human service professionals. *Human Service Education, 20*(1), 61–68.

Siegel, M. (1979). Privacy, ethics, and confidentiality. *Professional Psychology, 10,* 249–258.

Swoboda, J. S., Elwork, A., Sales, B. D., & Levine, D. (1978). Knowledge of a compliance with privileged communication and child-abuse reporting laws. *Professional Psychology, 9,* 448–457.

CHAPTER 12   Organizational Structures of Human Services Agencies and Macro-Level Practice

Alle-Corliss, L., & Alle-Corliss, R. (1999). *Advanced practice in human service agencies.* Pacific Grove, CA: Brooks/Cole.

Blake, R. R., & Mouton, J. S. (1968). *Corporate excellence through grid organization development.* Houston, TX: Gulf Publishing.

Brueggemann, W. G. (1996). *The practice of macro social work.* Chicago: Nelson-Hall.

Etzioni, A. (1965). Dual leadership in complex organizations. *American Sociological Review, 30,* 5.

Guba, E. G., & Bridwell, C. E. (1957). *Administrative relationships.* Chicago: Midwest Administration Center, University of Chicago.

Homan, M. S. (1994). *Promoting community change: Making it happen in the real world.* Pacific Grove, CA: Brooks/Cole.

Kanel, K. (2007). *A guide to crisis intervention* (3rd ed.). Pacific Grove, CA: Brooks/Cole.

Kirst-Ashman, K. K., & Hull, G. H., Jr. (1993). *Understanding generalist practice.* Chicago: Nelson Hall.

Maxwell, A. D. (1973). Number numbness. *Liberal Education, 59* (3), 405–416.

McAdam, T. W. (1986). *Careers in the nonprofit sector: Doing well by doing good.* Farmington Hill, MI: Taft Group.

McGregor, D. (1960). *The human side of enterprise.* New York: McGraw-Hill.

Mental Health Center of North Iowa., *Background phases of disaster* [Online]. Mason City, IA: Author. Available at www.mhconi.org/Topic-disasterBkgrd.htm

Natl. Center for Posttraumatic Stress Disorder. (2005). *Treatment of PTSD* [Online Fact Sheet]. White River Junction, VT: Author. Available at www.ncptsd.org/facts/treatment/fs_treatment.html

Netting, E. F., Kettner, P. M., & McMurtry, S. (1993). *Social work macro practice.* New York: Longman.

Parson, T., Bales, R., & Shills, E. (1955). *Family socialization and interaction process.* Glencoe, IL: Free Press.

Russo, J. R. (1980). *Serving and surviving as a human service worker.* Prospect Heights, IL: Waveland Press.

Weinstein, B. (1994). *I'll work for free: A short-term strategy with a long-term payoff* [audiocassette]. New York: Henry Holt.

Appendix

Human Services Career Inventor

1. Do I want to deal directly with clients?

   _____

   _____

2. What types of clients do I want to work with?

   _____

   _____

3. If I don't want to work with clients directly, for what client population am I interested in providing indirect services?

   _____

   _____

4. What specific duties do I want to engage in at work? (Reread Chapter 3. You may select more than one, of course.)

   _____

   _____

5. Do I need to engage in some type of self-awareness process to do my job effectively? What areas do I need to develop or eliminate in order to provide service appropriately?

   _____

   _____

6. Do I want to work for a public or a nonprofit agency? Why?

_____

_____

7. Do I want to work at a residential or an outpatient facility?

_____

_____

8. Do I want to participate in lobbying and coalition building?

_____

_____

9. Do I want to write program proposals?

_____

_____

10. How much money do I need to make to live satisfactorily ?

_____

_____

11. Are my career plans realistic for these financial desires?

_____

_____

12. How much education am I willing to obtain?

_____

_____

13. What are the realistic options for me at my educational attainment goal?

_____

_____

14. What am I going to do to ensure that I don't become burnt out as a human services worker?

_____

_____

15. Do I still want to go into the field of human services?

_____

_____

Good luck! Kristi Kanel

Name Index

Subject Index